TOPICS IN PARAPLEGIA

Edited by **Yannis Dionyssiotis**

Topics in Paraplegia
http://dx.doi.org/10.5772/56986
Edited by Yannis Dionyssiotis

Contributors

Stamatios Papadakis, Spyros Galanakos, Kleio Apostolaki, Konstantinos Kateros, Olga Antoniadou, George Machairas, George Sapkas, Anisha Perera, Richard Gibbs, Sean Christie, Venkataramana Neelam, Rakhi Pal, Yannis Dionyssiotis, Vafa Rahimi-Movaghar, Jennifer Lee, Giorgio Brunelli, Farhad Abbasi, Ari Papachristos

Published by InTech

Janeza Trdine 9, 51000 Rijeka, Croatia

Publishing Process Manager Iva Lipovic
Technical Editor InTech DTP team
Cover InTech Design team

First published July, 2014
Printed in Croatia

Additional hard copies can be obtained from orders@intechopen.com

Topics in Paraplegia, Edited by Yannis Dionyssiotis
p. cm.
ISBN 978-953-51-1621-9

For EU product safety concerns:
IN TECH d.o.o., Prolaz Marije Krucifikse Kozulić 3, 51000 Rijeka, Croatia,
info@intechopen.com or visit our website at intechopen.com.

Meet the editor

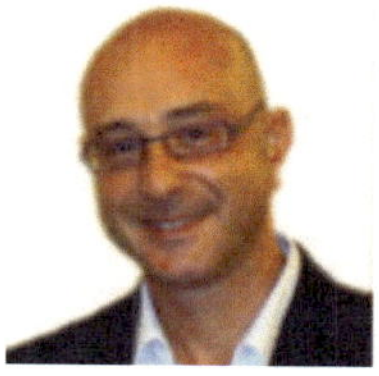

Dr. Yannis Dionyssiotis is specialized in Physical Medicine and Rehabilitation. He worked in the Laboratory for Research of the Musculoskeletal System at the University of Athens, in the Rehabilitation Department of KAT Hospital in Athens, Head of Physical Medicine and Rehabilitation Department in Rhodes General Hospital and Medical Director of Rehabilitation Center Amyntaio of Florina General Hospital in Greece and as Stationsarzt in the Klinik für neurochirourg.-neurologische Frührehabilitation, Westpfalz-Klinikum, Germany. Currently, he is the Medical Director of Physical Medicine and Rehabilitation Department of European Interbalkan Medical Center in Thessaloniki and is also working as Research Fellow in the 1st Department of Orthopaedics in General University Hospital ATTIKON. Dr. Dionyssiotis has clinical experience as physiatrist including experience in a variety of clinical settings as clinician, researcher, clinical instructor and consultant. He also holds a Thesis in Osteoporosis and Metabolic Bone Diseases from National and Kapodistrian University of Athens. Dr. Dionyssiotis has an extensive list of professional presentations and publications in the areas of rehabilitation, spinal cord injury, multiple sclerosis and osteoporosis. He has served as reviewer for several international journals and has written books and papers for osteoporosis in spinal cord injury, exercise, spinal orthoses, jumping mechanography, falls, and botulinum toxin.

Contents

Preface

Dear colleagues!

It was my great pleasure to be the Editor of this project published by InTech. All authors were enthusiastic to present their work which resulted in a high quality scientific project. It was impossible to cover all aspects of paraplegia, but this attempt brought together scientists and experts from various disciplines related to the field. This project could be a start for the development of a network in the field of spinal cord injuries in general and for exchanging scientific knowledge.

I would like to thank all authors who participated in this book project and the company InTech which produces continually high education free access publications.

Warm regards

Yannis Dionyssiotis, MD, PhD, FEBPRM
Rehabilitation Center "Aghios Loukas o Iatros",
Trikala Thessaly, Greece

University of Athens,
1st Department of Orthopaedics,
General University Hospital Attikon,
Athens, Greece

Section 1

Introduction-Epidemiology - Classification - Prognosis of Paraplegia

Chapter 1

Paraplegia Caused by Infectious Agents; Etiology, Diagnosis and Management

Farhad Abbasi and Soolmaz Korooni Fardkhani

Additional information is available at the end of the chapter

http://dx.doi.org/10.5772/56989

1. Introduction

Paraplegia or paralysis of lower extremities is caused mainly by disorders of the spinal cord and the cauda equina. They are classified as traumatic and non traumatic. Traumatic paraplegia occurs mostly as a result of traffic accidents and falls caused by lateral bending, dislocation, rotation, axial loading, and hyperflexion or hyperextension of the cord. Non-traumatic paraplegia has multiple causes such as cancer, infection, intervertebral disc disease, vertebral injury and spinal cord vascular disease [1, 2]. Although the incidence of spinal cord injury is low, the consequences of this disabling condition are extremely significant for the individual, family and community [3]. A spinal cord injury not only causes paralysis, but also has long-term impact on physical, psychosocial, sexual and mental health. The consequences of spinal cord injury require that health care professionals begin thinking about primary prevention. Efforts are often focused on care and cure, but evidence-based prevention should have a greater role. Primary prevention efforts can offer significant cost benefits, and efforts to change behavior and improve safety can and should be emphasized. Primary prevention can be applied to various etiologies of injury, including motor vehicle crashes, sports injuries, and prevention of sequelae of infectious diseases and prompt and correct diagnosis and treatment of infections involving spinal cord and vertebrae [4]. Infections are important causes of paraplegia. Several infections with different mechanisms can lead to paraplegia.

2. Infectious diseases and paraplegia

Several infections may cause paraplegia. They are classified into two categories: those that involve the spinal cord directly and those that involve vertebral column and cause pressure effect on the spinal cord that eventually leads to paraplegia. In fact paraplegia can arise from a lesion either within or outside the spinal cord or cauda equina. These are classified as compressive and non compressive. Compression is caused either by bone or other masses. The main compressive causes are Pott's disease (tuberculosis of spine). The main non-compressive causes are transverse myelitis secondary to viral infections, HIV, TB and very occasionally syphilis [1]. Several bacterial, viral, mycobacterial, fungal and parasitic infections can cause paraplegia. Infectious myelitis is usually caused by neurotropic viruses or mycoplasma in conjunction with concomitant meningitis or encephalitis; these in turn either induces transverse myelitis accompanied by severe sensorimotor deficits or chiefly affect the gray matter [5].

2.1. Bacterial infection

One of the most important causes of paraplegia among infectious causes is bacterial infection. These organisms can produce subdural empyema, epidural abscesses, radiculomyelitis or cause spondylitis with bony destruction or pressure effect.

2.1.1. Subdural empyema

Subdural empyema refers to a collection of pus in the space between the dura and arachnoid [6]. Spinal subdural empyema is a rare condition [7] that usually occurs secondary to metastatic infection from a distant site. The clinical presentation of spinal subdural empyema is usually radicular pain and symptoms of spinal cord compression, which may occur at multiple levels. The clinical presentation is difficult to distinguish from that of spinal epidural abscess [6]. Spinal subdural space remains the least common area of localized infection in the central nervous system (CNS). Infectious processes of the subdural spinal space include subdural spinal empyema, subdural spinal abscess, infected spinal subdural cyst, and infectious spinal subdural cyst [8]. Etiologies of spinal subdural empyema include hematogenous spread from skin lesions, sepsis, direct spread from spinal osteomyelitis, complications of discography and rarely iatrogenic after spinal anesthesia, spinal epidural insertion or acupuncture [9-11]. The most affected region is the thoraco-lumbar spine [12] and the most frequent microbial isolate is Staphylococcus aureus, followed by streptococci and coagulase-negative staphylococci. Gram-negative bacilli are less frequently isolated cause [6]. Mycoplasma hominis has been isolated from subdural empyema although it is very rare [13].

2.1.2. Epidural abscess

Epidural abscess refers to a localized collection of pus between the dura mater and vertebral column. Epidural abscess of the spinal column is a rare condition that can be fatal if left untreated. It promptly progresses and can cause neurologic paralysis, urinary retention or cauda equina syndrome [14]. It usually occurs secondary to hematogenous dissemination from foci elsewhere in the body to the epidural space or by local extension from vertebral osteomyelitis. Compromised immune system that occurs in patients with diabetes mellitus, AIDS, chronic renal failure, alcoholism, or cancer is a predisposing factor [6, 15]. Paraplegia and paralysis in spinal epidural abscess may be the result of spinal cord compression, spinal cord arterial or venous ischemia and thrombophlebitis or a combination of these. The most common

http://dx.doi.org/10.5772/56989

Etiology/ disease	Diagnosis	Medical treatment	Surgical intervention	Comment
Subdural empyema	MRI, CT Scan	Antibiotic	Yes	Combination antibiotic therapy is necessary
Epidural abscess	MRI, CT Scan	Antibiotic	Yes	Combination antibiotic therapy is necessary
Tuberculosis	MRI, CT-guided biopsy	Anti TB drugs	Yes	Four drugs combination is necessary
Syphilis	MRI, CSF analysis, VDRL, FTA-ABS	Penicillin, Doxycicline, amoxicillin, ceftriaxone	May be needed	-
Lyme	ELISA, PCR, CSF analysis	Doxycycline, amoxicillin, cefuroxime, ceftriaxone, cefotaxime	Usually not necessary	-
Brucellosis	MRI, Wright, 2ME, IFA, ELISA	Doxycycline, rifampin, trimethoprim-sulfamethoxazole, streptomycin, gentamicin, ciprofloxacin, ceftriaxone	Yes	Combination antibiotic therapy is necessary (usually 3 antibiotics)
HIV	ELISA, Western blot, P24 antigen, IFA, RIPA	ART	Usually not necessary	ART is used if HIV treatment is indicated
HTLV-I	Serology, antigen detection, PCR	Zidovudine and lamivudine may be used	Usually not necessary	-
Herpes zoster	Serology, PCR, IHC	Aciclovir	Usually not necessary	-
CMV	PP65 antigen, PCR	Ganciclovir, foscarnet, cidofovir	Usually not necessary	Combination therapy may be considered
Aspergillus	Histopathology, serology, antigen detection and PCR, culture	Amphotericin B, voriconazole, itraconazole	Yes	Voriconazole is treatment of choice
Candida	Histopathology, culture	Amphotericin B, fluconazole, echinocandins	Yes	-
Zygomycosis	Histopathology, culture	Amphotericin B, posaconazole, caspofungin	Yes	Posaconazole is treatment of choice
Schistosomiasis	Stool exam, IFA, ELISA	Praziquantel	May be needed	Steroid is usually used for treatment

Table 1. Summary of ethologic agents, diagnosis and treatment of paraplegia

organisms are Staphylococcus aureus, aerobic and anaerobic Streptococcus, Escherichia coli and Pseudomonas aeruginosa. Other organisms like Klebsiella pneumonia, Bacteroides fragilis, Enterococcus faecalis, Salmonella, Nocardia, etc. can cause spinal epidural abscess [6]. Paralysis in spinal epidural abscess may be the result of spinal cord compression, spinal cord arterial or venous ischemia and thrombophlebitis or a combination of these [16].

2.1.3. Tuberculosis

Tuberculosis is one of the most common infections worldwide [17]. Extrapulmonary sites most commonly involved by tuberculosis are lymph nodes, pleura, genitourinary tract, bones and joints, meninges, peritoneum and pericardium. However all organ systems may be involved [18]. There are reports about disseminated tuberculosis involving CNS and spine [19]. Tuberculosis may involve any part of CNS. Meningitis, CNS tuberculoma [20] and spinal cord involvement are neurologic presentation of tuberculosis. In some cases one, several or all presentation may be present [21]. In developing countries, a recognized etiology of paraplegia can be tuberculous radiculomyelitis or tuberculomas, especially in patients with evidence of either active or latent tuberculosis. Spinal deformity arises from tuberculosis is the leading cause of paraplegia [22]. It arises from hematogenous spread of the tubercle bacillus from pulmonary infection. The paraplegia occurs either at the time of the primary infection or more commonly 3-5 years later by reactivation [1]. Spinal tuberculosis can present with wide spectrum of symptoms, with back pain being the most common symptom. It is the leading cause of non-traumatic paraplegia in developing countries [23]. Spine is affected in 50% of skeletal tuberculosis patients. Tuberculous infection of the spine causes a bony destruction and collapse of the vertebra, with a gibbus deformity, skip lesion, intervertebral disc involvement, epidural abscess, paravertebral abscess and edema in the soft tissue planes [17]. Characteristically, there is destruction of the intervertebral disk space and the adjacent vertebral bodies, collapse of the spinal elements, and anterior wedging leading to kyphosis and gibbus formation. The thoracic region of vertebral column is most frequently affected. Formation of a 'cold' abscess around the lesion is another characteristic feature. The incidence of multi-level noncontiguous vertebral tuberculosis occurs more frequently than previously recognized. Common clinical manifestations include constitutional symptoms, back pain, spinal tenderness, paraplegia and spinal deformities [24]. In Abbasi's study on tuberculosis spondylitis in Iran, back pain was detected in 100%, anorexia in 100%, fever in 90%, cough in 50% and limb paralysis in 2.5% of patients [25]. These entities should also be considered in high-risk patients or in patients who have emigrated from regions with a high prevalence of tuberculosis [22]. Neurological complications in spinal tuberculosis occur in active stage of disease by mechanical compression, instability and inflammation changes, while in healed disease, these occur due to intrinsic changes in spinal cord secondary to internal salient in long standing kyphotic deformity [26]. Tuberculomas are rare tumorlike growth of tuberculous tissue in the central nervous system, characterized by symptoms of expanding these lesions. They result from enlargement of a caseated tubercle. Intramedullary tuberculomas can cause paraplegia although it is a rare event [27].

2.1.4. Syphilis

Syphilis is a sexually transmitted disease caused by the spirochete Treponema pallidum. The involvement of the CNS by Treponema pallidum has increased in the past 20 years, particularly as a result of HIV pandemic. However, tertiary forms, and especially syphilitic gumma, are rare as a result of the widespread use of penicillin. Spinal cord compression due to syphilitic gumma is an exceptional event that may cause paraplegia [28]. Syphilitic myelitis is a very rare manifestation of neurosyphilis that may lead to paraplegia [29]. There are several reports in literature about syphilitic aortic aneurysm with destructive spinal erosion that cause paraplegia [30, 31].

2.1.5. Lyme

Lyme disease is a tick-borne infection caused by Borrelia burgdorferi [32]. It is one of the most important arthropod-borne zoonosis-pathogen [33] and is transmitted from infected Ixodes ticks to a mammalian host following a tick bite [34]. Lyme borreliosis causes a multisystemic disease which may result in dermatologic, musculoskeletal, cardiovascular, and neurologic manifestations [35]. Lyme borreliosis is a multisystem disease and when involve neurologic system is named neuroborrelosis. Each part of neurologic system may be involved. A broad range of neurologic disorders have been described in Lyme disease, of which peripheral facial nerve palsy and aseptic meningitis are more prevalent [36]. The most common clinical picture of neuroborreliosis is meningitis with cranial or peripheral neuropathies connected with radiculalgia. Encephalitis, myelitis, neuropathies, polyneuropathies, encephalopathies and cerebellar involvement are less common presentation [36, 37]. Acute transverse myelitis is a rare Borellia burgdorferi-related neurologic complication [36]. Encephalomyelitis is the most serious form of neuroborreliosis. Encephalopathy is due to neuroimmunomodulators, like lymphokines and by toxico-metabolic effect could be connected with each form of systemic borreliosis [37]. Neuroborreliosis can cause paraplegia. In Salonen's study paraplegia caused by lyme was complete, flaccid and upper motor neurone type [38].

2.1.6. Brucellosis

Brucellosis is a systemic infectious disease caused by Brucella and a is common zoonosis that still remains a major health problem in certain parts of the world such as the Mediterranean region, the Middle East, and Latin America. It may involve multiple organs and tissues. Osteoarticular involvement is the most frequent complication of brucellosis, in which the diagnosis of brucella spondylitis is often difficult since the clinical presentation may be obscured by many other conditions [39]. Brucellosis can cause multisystemic involvement [40]. One of the most common complications is bone and joint involvement, particularly sacroilitis and spondylitis [41]. Brucella spondylitis may be complicated with paravertebral or epidural abscess, radiculitis and psoas abscess [42]. Rarely CNS involvement causes serious manifestations. Neurobrucellosis occurs less than 5% of patients and presents with meningitis, encephalitis, myelitis, myelopathy, stroke, paraplegia, radiculoneuritis, intracerebral abscess, epidural abscess, demyelination and cranial nerve involvement or any combination of these manifestations [40, 43]. Spinal epidural abscess may be caused due to brucellosis [44]. It is a very rare disease which is usually a consequence of spondylodiscitis. The spinal column can be affected at any joint; however, the lumbar spine is the most common region, especially at the level of the L4-5 and L5-S1. Spinal involvement may be seen at the lumbar, thoracic and cervical spine [45]. There are several reports about paraplegia caused by brucellosis [46, 47].

2.2. Viral infection

Several viral infections can cause paraplegia. Paraplegia is a major neurological disorder in HIV infection. It can occur during the asymptomatic stage of HIV infection when CD4 counts are $>200/cm^3$ and more commonly during the symptomatic stage when CD4 counts are low ($<100/cm^3$). The main causes are opportunistic processes and direct HIV involvement of the spinal cord. Opportunistic infections include tuberculosis, herpes zoster, herpes simplex, cytomegalovirus (CMV), syphilis and co-infection with human T-lymphotropic virus-1 (HTLV-I) in endemic areas [1]. In developed countries, the most prominent reported spinal cord disease in HIV/AIDS patients is vacuolar myelopathy. Other causes of myelopathy in HIV/AIDS patients include opportunistic infections, neoplasms, vascular lesions and metabolic disease. In developing regions, opportunistic infections are more common [48]. In patients with HIV infection, chronic inflammation can lead to a lesion that compresses the spinal cord and should be considered in differential diagnosis [49]. HTLV-I is a retrovirus which is endemic in some areas of western, southern and central Africa with just a few clusters reported in eastern Africa. It is endemic in areas of Japan, the Caribbean and South America. It is transmitted perinatally, sexually and by blood transfusion. Chronic infection for up to 20-30 years can result in a slow progressive form of tropical spastic paraplegia known as HTLV-I associated myelopathy [1]. This diagnosis should be considered in every patient with progressive spastic paraplegia [50]. Herpes zoster myelitis may cause paraplegia especially in HIV positive patients. Subacute onset paraplegia with a sensory level, which developed 10 days after herpes zoster dermatomal rash, is typical presentation of disease [51]. Extensive necrotic and hemorrhagic changes with marked necrotizing vasculitis involved the entire spinal cord and spinal roots, may be seen [52]. Neurological syndromes attributed to CMV include encephalitis, myelitis, and peripheral neuropathy [53]. Acute lumbosacral polyradiculopathy caused by the CMV infection is a rare neurological complication usually is seen in immunocompromised patients especially in AIDS. Progressive flaccid paraplegia with sensory disturbance, radicular pain, or bladder dysfunction are characteristic symptoms [54]. CMV may cause a severe motor polyradiculopathy by selective destruction of the motor neurons of ventral spinal roots and motor cranial nerves [55]. Several other viruses like Poliovirus, Entroviruse 71, Echovirus, Cocksackie B, Cocksackie A, etc can cause myelitis and paralysis.

2.3. Fungal infection

Aspergillosis of the spine has been reported infrequently. It has usually been attributed to hematogenous infection or spread from an adjacent pulmonary infection. Acute paraplegia may develop after aspergillus infection. Direct extension of aspergillus infection can cause spondylitis, vertebral destruction, spinal cord compression and paraplegia [56, 57]. Vertebral osteomyelitis caused by Aspergillus is rare and usually affects immunocompromised patients.

http://dx.doi.org/10.5772/56989

Aspergillus may lead to epidural abscesses [58, 59], kyphosis, discharging sinus in the back, vertebral destruction and paraplegia [60]. Spondylodiscitis has been reported due to candida [61]. Zygomycosis may be the cause of epidural abscess and paraplegia usually in immunocompromised patients [62]. Spinal cord histoplasmomosis with flaccid paralaysis has been reported [63].

2.4. Schistosomiasis

Schistosomiasis is a parasitic disease caused by blood flukes of the genus Schistosoma. Currently more than 200 million people worldwide are affected. Neuroschistosomiasis constitutes a severe presentation of the disease. Neurological symptoms result from the inflammatory response of the host to egg deposition in the brain and spinal cord. Neurological complications of cerebral schistosomiasis include delirium, loss of consciousness, seizures, dysphasia, visual field impairment, focal motor deficits and ataxia [64]. Transverse myelitis and myeloradiculopathy affecting the conus medullaris and cauda equina are the most common spinal cord syndromes. Transverse myelitis can present as flaccid areflexic paraplegia with sensory level and sphincter dysfunction [65]. Schistosomal myelopathy tends to occur early after infection and is more likely to be symptomatic than cerebral schistosomiasis [64]. Involvement of the spinal cord is considered to be uncommon, although 1-5% of all cases of non traumatic paraplegia in endemic parts of Africa are reported to be caused by schistosomiasis. Paraplegia occurs mostly with S. mansoni and occasionally with S. haematobium [1].

2.5. Other microorganism

Rarely some other organisms like non-tuberculosis mycobacteria [66, 67], Nocardia [68], pasturella [69], etc may involve spinal column, cause spondylitis, epidural or subdural abscess that may lead to paraplegia.

3. Diagnosis

3.1. Subdural empyema

Spinal subdural empyema is an unpredictable disease, with an unfavorable outcome if left untreated. If there is suspicion of a spinal subdural abscess, urgent radiological examination followed by immediate surgical drainage and appropriate antibiotic therapy is warranted [70]. Morbidity and mortality in intracranial and spinal subdural empyema directly relate to the delay in diagnosis and therapy [71]. The diagnostic procedure of choice for spinal subdural empyema is magnetic resonance imaging (MRI) with gadolinium enhancement. Occasionally spinal subdural empyemas may be detected by computed tomography (CT) myelography where MRI is negative [72]. The timing of performing MRI is very important in these patients. Early diagnosis and emergent treatment is necessary to prevent neurologic deficits [12].

3.2. Epidural abscess

A high level of clinical suspicion is necessary for rapid diagnosis and treatment initiation [73]. MRI with gadolinium enhancement is the diagnostic procedure of choice for diagnosis. MRI is recommended over CT scan because it can better visualize the spinal cord and epidural space in both sagittal and transverse sections and can also identify accompanying osteomyelitis, intramedullary spinal cord lesions, and discitis [6].

3.3. Tuberculosis

The diagnosis of Pott's disease is usually made by clinical suspicion, in combination with an elevated ESR and typical radiologic findings. Biopsy may be necessary for confirmation [1]. The awareness and suspicion of an atypical presentation of spinal tuberculosis should be high in order to obtain a good outcome [74]. MRI is the most valuable investigation in the patients with spinal tuberculosis. It is highly sensitive in detection of various pathological processes of Pott's disease [17]. For the diagnosis of spinal tuberculosis MRI is more sensitive imaging technique than x-ray and more specific than CT scan [24]. MRI allows the diagnosis of a tuberculous lesion, with a sensitivity of about 100% and specificity of 88%, well before deformity develops [74]. MRI frequently demonstrates involvement of the vertebral bodies on either side of the disk, disk destruction, cold abscess, vertebral collapse and presence of vertebral column deformities [24]. Marrow edema, preservation of disc space, subligamentous extension of abscess, paravertebral abscess, epidural extension, endplate erosions and discitis were consistently observed in 83% cases of spine tuberclusis on MRI [75]. If pus exists, the diagnosis may be confirmed by histopathological demonstration of Mycobacterium tuberculosis in drained pus [76]. CT-guided needle biopsy from the affected site in the center of the vertebral body is the gold standard technique for early histopathological diagnosis [24].

3.4. Syphilis

The diagnosis of neurosyphilis depends on the serological detection of antibodies in both blood and cerebrospinal fluid (CSF). The Venereal Disease Research Laboratory (VDRL) is the screening test most commonly used. More sensitive and specific diagnostic antibody tests include the fluorescent treponemal antibody absorption (FTA) and the treponemal antibody immobilization test (TPI) [1]. CSF study confirms the diagnosis of neurosyphilis [77]. CSF pleocytosis with positive CSF VDRL often is obvious [78]. MRI appearance of syphilitic myelitis is not well documented and only a few cases have been reported. MRI of the spine shows diffuse high signal intensity in the whole spinal cord on T2-weighted images. Focal enhancement may be observed in the dorsal aspect cord on T1-weighted gadolinium-enhanced images [29]. MRI imaging provides documentation of spinal cord involvement and is useful in monitoring recovery [77]. Marked sclerosis and osteophytes restricted to lumbo-dorsal spine, absence of ligamentous calcification and lack of long standing spinal symptoms may be seen in patients with syphilitic paraplegia [79].

3.5. Lyme

Serological tests, including enzyme linked immunosorbent assay (ELISA) and Western blot analysis can be used for diagnosis. B. burgdorferi polymerase chain reaction (PCR) may be used to confirm the diagnosis. Different techniques have been developed to aid in laboratory diagnosis of Lyme disease. Detection of serum antibodies is currently the most practical means of confirming B. burgdorferi infections. Although most assays may not detect low amounts of IgM antibody during the initial weeks of infection, application of a capture ELISA method has been reported to improve test sensitivity [80]. Detection of large amounts of IgM and IgG borrelia antibodies in the acute phase and complete disappearance of IgM antibody during the review period confirms the diagnosis [38]. Diagnosis of neuroborreliosis is based on culturing of B. burgdorferi from CSF, detection of specific antispirochaetal antibodies produced in subarachnoid space, detection of activated lymphocytes and antigens or borrelial DNA detection in CSF [37].

3.6. Brucellosis

In endemic regions brucella spondylitis should always be considered in the differential diagnosis especially in older patients with back pain and constitutional symptoms. An early diagnosis will help to prevent the development of more severe complications such as spinal cord compression [47]. Rose Bengal, standard agglutination, indirect immunofluorescent assay (IFA) and ELISA tests usually used for diagnosis [41, 46]. Serologic tests provide valuable information but always point to a generic and not a specific diagnosis [81]. ESR and CRP are usually highly positive [82]. Imaging studies, including radiography, computed tomography, magnetic resonance imaging and bone scintigraphy have been used for diagnosis. Radiography is limited to evaluating the focal form of spinal brucellosis. CT and bone scintigraphy have limited value because of their inadequate soft tissue resolution. MRI is the method of choice to assess the extent of disease and follow up the treatment response. However, MRI has a low specificity to predict the exact cause spondylodiscitis, the index of suspicion should be high in regions where the disease is endemic [83].Serological test for Brucella is usually positive and MRI may reveal epidural abscess or spondylodiscitis [44]. Early diagnosis and specific treatment are important to prevent later complications [41].

3.7. Viral infection

HIV is diagnosed by serological tests, including ELISA and Western blot. Several other tests such as P24 antigen, IFA, radioimmunoprecipitation assay (RIPA) and PCR may be used. Serologic assays, antigen detection and viral Isolation are used to diagnosis of HTLV infection. Serologic tests, PCR and Immunocytochemistry method are used for diagnosis of Varicella zoster virus (VZV) [52]. CMV infection should be included in the differential diagnosis of transcers myelitis of uncertain etiology [84]. CMV-DNA amplification in PCR method or immunohistochemical approach from CSF is a useful procedure for diagnosis of CMV infection [54]. If viremia exists PP65 antigen detection enables early and rapid diagnosis of CMV [85].

3.8. Fungal infection

In the era of transplantation and increase in use of immunosuppressive medications, spinal fungal infection should be considered in differential diagnosis of spinal infectious involvement [60]. The best method for diagnosis of fungal infection is biopsy and visualization of hyphae. Histopathologic findings confirm the diagnosis. Several serologic tests, antigen detection and PCR method for different fungal infection exist. Aspergillus can be identified by fungal culture and PCR [58]. Rhizopus may be identified by smear or culture from tissue biopsy [86].

3.9. Schistosomiasis

The diagnosis is difficult because the paraplegia mainly occurs during the early invasive phase of the adult worms, when there is little clinical or laboratory evidence of underlying schistosome infection. Stool examination for eggs and rectal snips are used for diagnosis [1]. Although laboratory investigations, including serological tests are of limited diagnostic value [87] Immunofluorescence assay and ELISA has been used for diagnosis [88].

4. Treatment

4.1. Subdural empyema

Treatment in virtually all cases of spinal subdural empyema requires prompt surgical drainage and antibiotic therapy [72] although a more expectant approach consisting of antibiotics and observation has also been proposed [8]. Provisional antibiotic therapy of spinal subdural empyemas should be directed against S. aureus and streptococci, and should include nafcillin, oxacillin, or vancomycin [72]. In some cases treatment with intravenous antibiotics and drainage is not enough and complete surgical excision of the lesion may be necessary [89].

4.2. Epidural abscess

The principles of therapy for spinal epidural abscess are prompt surgical decompression, drainage of the abscess, and long-term antimicrobial therapy. Empirical antimicrobial therapy for spinal epidural abscess must include antistaphylococcal agent plus coverage for aerobic gram-negative bacilli [6]. Recent reports have advocated for conservative, non-operative management of this devastating disorder with appropriate risk stratification. Crucial to a successful management strategy are definitive diagnosis, prompt intervention, and consistent follow-up care [90]. Although there are some case reports that present spinal epidural abscess treated with antibiotics alone [91] result of several studies strongly support immediate surgical decompression combined with appropriately tailored antibiotic therapy for the treatment of symptomatic spinal epidural abscess presenting with focal neurological deficit [90]. Recent evidence indicates the following areas of investigation and management can improve outcome in spinal epidural abscess: minimally invasive surgery early versus medical management when there are no significant neurological deficits, neuroradiologic arterial evaluation with therapies directed at vascular ischemia and thrombosis and aggressive rehabilitation [16].

4.3. Tuberculosis

Four anti tuberculosis drugs plus surgical intervention when indicated are cornerstones of treatment. In patients with multi drug resistant tuberculosis antibiogram and more prolong course of treatment is necessary. Anti tuberculosis therapy should be considered for at least 12 months [17]. A combination of conservative therapy and operative decompression when needed should form a comprehensive integrated course of treatment for spinal tuberculosis with neurological complications. The patients showing relatively preserved cord with evidence of edema or myelitis with predominantly fluid collection in extradural space on MRI may be managed by non-operative treatment, while the patients with extradural compression of mixed or granulomatous nature showing entrapment of spinal cord should be candidate for early surgical decompression. The disease focus should be debrided with removal of pus and sequestra. The viable bone should only be removed to decompress the spinal cord and resultant gap should be bridged by bone graft. The preserved volume of spinal cord with edema or myelitis and wet lesion on MRI usually would show good neural recovery. The spinal cord showing myelomalacia with reduced cord volume and dry lesion likely to show a poor neural recovery. The internal kyphectomy is indicated for paraplegia with healed disease. The best form of treatment of late onset paraplegia is the prevention of development of severe kyphosis in initial active stage of disease [26]. Surgery may be required in selected cases, e.g. large abscess formation, severe kyphosis, neurological deficit or lack of response to medical treatment [24].

4.4. Syphilis

Recognition of unusual complication of neurosyphilis is important, because it is a treatable cause of parapalegia with good recovery [77]. Greater alertness to diagnosis may result in earlier therapy and thus possibly lead to improved prognosis [78]. Aqueous crystalline penicillin G 3-4 million units intravenous every 4 hours for 10-14 days is treatment of choice. For patients with penicillin allergy other regimens may be used. Docycicline, amoxicillin and ceftriaxone are alternative treatments [92].

4.5. Lyme

The tick-borne spirochete responsible for Lyme disease is highly antibiotic-sensitive. Treatment is highly effective in the vast majority of patients, including those with nervous system disease. Nervous system infection, most typically meningitis, cranial neuritis, radiculoneuritis, and other forms of mononeuropathy multiplex, is highly antibiotic responsive. In patients with infection not involving the CNS, oral treatment with amoxicillin, cefuroxime axetil, or doxycycline for 2-4 weeks is almost always curative. Despite historic preferences for parenteral treatment with ceftriaxone, cefotaxime, or meningeal dose penicillin, patients with the forms of nervous system involvement listed above are highly responsive to oral doxycycline. Parenteral regimens can be reserved for those very rare patients with parenchymal CNS involvement, other severe forms of infection or the approximately 5% of patients who fail to respond to oral regimens [93].

4.6. Brucellosis

Neurobrucellosis, if not treated early, can result in severe neurological morbidity and sequelae, which may be irreversible. Hence it is important to consider the possibility of neurobrucellosis in endemic region and treat aggressively (94). Treatment with streptomycin, rifampicin and doxycyclin significantly improve the symptoms [44]. Doxycycline, rifampin, trimethoprim-sulfamethoxazole, streptomycin, gentamicin, ciprofloxacin and ceftriaxone are used for treatment of neurobrucellosis [95]. The mean duration of antimicrobial therapy is 18 weeks with range of 12-56 weeks. Prolonged duration of treatment especially in complicated cases in order to avoid possible sequelae is necessary [42]. In Gul's study duration of antibiotic therapy was ranged from 2 to 15 months (median 5 months) [96]. Neurobrucellosis and brucella spondylitis usually are treated with 3 drugs combination [46, 97]. The standard treatment of brucella spondylitis with a combination of two antibiotics for 6-12 weeks is associated with high rates of treatment failure and relapse. Prolonged administration of a triple combination of suitable antibiotics appears to be an effective treatment for brucella spondylitis [98]. The most commonly-used antibiotics are combinations of rifampin, doxycycline and trimethoprim-sulfamethoxazole [99].

4.7. Viral infection

For treatment of HIV usually 2 nucleoside analogue plus one protease inhibitor or one non-nucleoside reverse transcriptase inhibitor are used. Although nucleoside analogues, such as zidovudine and lamivudine, have long been recognized to have activity against HTLV reverse transcription in vitro, there is little clinical evidence of their efficacy in vivo, so treatment of asymptomatic HTLV carriers is not indicated. A combination of zidovudine and lamivudine has been used for treatment, but no clinical improvement was seen, and there was no effect on HTLV-I proviral load or immunologic markers [100]. The most commonly antiviral agents used for treatment of CMV are: ganciclovir, foscarnet, cidofovir, valganciclovir and valaciclovir [101]. Ganciclovir has been used in patients with CMV polyradiculopathy successfully [53].

4.8. Fungal infection

Depending on fungal infection, antifungal regimen such as amphotericin B, posaconazol, voriconazol, etc may be used with surgical intervention. Voriconazole has been used to treat aspergillosis [58]. The gold standard of systemic antifungal treatment is voriconazole, which has been proved to be significantly superior to conventional amphotericin B. Liposomal amphotericin B appears to be a suitable alternative for primary treatment, while caspofungin, amphotericin B lipid complex or posaconazole have shown partial or complete response in patients who had been refractory to or intolerant of primary antifungal therapy [101]. Itraconazole is more frequently used in immunosuppressed patients who are able to take oral therapy and for use as sequential oral therapy [102]. Options for initial therapy for invasive Candida infections include fluconazole, echinocandin compounds or liposomal amphotericin B. Voriconazole is the secondary alternative treatment [101]. Amphotericin B, caspofungin or posaconazole are used for treatment of Zygomycosis [103, 104].

4.9. Schistosomiasis

Praziquantel and corticoids have been successfully used to treat neuroschistosomiasis [65]. Surgery has been tried for acute cases of failed medical treatment [1].

5. Conclusion

Infectious diseases are important causes of non-traumatic paraplegia. High index of suspicion, precise history taking, exact physical examination and proper use of laboratory tests and radiologic studies are necessary for making accurate diagnosis. Sometimes the diagnosis is dependent to invasive procedure such as CT guided biopsy and subsequent histopathologic study, without them appropriate diagnosis may be impossible. Sometimes for accurate diagnosis using several laboratory and radiologic modalities, simultaneously, may be needed. Paying attention to specific treatment and its duration is very important. Sometimes combination antibiotic therapy is needed. If treatment or its duration is not appropriate, relapse may occur. Although paraplegia due to infectious diseases can be with high mortality rate, early diagnosed and successful treatment can prevent neurological sequelae.

Acknowledgements

With special thanks to Dr Katayoun Vahdat and Dr Mohammad Javadi

Author details

Farhad Abbasi[1] and Soolmaz Korooni Fardkhani[2]

1 Bushehr University of Medical Sciences, Iran

2 Shiraz University of Medical Sciences, Iran

References

[1] Howlwtt W.P. Paraplegia non traumatic. In: Howlwtt W. Neurology in Africa. Bergen, Norway: Bodoni; 2012.p.231.

[2] Chen Y, Tang Y, Vogel LC, Devivo MJ. Causes of spinal cord injury. Top Spinal Cord Inj Rehabil. 2013;19(1):1-8.

[3] Sandin KJ, Klaas SJ. Assessment and evaluation of primary prevention in spinal cord injury. Top Spinal Cord Inj Rehabil. 2013;19(1):9-14.

[4] Bellon K, Kolakowsky-Hayner SA, Chen D, McDowell S, Bitterman B, Klaas SJ. Evidence-based practice in primary prevention of spinal cord injury. Top Spinal Cord Inj Rehabil. 2013;19(1):25-30.

[5] Hess ChW. Non-traumatic acute transverse spinal cord syndromes. Praxis. 2005;94(30-31):1151-9.

[6] Tunkel A.R. Subdural empyema, epidural abscess and suppurative intracrainial thrombophelebitis. In: Mandell G.L, Benett J.E, Dolin R. Principle and practice of infectious diseases. 7th edition. Philadelphia, USA: Elsevier; 2010.p.1279-82.

[7] Coumans JV, Walcott BP. Rapidly progressive lumbar subdural empyema following acromial bursal injection. J Clin Neurosci. 2011;18(11):1562-3.

[8] Sandler AL, Thompson D, Goodrich JT, van Aalst J, Kolatch E, El Khashab M, Nejat F, Cornips E, Mohindra S, Gupta R, Yassari R, Daniels LB, Biswas A, Abbott R. Infections of the spinal subdural space in children: a series of 11 contemporary cases and review of all published reports. A multinational collaborative effort. Childs Nerv Syst. 2013;29(1):105-17.

[9] Chen MH, Chen MH, Huang JS. Cervical subdural empyema following acupuncture. J Clin Neurosci. 2004;11(8):909-11.

[10] Kalaycý M, Cadavi F, Altunkaya H, Gül S, Ackgöz B. Subdural empyema due to spinal anesthesia. Acta Anaesthesiol Scand. 2005;49(3):426.

[11] Volk T, Hebecker R, Ruecker G, Perka C, Haas N, Spies C. Subdural empyema combined with paraspinal abscess after epidural catheter insertion. Anesth Analg. 2005;100(4):1222-3.

[12] Vural M, Arslantaş A, Adapinar B, Kiremitçi A, Usluer G, Cuong B, Atasoy MA. Spinal subdural Staphylococcus aureus abscess: case report and review of the literature. Acta Neurol Scand. 2005;112(5):343-6.

[13] Delgado Tapia JA, Galera López J, Santiago Martín J, Galdo Abadín JR, Quirante Pizarro A, Cánovas Fernández E, García Villalba F. Subdural empyema due to Mycoplasma hominis after a cesarean section under spinal anesthesia. Rev Esp Anestesiol Reanim. 2005;52(4):239-42.

[14] Sales JG, Tabrizi A, Elmi A, Soleimanpour J, Gavidel E. Adolescence spinal epidural abscess with neurological symptoms: case report, a lesson to be re-learnt. Med J Islam Repub Iran. 2013;27(1):38-41.

[15] Ohyagi M, Ohkubo T, Taniyama T, Tomizawa S, Okawa A, Yokota T, Mizusawa H. Spinal epidural abscess caused by bacteroides fragilis group after dilation and curettage for incomplete abortion. J Glob Infect Dis. 2012;4(2):132-4.

[16] Shah NH, Roos KL. Spinal epidural abscess and paralytic mechanisms. Curr Opin Neurol. 2013;26(3):314-7.

[17] Gehlot PS, Chaturvedi S, Kashyap R, Singh V. Pott's Spine: Retrospective Analysis of MRI Scans of 70 Cases. J Clin Diagn Res. 2012;6(9):1534-8.

[18] Yadegarynia D, Abbasi F, Keshtkar-Jahromi M, Gholamin S. Gastrointestinal Tuberculosis with Cecum Involvement in a 33-Year-Old Woman. Iran J Med Sci. 2009;34(3): 213-16

[19] Goasdoué P, Dubayle P, Boyer B, Debord T, Le Clainche P, Pharaboz C. Disseminated tuberculosis of unusual locations. J Radiol. 1997;78(9):659-61.

[20] Beshart M, Abbasi F, Behzad H.R. Tuberculosis meningitis, mutiple brain tuberculoma and ocular involvement in a 20 year old man. Journal of medical council of I.R.I. 2008; 26(3);409-412.

[21] Beshart M, Abbasi F, Behzad H.R. A young Afghan man with prolonged fever and headache. Iran J Clin infect Dis. 2009;4(1):45-6.

[22] Hristea A, Constantinescu RV, Exergian F, Arama V, Besleaga M, Tanasescu R. Paraplegia due to non-osseous spinal tuberculosis: report of three cases and review of the literature. Int J Infect Dis. 2008;12(4):425-9.

[23] Abbas A, Rizvi SR, Mahesri M, Salahuddin HR. Conservative management of spinal tuberculosis: initial series from pakistan. Asian Spine J. 2013;7(2):73-80.

[24] Garg RK, Somvanshi DS. Spinal tuberculosis: a review. J Spinal Cord Med. 2011;34(5):440-54.

[25] Abbasi F, Besharat M. Tuberculosis Spondylitis (Pott's Disease) in Iran, Evaluation of 40 Cases. Iran J Clin infect Dis. 2011;6 suppl:30-32

[26] Jain AK, Kumar J. Tuberculosis of spine: neurological deficit. Eur Spine J. 2013 Jun;22 Suppl 4:624-33.

[27] Muthukumar N, Venkatesh G, Senthilbabu S, Rajbaskar R. Surgery for intramedullary tuberculoma of the spinal cord: report of 2 cases. Surg Neurol. 2006;66(1):69-7.

[28] Molina-Olier O, Tuñón-Pitalúa M, Alcalá-Cerra G, Niño-Hernández L, Moscote-Salazar L. Spinal cord compression due to intraspinal syphilitic gumma in one patient. Clinical case. Acta Ortop Mex. 2012;26(3):197-201.

[29] Tsui EY, Ng SH, Chow L, Lai KF, Fong D, Chan JH. Syphilitic myelitis with diffuse spinal cord abnormality on MR imaging. Eur Radiol. 2002;12(12):2973-6.

[30] Miura M, Kuraoka S, Kanazawa H, Oguma F, Irisawa H, Kasuya S, Sakashita I. Syphilitic thoracic aortic aneurysm with destruction of vertebral body, producing numbness of lower extremities and paraplegia. Kyobu Geka. 1995;48(11):953-6.

[31] Leung JS, Mok CK, Leong JC, Chan WC. Syphilitic aortic aneurysm with spinal erosion. Treatment by aneurysm replacement and anterior spinal fusion. J Bone Joint Surg Br. 1977;59(1):89-92.

[32] Brangulis K, Tars K, Petrovskis I, Kazaks A, Ranka R, Baumanis V. Structure of an outer surface lipoprotein BBA64 from the Lyme disease agent Borrelia burgdorferi which is critical to ensure infection after a tick bite. Acta Crystallogr D Biol Crystallogr. 2013;69(Pt 6):1099-107.

[33] Büker, Picozzi, Kolb, Hatt. First detection of Borrelia burgdorferi-antibodies in free-living birds of prey from Eastern Westphalia, Germany. Schweiz Arch Tierheilkd. 2013;155(7):411-6.

[34] Brangulis K, Petrovskis I, Kazaks A, Baumanis V, Tars K. Structural characterization of the Borrelia burgdorferi outer surface protein BBA73 implicates dimerization as a functional mechanism. Biochem Biophys Res Commun. 2013;434(4):848-53.

[35] Potok OV, Brassard A. Lyme borreliosis: an update for Canadian dermatologists. J Cutan Med Surg. 2013;17(1):13-21.

[36] Erol I, Kılıçarslan B, Saygi S, Demir S, Alehan F. Acute transverse myelitis in a child with lyme disease and a review of literature. Pediatr Neurol. 2013;48(4):325-8.

[37] Zajkowska JM, Hermanowska-Szpakowicz T, Kondrusik M, Pancewicz SA. Neurologic syndromes in Lyme disease. Pol Merkur Lekarski. 2000;9(50):584-8.

[38] Salonen R, Rinne JO, Halonen P, Puusa A, Marttila R, Viljanen MK. Lyme borreliosis associated with complete flaccid paraplegia. J Infect. 1994;28(2):181-4.

[39] Lim KB, Kwak YG, Kim DY, Kim YS, Kim JA. Back pain secondary to Brucella spondylitis in the lumbar region. Ann Rehabil Med. 2012;36(2):282-6

[40] Baykal T, Baygutalp F, Senel K, Levent A, Erdal A, Ugur M, Ozgocmen S. Spastic paraparesis and sensorineural hearing loss in a patient with neurobrucellosis. J Back Musculoskelet Rehabil. 2012;25(3):157-9

[41] Köse Ş, Senger SS, Çavdar G, Yavaş S. Case report on the development of a brucellosis-related epidural abscess. J Infect Dev Ctries. 2011;5(5):403-5.

[42] Ulu-Kilic A, Sayar MS, Tütüncü E, Sezen F, Sencan I. Complicated brucellar spondylodiscitis: experience from an endemic area. Rheumatol Int. 2012; DOI: 10.1007/s00296-012-2555-5

[43] Tappe D, Melzer F, Schmoock G, Elschner M, Lâm TT, Abele-Horn M, Stetter C. Isolation of Brucella melitensis biotype 3 from epidural empyema in a Bosnian immigrant in Germany. J Med Microbiol. 2012;61(Pt 9):1335-7.

[44] Lampropoulos C, Kamposos P, Papaioannou I, Niarou V. Cervical epidural abscess caused by brucellosis. BMJ Case Rep. 2012 Nov 27;2012. pii: bcr2012007070. doi: 10.1136/bcr-2012-007070.

[45] Ekici MA, Ozbek Z, Gökoğlu A, Menkü A. Surgical management of cervical spinal epidural abscess caused by Brucella melitensis : report of two cases and review of the literature. J Korean Neurosurg Soc. 2012;51(6):383-7

[46] Mousa AR, Koshy TS, Araj GF, Marafie AA, Muhtaseb SA, Al-Mudallal DS, Busharetulla MS. Brucella meningitis: presentation, diagnosis and treatment--a prospective study of ten cases. Q J Med. 1986;60(233):873-85.

[47] Tur BS, Suldur N, Ataman S, Ozturk EA, Bingol A, Atay MB. Brucellar spondylitis: a rare cause of spinal cord compression. Spinal Cord. 2004;42(5):321-4.

[48] Modi G, Ranchhod J, Hari K, Mochan A, Modi M. Non-traumatic myelopathy at the Chris Hani Baragwanath Hospital, South Africa--the influence of HIV. QJM. 2011;104(8):697-703

[49] Grasso G, Meli F, Graziano F, Stagno V, Imbrucè P, Florena AM, Maugeri R, Iacopino DG. Chronic inflammation causing spinal cord compression in human immunodeficiency virus infection. Med Sci Monit. 2008;14(11):CS134-7.

[50] Gonzalez LA, Villa AM, Kohler G, Garcea O, Kremenchutzky M, Caceres F, Sanz OP, Sica RE. Further studies on HTLV-I associated myelopathy in Argentina. Medicina (B Aires). 1998;58(4):411-4.

[51] Amayo EO, Kwasa TO, Otieno CF. Herpes zoster myelitis: report of two cases. East Afr Med J. 2002;79(5):279-80.

[52] Chrétien F, Gray F, Lescs MC, Geny C, Dubreuil-Lemaire ML, Ricolfi F, Baudrimont M, Levy Y, Sobel A, Vinters HV. Acute varicella-zoster virus ventriculitis and meningo-myelo-radiculitis in acquired immunodeficiency syndrome. Acta Neuropathol. 1993;86(6):659-65.

[53] Kim YS, Hollander H. Polyradiculopathy due to cytomegalovirus: report of two cases in which improvement occurred after prolonged therapy and review of the literature. Clin Infect Dis. 1993;17(1):32-7.

[54] Matsumoto R, Nakagawa S, Nakayama J, Hashimoto T, Shindo M. A case of acquired immune deficiency syndrome presenting acute lumbosacral polyradiculopathy due to opportunistic infection of cytomegalovirus. Rinsho Shinkeigaku. 1998;38(7):653-7.

[55] Behar R, Wiley C, McCutchan JA. Cytomegalovirus polyradiculoneuropathy in acquired immune deficiency syndrome. Neurology. 1987;37(4):557-61.

[56] López-Cortés LE, Garcia-Vidal C, Ayats J, Gudiol C, Bodro M, Sánchez-Ortega I, Peña C, Carratalá J. Invasive aspergillosis with extrapulmonary involvement: pathogenesis, clinical characteristics and prognosis. Rev Iberoam Micol. 2012;29(3):139-43.

[57] Kim CH, Kim MO, Yoon JS. Paraplegia Caused by Infection Extending to Spine Due to Aspergillosis: A Case Report. J Korean Acad Rehabil Med. 2001;25(3):519-522.

[58] Jiang Z, Wang Y, Jiang Y, Xu Y, Meng B. Vertebral osteomyelitis and epidural abscess due to Aspergillus nidulans resulting in spinal cord compression: Case report and literature review. J Int Med Res. 2013;41(2):502-10.

[59] Chang HM, Yu HH, Yang YH, Lee WI, Lee JH, Wang LC, Lin YT, Chiang BL. Successful treatment of Aspergillus flavus spondylodiscitis with epidural abscess in a patient with chronic granulomatous disease. Pediatr Infect Dis J. 2012;31(1):100-1.

[60] Karthik K, Shetty AP, Rajasekaran S. Spontaneous cord transection due to invasive aspergillus spondylitis in an immunocompetent child. Eur Spine J. 2011;20 Suppl 2:S188-92.

[61] Werner BC, Hogan MV, Shen FH. Candida lusitaniae discitis after discogram in an immunocompetent patient. Spine J. 2011;11(10):e1-6.

[62] Tuyumu K, Nakaya A, Miyauchi J, Okamoto S. Epidural abscess in the spine extended from pulmonary zygomycosis during consolidation chemotherapy for acute lymphoblastic leukemia. Rinsho Ketsueki. 2011;52(8):718-21.

[63] Rivierez M, Heyman D, Brebion A, Landau-Ossondo M, Desbois N, Vally P. Spinal cord histoplasmoma. A case report. Neurochirurgie. 2002;48(1):44-8.

[64] Carod-Artal FJ. Neurological complications of Schistosoma infection. Trans R Soc Trop Med Hyg. 2008;102(2):107-16.

[65] Carod-Artal FJ. Neuroschistosomiasis. Expert Rev Anti Infect Ther. 2010;8(11): 1307-18.

[66] II. Kim SH, Son DW, Lee SW, Song GS. An unusual case of post-operative spondylitis caused by mycobacterium intracellulare in an immunosuppressed patient. J Korean Neurosurg Soc. 2011;50(5):460-3.

[67] Edwards C, Diveronica M, Abel E. Epidural abscess caused by Mycobacterium abscessus. Am J Case Rep. 2012;13:180-2.

[68] West KR, Mason RC, Sun M. Nocardia spinal epidural abscess: 14-year follow-up. Orthopedics. 2012;35(1):e128-31.

[69] Fernández-Fernández FJ, Puerta-Louro R, Rodríguez-Conde I, de la Fuente-Aguado J. Epidural abscess caused by Pasteurella pneumotropica. Enferm Infecc Microbiol Clin. 2011;29(8):637-8.

[70] Bartels RH, de Jong TR, Grotenhuis JA. Spinal subdural abscess. Case report. J Neurosurg. 1992;76(2):307-11.

[71] De Bonis P, Anile C, Pompucci A, Labonia M, Lucantoni C, Mangiola A. Cranial and spinal subdural empyema. Br J Neurosurg. 2009;23(3):335-40.

[72] Greenlee JE. Subdural Empyema. Curr Treat Options Neurol. 2003;5(1):13-22.

[73] Araújo F, Ribeiro C, Silva I, Nero P, Branco JC. Klebsiella pneumoniae Spinal Epidural Abscess treated conservatively: case report and review. Acta Reumatol Port. 2012;37(3):260-3.

[74] Jain AK. Tuberculosis of the spine: a fresh look at an old disease. J Bone Joint Surg Br. 2010;92(7):905-13.

[75] Jain AK, Sreenivasan R, Saini NS, Kumar S, Jain S, Dhammi IK. Magnetic resonance evaluation of tubercular lesion in spine. Int Orthop. 2012;36(2):261-9.

[76] Arora S, Kumar R. Tubercular spinal epidural abscess involving the dorsal-lumbar-sacral region without osseous involvement. J Infect Dev Ctries. 2011 Jul 27;5(7):544-9.

[77] Jacquemin GL, Proulx P, Gilbert DA, Albert G, Morcos R. Functional recovery from paraplegia caused by syphilitic meningomyelitis. J Spinal Cord Med. 2002;25(2): 133-7.

[78] Silber MH. Syphilitic myelopathy. Genitourin Med. 1989;65(5):338-41.

[79] Barón M, Heredero J, Prieto I, Lousa M, Masjuán J, Gobernado JM. Dorsal subdural spinal abscess after epidural anesthesia. Neurologia. 1997;12(6):262-4.

[80] Magnarelli LA. Laboratory diagnosis of Lyme disease. Rheum Dis Clin North Am. 1989;15(4):735-45.

[81] Bodmer K. Brucella spondylodiskitis. Schweiz Med Wochenschr. 1985;115(34):1160-5.

[82] Besharat M, Abbasi F, Korooni Fardkhani S. Epidemiological features, hematologic characteristics and clinical manifestations in adult patients with brucellosis. Iran J Clin infect Dis.2010;5(3):189-190.

[83] Arkun R, Mete BD. Musculoskeletal brucellosis. Semin Musculoskelet Radiol. 2011;15(5):470-9.

[84] Karacostas D, Christodoulou C, Drevelengas A, Paschalidou M, Ioannides P, Constantinou A, Milonas I. Cytomegalovirus-associated transverse myelitis in a non-immunocompromised patient. Spinal Cord. 2002;40(3):145-9.

[85] Yadegarynia D, Abbasi F, Haghighi M, Korooni Fardkhani S, Yadegarynia S. Pneumonitis due to cytomegalovirus in an immunocompromised patient. Iran J Clin infect Dis. 2009;4(4):238-240.

[86] Mardani M, Abbasi F, Aghahasani M, Aghazade Sarhangipour K,Hoseinishokouh S.J, Talebzade A. Report of four cases of Rhinocerebral mucormycosis in Loghman hospital. Journal of army university of medical sciences. 2009; 7(2): 143-6.

[87] Scrimgeour EM, Gajdusek DC. Involvement of the central nervous system in Schistosoma mansoni and S. haematobium infection. A review. Brain. 1985;108 (Pt 4): 1023-38.

[88] Peregrino AJ, Puglia PM, Nobrega JP, Livramento JA, Marques-Dias MJ, Scaff M. Schistosomiasis of the spinal cord: analysis of 80 cases. Arq Neuropsiquiatr. 2002;60(3-A):603-8.

[89] Barón M, Heredero J, Prieto I, Lousa M, Masjuán J, Gobernado JM. Dorsal subdural spinal abscess after epidural anesthesia. Neurologia. 1997;12(6):262-4.

[90] Connor DE Jr, Chittiboina P, Caldito G, Nanda A. Comparison of operative and non-operative management of spinal epidural abscess: a retrospective review of clinical and laboratory predictors of neurological outcome. J Neurosurg Spine. 2013;19(1): 119-27.

[91] Pathak A, Singh P, Gehlot P, Dhaneria M. Spinal epidural abscess treated with antibiotics alone. BMJ Case Rep. 2013 Apr 30;2013. pii: bcr2013009285. doi: 10.1136/bcr-2013-009285.

[92] Tramont E.C. Treponoma pallidum (Syphilis). In: Mandell G.L, Benett J.E, Dolin R. Principle and practice of infectious diseases. 7th edition. Philadelphia, USA: Elsevier; 2010.p.3035-53

[93] Halperin JJ. Nervous System Lyme Disease: Diagnosis and Treatment. Curr Treat Options Neurol. 2013 May 12.

[94] Vajramani GV, Nagmoti MB, Patil CS. Neurobrucellosis presenting as an intra-medullary spinal cord abscess. Ann Clin Microbiol Antimicrob. 2005 16;4:14.

[95] Asadipooya K, Dehghanian1 AR, Ranjbar Omrani1 GH, Abbasi F. Short-course treatment in neurobrucellosis: A study in Iran. Neurology India. 2011;59 (1):101-3

[96] Gul HC, Erdem H, Bek S. Overview of neurobrucellosis: a pooled analysis of 187 cases. Int J Infect Dis. 2009;13(6):e339-43.

[97] Bucher A, Gaustad P, Pape E. Chronic neurobrucellosis due to Brucella melitensis. Scand J Infect Dis. 1990;22(2):223-6.

[98] Ioannou S, Karadima D, Pneumaticos S, Athanasiou H, Pontikis J, Zormpala A, Sipsas NV. Efficacy of prolonged antimicrobial chemotherapy for brucellar spondylodiscitis. Clin Microbiol Infect. 2011;17(5):756-62.

[99] Haji-Abdolbagi M, Rasooli-Nejad M, Jafari S, Hasibi M, Soudbakhsh A. Clinical and laboratory findings in neurobrucellosis: review of 31 cases. Arch Iran Med. 2008;11(1):21-5.

[100] Murphy E.L, Biswas H.H. Human T-Cell Lymphotropic Virus Types I and II. In: In: Mandell G.L, Benett J.E, Dolin R. Principle and practice of infectious diseases. 7th edition. Philadelphia, USA: Elsevier; 2010.p. 2303-32

[101] Abbasi F. Infectious diseases and clinical complications during treatment in CLL. In: Oppezzo P. Chronic lymphocytic leukemia. 1st edition. Rijeka, Croatia: InTech; 2012. p 367-382.

[102] Yadegarynia D, Haghighi M, Abbasi F, Gholamin S, Yadegarynia S. Invasive aspergillosis of pituitary gland in an immunocompetent patient. Iran J Clin infect Dis. 2008;3(3):163-165

[103] De Pasqual A, Deprez M, Ghaye B, Frère P, Kaschten B, Hayette MP, Radermecker M, Martin D, Canivet JL. Invasive pulmonary mucormycosis with invasion of the thoracic spine in a patient with myelodysplastic syndrome. Rev Med Liege. 2008 Dec; 63(12):702-6.

[104] Gurevich M, Levi I, Steinberg R, Shonfeld T, Shapiro R, Israeli M, Sprecher H, Shalit I, Mor E. Mucormycosis in a liver allograft: salvage re-transplantation and targeted immunosuppressive management. Transpl Infect Dis. 2012;14(5):E97-101.

Chapter 2

Paraplegia as a Complication of Thoracic and Thoracoabdominal Aortic Interventions

Anisha H. Perera and Richard G.J. Gibbs

Additional information is available at the end of the chapter

http://dx.doi.org/10.5772/57528

1. Introduction

1.1. The thoracic aorta, its conditions and their management

The thoracic aorta The thoracic aorta comprises the ascending aorta, transverse aortic arch and descending thoracic aorta (Figure 1). The aortic arch is the segment from where the carotid and subclavian vessels arise. The descending thoracic aorta begins immediately distal to the left subclavian artery and extends up to the diaphragm. A thoracic aortic aneurysm (TAA) is defined as dilatation of the thoracic aorta to a diameter at least 1.5 times greater than is normal at a given aortic level (Figure 2). Thoracoabdominal aortic aneurysms (TAAA) involve the thoracic aorta and extend into the abdominal aorta. They are classified according to the Crawford classification as types I to IV. Due to their extent and frequent involvement of the visceral vessels, management is invariably complex. TAAs often result from cystic medial degeneration weakening of the aortic wall, though the majority are associated with atherosclerosis and risk factors such as hypertension, hypercholesterolemia and smoking. These aneurysms occur most frequently in the 6th and 7th decade of life. In younger patients TAA is commonly associated with connective tissue disorders such as Marfan, Ehlers-Danlos and Loeys-Dietz syndromes. Acute aortic syndrome comprises a spectrum of emergency conditions caused by disruption of the medial layer of the aortic wall, which includes aortic dissection, intramural haematoma and penetrating atherosclerotic ulcers. Thoracic aortic dissection (TAD) is defined as separation of the aortic media, with the presence of extraluminal blood within the layers of the aortic wall (Figure 3).

Asymptomatic and small TAAs are initially managed medically, whilst symptomatic (usually pain or compression symptoms) or rapidly expanding aneurysms as well as those greater than 6cm in diameter necessitate surgical intervention to prevent rupture. TADs many also be

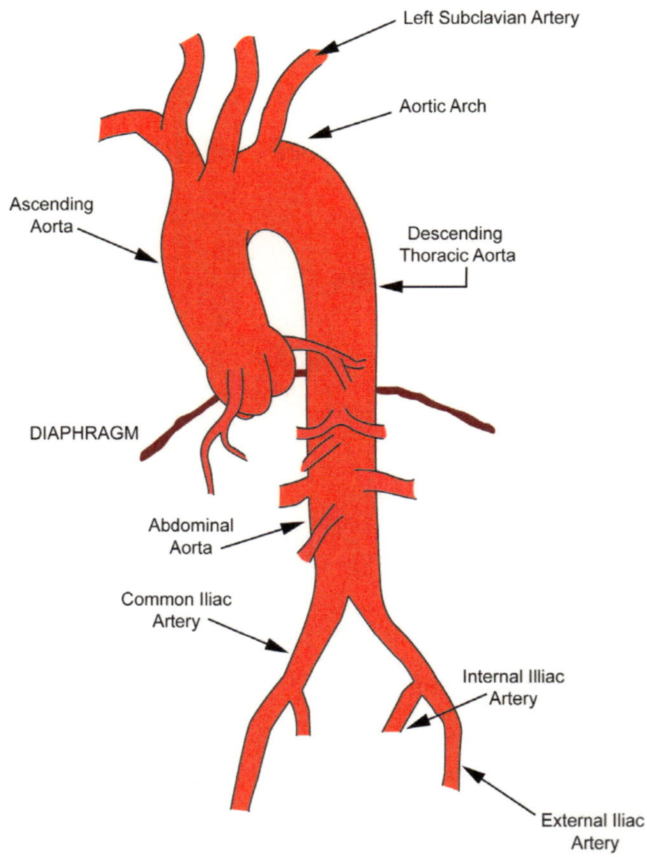

Figure 1. The aorta (*Image by Miss S. M. Perera*)

initially managed medically with the focus on blood pressure control, although immediate surgical intervention is required in patients with visceral, renal or limb malperfusion or for complications such as secondary dilatation and aneurysm formation. Historically, open surgical repair was the treatment for both TAA and TAD. In recent years, the advent of the endovascular stent-graft has resulted in minimally invasive treatment options. Thoracic endovascular aortic repair (TEVAR) is the placement of an endovascular stent to treat pathology of the thoracic aorta (Figure 4), and there has been a dramatic increase in the number of thoracic endografts placed in the recent years. TEVAR has now been adopted as the surgical approach of choice (particularly in the developed world), and in many countries it exceeds the number of open procedures performed for thoracic aortic pathologies.

Open surgical repair (Figure 5) Open surgery of TAA involves a left thoracotomy or thoracoabdominal incision, and the choice of specific surgical technique is dependent on aneurysm morphology, aortic anatomy and surgeon preference. The aorta is cross-clamped and minimizing ischemia time is vital to ensure adequate perfusion of the bowel, kidneys and lower limbs. The two most commonly applied approaches include a clamp-and-sew technique or the

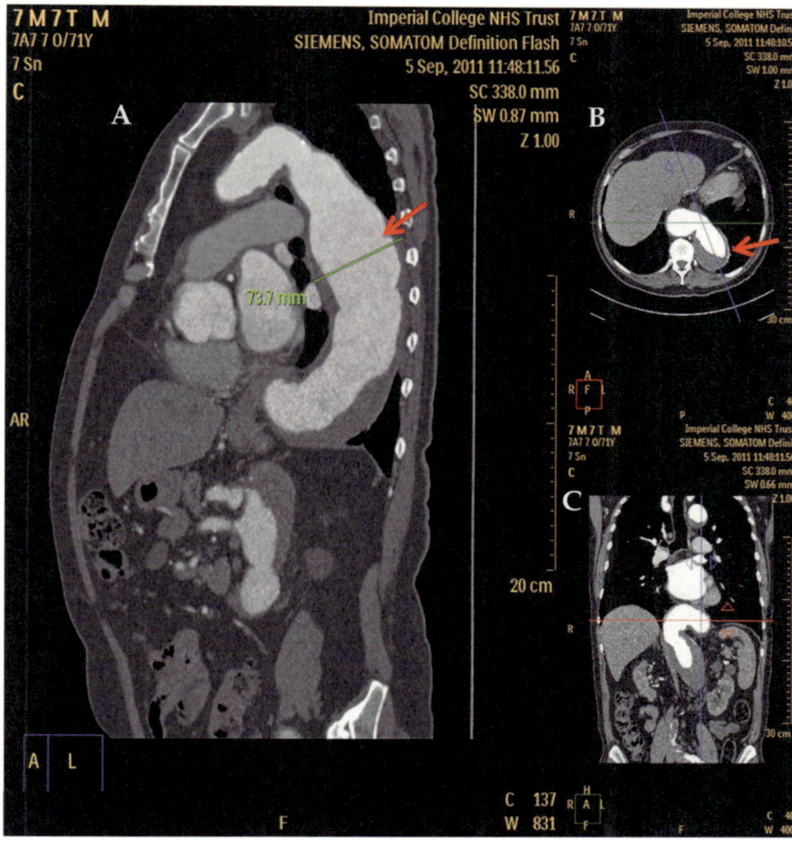

Figure 2. Thoracic aortic aneurysm CT angiogram of 7cm thoracic aortic aneurysm (arrow) in A) sagittal B) axial and C) coronal planes

use of distal aortic perfusion usually provided with an atrio-femoral bypass circuit, although total cardiopulmonary bypass with deep hypothermic circulatory arrest can also be utilized [1]. The aneurysmal aorta is replaced with a Dacron graft using a hand-sewn anastomosis, and vessels (visceral or head and neck) involved in the aneurysm are revascularized. Complications include mortality, cardiovascular and respiratory compromise, bleeding, acute renal failure, stroke and paraplegia. For thoracic and thoracoabdominal aneurysm repair, operative mortality is significant and varies from 2.7 to 8.8% and 7.6 to 14 respectively [2-5]. Paraplegia/paraparesis occurs in 2.7 to 12% in thoracic and 3.6 to 16% in thoracoabdominal open surgical procedures [2, 3, 5, 6].

Thoracic endovascular aortic repair TEVAR allows aneurysm exclusion without the need for thoracotomy and aortic cross-clamping. A pre-sized covered stent-graft is inserted through the common femoral artery via a surgical groin incision and deployed under fluoroscopic guidance (Figure 4). Additional percutaneous access via the contralateral femoral or left brachial artery is obtained for placement of an imaging catheter. Similar to open techniques, any vessels involved in the aneurysm or dissection, both visceral and head and neck, are

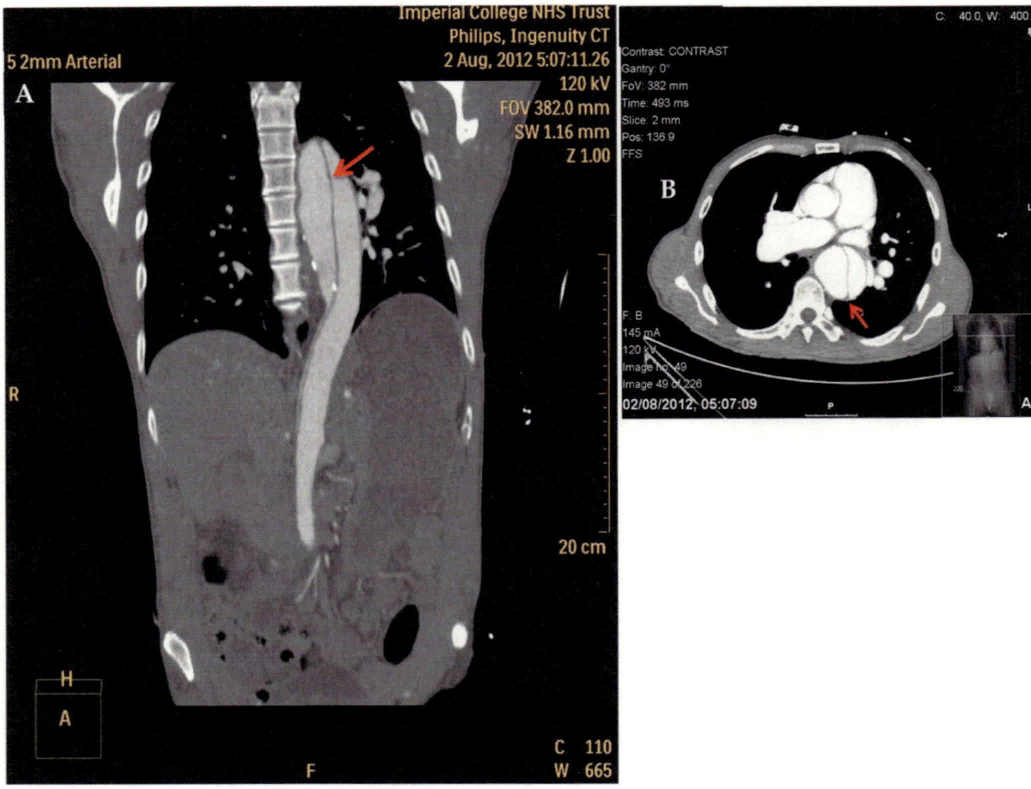

Figure 3. Aortic dissection CT angiogram of type B aortic dissection in A) coronal and B) axial planes. Arrow indicates dissection flap caused by separation of the layers of the aortic wall, with blood within the layers forming a true and false lumen

revascularized prior to stent-graft deployment. In instances of extensive arch or visceral open revascularization prior to stenting, the procedure is termed a hybrid procedure, denoting the combined open and endovascular approach. Recent advances in stent-graft technology have now allowed options for scalloped, fenestrated and branched grafts, mitigating the need for open surgical revascularization in suitable cases. Several challenges remain with TEVAR however, including narrow iliac diameter, vessel tortuosity, aortic arch angulation and the need for adequate sealing zones to ensure stable stent fixation. Complications include stroke, paraplegia, endoleak (persistent blood flow outside the lumen of the stent-graft and within the aneurysm sac due to incomplete sealing or exclusion of aneurysm sac, usually requiring further intervention), the need for re-intervention and less frequently mortality and conversion to open procedure. The global incidence for paraplegia post thoracic stenting varies from 0 to 9.8%, with a permanent paraplegia risk of 5.5%. The paraplegia risk for isolated descending thoracic stents is 0.9%, with poorer outcomes for more complex procedures involving fenestrated and branched stents (7.1%) and visceral hybrid procedures (11.3%) [7]. Both immediate and delayed onset paraplegia have been observed following TEVAR, with cases of delayed neurological deficit occurring from twelve hours up to one month postoperatively [8].

http://dx.doi.org/10.5772/57528

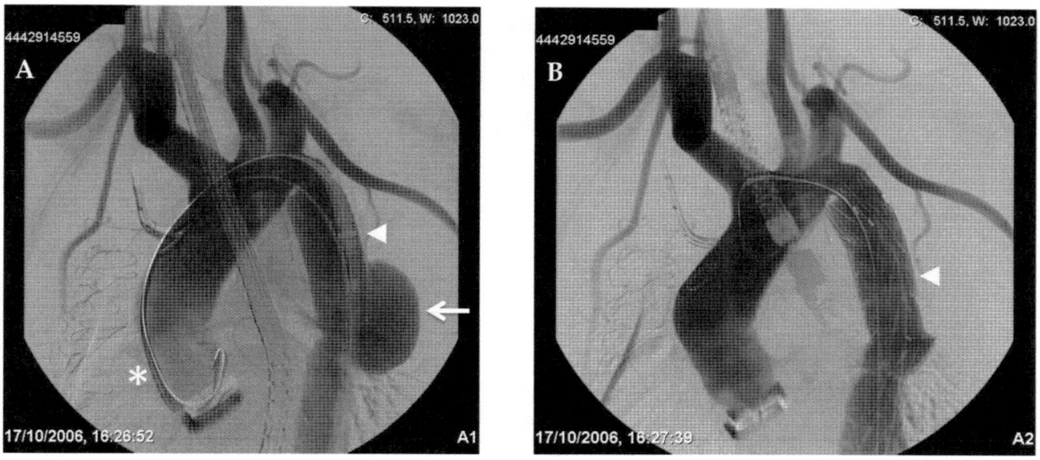

Figure 4. Thoracic endovascular aortic repair (TEVAR) Angiogram images outlining procedural steps A) Guidewire and catheter in aortic arch (star). Stent-graft ensheathed within delivery device advanced up descending thoracic aorta (arrow head). Placed under fluoroscopic guidance and contrast angiogram performed. Arrow indicates thoracic aortic aneurysm B) Stent-graft deployed (arrow head). Contrast angiogram performed to confirm exclusion of aneurysm, correct position of stent and patency of all arch vessels

Epidemiology Between 1999 and 2010, hospital admissions for total (ascending and descending) thoracic aortic disease in the UK rose steadily from 7.2 to 8.8 per 100,000 of population (p=0.0001) for TAD, and from 4.4 to 9.0 (p<0.0001) for TAA [9]. Since separate coding for open repair and TEVAR was initiated in 2006, the rate of repairs for descending TAAs have more than doubled from 0.7 in 2005 to 1.9 per 100,000 population in 2010. The rates for open repair have been steady, and the observed increase is entirely attributable to the increased rate of TEVAR. The changes for type B aortic dissection are even more remarkable, where overall repair rates have increased from 0.1 per 100,000 in 2000 to 0.5 per 100,000 population (p=0.0001) in 2010. Data is from Hospital Episodes Statistics (HES) (England) and Health Solutions Wales PEDW Statistics (Wales). The changing trends indicate a likely increase in thoracic vascular workload in the future. Therefore recognizing, managing and reducing the incidence of spinal cord ischemia (SCI) as a complication of thoracic and thoracoabdominal aortic intervention is essential.

1.2. The spinal cord

Anatomy The blood supply to the thoracic spinal cord comes from a single anterior spinal artery (formed by the union of two branches from the vertebral arteries) and two paired posterior spinal arteries (also derived from the vertebral arteries), which run the length of the spinal cord [10]. The vascular anatomy is variable however, and these arteries may not be continuous along their course. Both the anterior and posterior spinal arteries are supplemented by segmental radicular arteries, which are small branches of the cervical, thoracic and lumbar vessels. The largest of the radicular arteries is the artery of Adamkiewicz, often given off at the level of T10 but it can vary in position from T7 to L4 [11]. This artery supplies the conus, but has a poor connection with the superior portion of the spinal cord. It is given off by the left

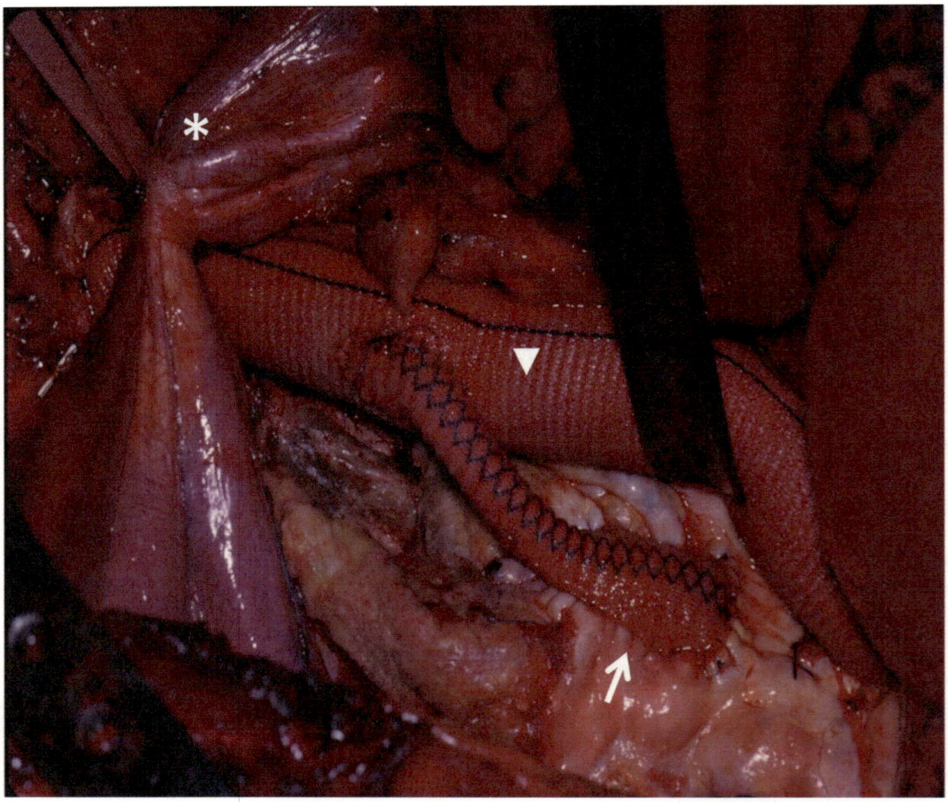

Figure 5. Open repair Retraction of the diaphragm (star) with open repair of thoracoabdominal aortic aneurysm with Dacron graft (arrow head) and reimplantation of an intercostal artery (arrow) (*Image courtesy of Mr J. H. Wolfe)*

intercostal or lumbar artery in over 75% of patients and is recognized by its characteristic hairpin bend. Another important radicular artery is the mid-thoracic radicular branch, which arises from the T7 posterior intercostal artery and supplements the blood supply of the fourth to eighth segments of the thoracic spinal cord.

Previous consensus has been that identification and reimplantation of the artery of Adamkiewicz during TAAA repair is the best strategy for preserving spinal cord blood supply and thereby preventing paraplegia. SCI remains a problem however and re-anastomosis of arteries, a difficult enough undertaking in the context of an open repair, is not possible with current endovascular techniques. Anatomic studies have been undertaken to establish the presence of an extensive collateral network that supports spinal cord perfusion and explains preservation of spinal cord perfusion when segmental vessels are interrupted [12]. It is reported that the thoracic and lumbar segmental arteries give rise to three major vessel groups which anastomose with one another and with the nutrient arteries of the spinal cord: 1) the intrathecal vessels; the anterior spinal artery and the longitudinal chain of epidural arcades lying between the spinal cord and the vertebral bodies, 2) the interconnecting vessels lying outside the spinal canal along the dorsal processes of the vertebral bodies and paravertebral tissues, 3) a large collection of interconnecting vessels supplying the paraspinous muscles including the iliopsoas anteriorly and erector spinae posteriorly (Figure 6). The configuration of the arterial network includes inputs not only from the intercostal and lumbar segmental vessels, but also from the subclavian and hypogastric arteries. The presence of this extensive network implies a considerable reserve to ensure spinal cord perfusion when some inputs are compromised. It also highlights the threat of steal phenomenon, as a significant finding of the study was how dramatically the muscular arterial component dominates the anatomy of the network when compared with the small arteries that feed the spinal cord directly. The studies reinforce the idea that the spinal cord circulation is a longitudinally continuous and flexible system, so that input from any single segmental artery along its length is unlikely to be critical. Various studies have already demonstrated that the total loss of segmental arteries sacrificed during TAAA repair is a more powerful predictor of the risk of paraplegia than loss of any individual segmental artery.

Physiology Cerebrospinal fluid (CSF) is secreted by the central nervous system and fills the ventricles and subarachnoid space of the brain and the spinal column. It protects the brain from physical impact, circulates nutrients and has a role in waste management. Spinal cord perfusion pressure is a balance between the inflow and outflow pressures within the closed confines of the spinal canal, calculated as mean arterial pressure (MAP) minus CSF pressure. The inflow depends principally on arterial pressure, which is largely determined by cardiac output, blood volume, and the competing demands of viscera and muscle tissue connected to the same collateral network. Theoretically therefore, decreasing the CSF pressure or increasing the blood pressure/MAP will improve spinal cord perfusion pressure. CSF pressure can be decreased by insertion of a lumbar CSF drain and allowing free drainage by gravity (Figure 7). The drain is transduced to obtain pressure measurements and the rate of CSF drainage is altered by adjusting the height of the drip chamber from the ground until the desired drainage rate and pressure is achieved. MAP is increased and maintained with the use of vasopressors, which induce vasoconstriction and thereby increase the MAP. The MAP is monitored with an arterial line to provide invasive blood pressure readings.

1.3. Risk factors for spinal cord ischemia

Blood supply Given that spinal cord blood supply is often segmental and dependent upon contribution from collateral arteries, the need for more extensive aortic replacement requires interruption of an increasing number of intercostal arteries providing spinal cord perfusion, thereby posing a higher risk of SCI [13]. Type II TAAAs have been reported to have a greater negative neurological outcome compared to less extensive type IV TAAAs. The increased risk of paraplegia with type I and type II TAAAs may also be due to interruption of intercostal arteries in the area of T9–L2 where the anterior spinal artery may be discontinuous and the spinal cord may be more dependent on collateral supply. Dissection and acute presentation have also been identified as variables associated with paralysis risk [14].

Perfusion pressure With open repair the placement of a proximal aortic clamp interferes with the autoregulatory response controlling cerebral perfusion with resulting fluctuations in cerebral blood flow [13]. Control of proximal hypertension following placement of an aortic

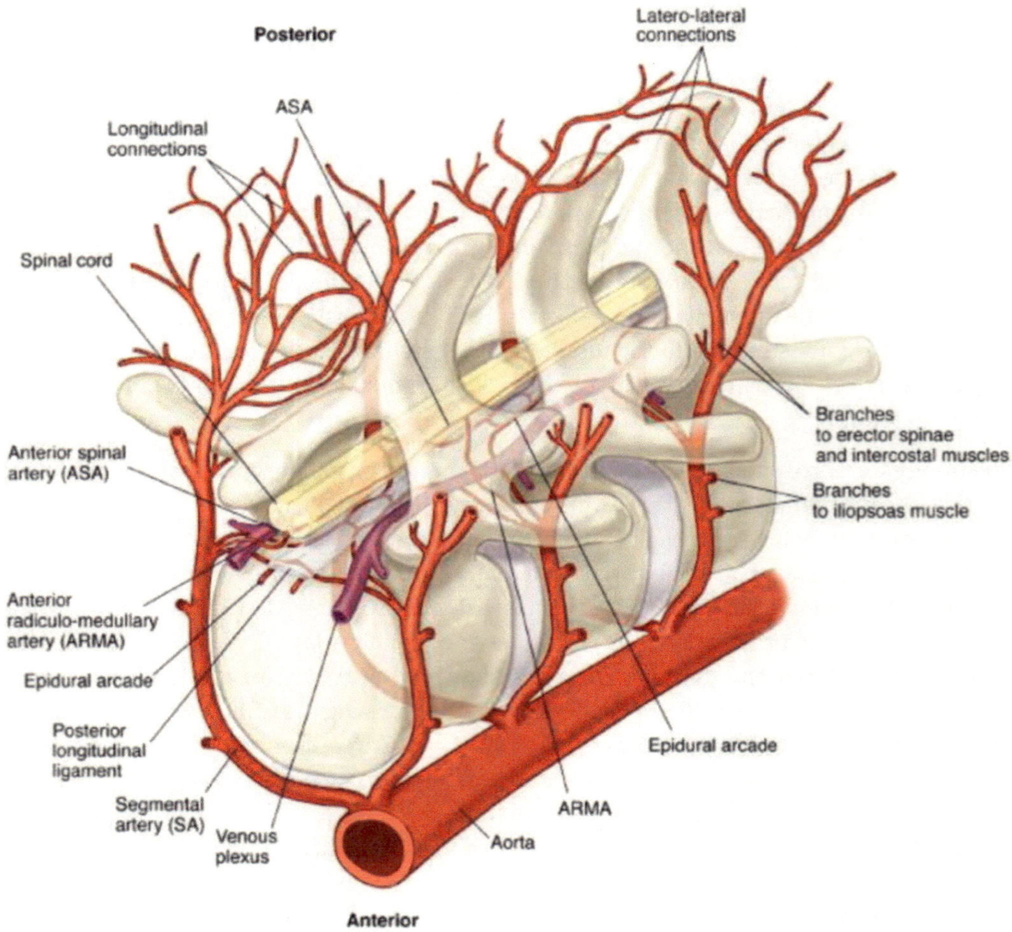

Figure 6. Blood supply to the spinal cord Schematic diagram demonstrating the relationships, relative sizes and interconnections among the segmental arteries (SA), the anterior radiculomedullary arteries (ARMA), the epidural arcades and the anterior spinal artery (ASA). Longitudinal anastomoses along the dorsal processes of the spine as well as dorsal communications (interstitial connections) between right and left branches of the segmental arteries are also shown. (*From Etz CD, Kari FA, Mueller CS, Silovitz D, Brenner RM, Lin HM, Griepp RB. The collateral network concept: a reassessment of the anatomy of spinal cord perfusion. J Thorac Cardiovasc Surg. 2011 Apr;141(4):1020-8. Reproduced with permission from Elsevier)*

cross-clamp maintains autoregulation in the coronary and cerebral circulation, often at the expense of adequate distal cord perfusion. Lowering proximal pressure decreases distal mean arterial pressure, which in the presence of an unchanged or possibly increased CSF pressure, results in decreased perfusion pressure of the distal cord. Thus, CSF drainage through insertion of a spinal drain (usually controlled to maintain a CSF pressure of less than 10-12mmHg) can reduce CSF pressure, thereby improving spinal cord perfusion.

Reperfusion injury Ischemia and reperfusion initiate neurochemical cellular responses that can exacerbate ischemia, which may in turn progress to infarction [14]. Restoration of blood

http://dx.doi.org/10.5772/57528

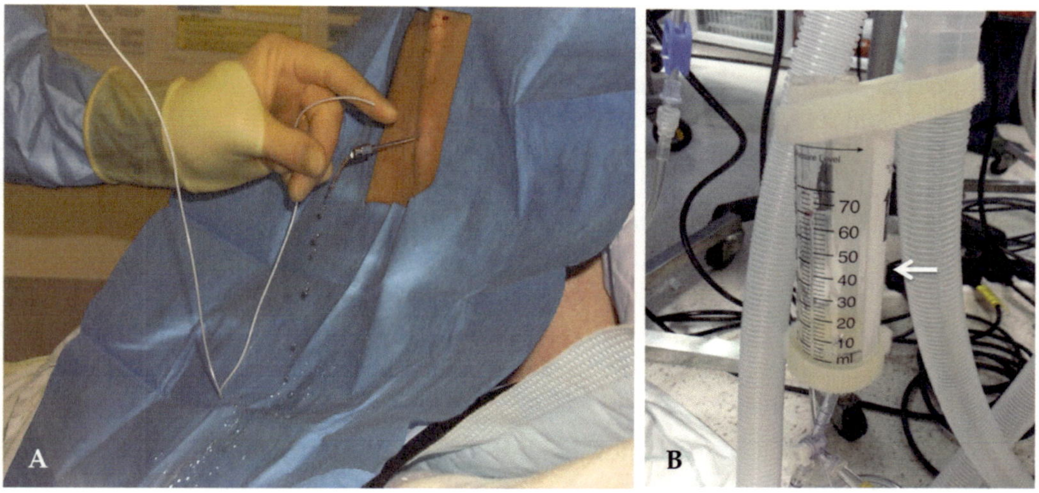

Figure 7. Insertion of lumbar cerebrospinal fluid (CSF) drain A) Performed by anesthetist under aseptic conditions. Spinal needle inserted at or below L3/4 intervertebral space. Position confirmed by free drainage of CSF. Flexible catheter inserted through needle, needle withdrawn and catheter connected to drip chamber, sterile drainage bag and pressure transducer. B) CSF drained passively by gravity by adjusting height of drip chamber (arrow) off the ground

flow to an already ischemic spinal cord introduces oxygen, which is rapidly metabolized to form oxygen radicals [13]. Through lipid peroxidation with cell membrane destruction, there is release of excitatory amino acids known to have a role in spinal cord ischemia. Reperfusion also introduces inflammatory cells including leukocytes, which adhere to the microvasculature and release cytotoxic mediators. The cellular damage induced by this reperfusion process functions as debris in further occluding the microvasculature and propagating the ischemic insult. Inflammatory cytokines derived from visceral ischemia, when introduced to the spinal cord following reperfusion, may compound this effect.

Critical intercostal artery coverage In contrast to open repair, cross-clamping of the aorta is not undertaken in endovascular repair, leaving blood pressure as a major determinant of spinal cord perfusion. With TEVAR, it is thought that stent-graft coverage of the critical thoracic intercostal arteries results in reduced perfusion of the thoracic spinal cord and watershed infarction. The mid-thoracic branch may also be more critical given that the artery of Adamkiewitz can originate below the area involved in graft coverage. Loss of the artery of Adamkiewitz in prior abdominal aortic repairs may explain why patients with prior repair are at higher risk of SCI during subsequent TAA repair. With the loss of thoracic radicular arteries due to occlusion, increased pressure is required through the anterior and posterior spinal arteries along with other collaterals to maintain adequate perfusion pressure of the spinal cord [10]. Given patients undergoing TEVAR are less susceptible to bleeding complications in comparison with open repair, they are able to tolerate higher intraoperative and postoperative systemic pressures.

Collateral circulation SCI following stent-graft deployment can also be dependent upon the extent of existing collateral circulation. Other collaterals to the spinal cord include the hypogastric artery, internal iliac arteries, internal thoracic artery and branches of the subclavian artery. Therefore where possible these should be revascularized or preserved, particularly in high-risk individuals. Where there is adequate collateral preservation following stent deployment, one would not expect to see clinical evidence of ischemia [13]. If collaterals are absent and critical intercostal arteries are covered, an ischemic event is more likely to occur. If the existing intercostal or lumbar artery collateral supply is marginal, tenuous cord perfusion results, which is more vulnerable to any postoperative hemodynamic insult. Incomplete or intermediate cord ischemia may exist in the regional distribution of the excluded intercostal arteries secondary to marginal collateralization. This may present as a delayed onset neurological deficit as the vulnerable cord is more sensitive to decreases in spinal artery perfusion pressure. These decreases may be the result of postoperative hemodynamic compromise or delayed thrombosis of previously patent yet now covered intercostal arteries.

Hypotension It has been demonstrated that hypotension that precipitates spinal cord injury within the first 48 hours after open surgical intervention is quite subtle and depends on interpreting postoperative blood pressure with preoperative values in mind [15]. The findings of this study support a policy of maintaining blood pressures at high levels not only intraoperatively, which has become practice with endovascular repair, but for at least 48 hours postoperatively. This should especially be emphasized in patients with antecedent hypertension, and this finding is likely to be valid following both open and endovascular repair. Following TEVAR, MAP should be maintained at greater than 80mmHg with the use of vasopressors when required. As a rule, at our unit following TEVAR, patients are monitored on a high dependency unit (HDU) environment for 24-48 hours, and maintained on a noradrenaline infusion of 0.01mcg/kg/minute. If the MAP drops below 80mmHg the infusion rate is increased and titrated in order to maintain an adequate MAP. Instigating timely management is crucial, and having a very low background infusion rate prevents common delays associated with initiating new treatment, particularly out of hours.

Delayed onset spinal cord ischemia The extent of neurological deficits attributed to SCI after TEVAR can range from mild paraparesis to flaccid paralysis [16]. At the most severe end of this clinico-pathologic spectrum, patients with complete paralysis are those who have suffered irreversible SCI due to spinal cord infarction. Patients at the opposite end of the spectrum represent a mild form of cord ischemia with the potential for reversibility and full neurological recovery. Delayed-onset SCI, which can occur up to several weeks after TEVAR, is also typically due to ischemia as opposed to infarction of the spinal cord, with the potential for recovery. Whereas a deficit noted immediately upon emergence from anesthesia would be attributed to an intraoperative cause, a delayed neurological deficit observed after a period of normal neurological function is secondary to a postoperative event. Indeed several postoperative events have been linked to the development of delayed-onset SCI, including hypotension, thrombosis, hematoma, embolization and elevated CSF pressures.

Length of aortic coverage The authors conducted a study to determine the incidence and risk factors for SCI following thoracic and thoracoabdominal aortic intervention using a prospective database of all interventions between 2001 and 2009, including both elective and emergency cases [7]. Logistic regression was used to investigate the factors associated with SCI. The results revealed 235 patients underwent thoracic aortic stent-grafting; 111 (47%) thoracic aortic stent-grafts alone, with an additional 14 (6%) branched or fenestrated thoracic grafts, 30 (13%) arch hybrids and 80 (34%) visceral hybrids. The global incidence of SCI for all procedures was 23/235 (9.8%), which included emergency indications (ruptured TAAA and complex acute dissections). The incidence varied considerably between types of procedures. Of the twenty-three cases of SCI, death occurred in four patients, recovery of function was seen in six and permanent paraplegia occurred in 13/235 patients (5.5%). Of the nine pre-specified factors investigated for association with SCI (age, sex, indication, urgency, type of procedure, duration of procedure, percentage of aorta covered, spinal drain usage and left subclavian artery coverage), only percentage of aortic coverage was significantly associated with the incidence of SCI on logistic regression; adjusted odds ratio per 10% increase in aorta covered=1.78[95% CI 1.18-2.71], p=0.007. In patients who developed SCI the operative time was increased (463.5 versus 307.2 minutes) and more stents were utilized (4 versus 2). Therefore the study concluded that SCI following thoracic and thoracoabdominal aortic endovascular intervention is significantly associated with the proportion of aorta covered. The degree of risk varies between different types of procedures, and visceral hybrids appeared to carry the highest risk of SCI. The study however included a heterogeneous group of conditions (atherosclerotic degenerative aneurysms, chronic type B dissections and acute aortic syndromes) with differences in the complexity of procedures performed (endovascular, arch and visceral hybrid solutions). No patient developed SCI with less than 54% coverage of the aorta. This work demonstrated a significant rise in the risk of SCI with increasing magnitude of procedure type; TEVAR (stent-graft confined to the thoracic aorta) was associated with the least risk at 1.8% SCI and 0.9% permanent paraplegia, arch hybrid 10% and 6.7%, fenestrated or branched graft 14.3% and 7.1% and visceral hybrid 20% and 11.3%.

Chronic renal insufficiency Ullery et al [16] also reported similar findings with an SCI rate of 2.8% with TEVAR (12 of 424), 14% with arch hybrid (6 of 43) and 17% with visceral hybrid (1 of 6), and a global incidence of 4% (9 of 473). The twelve patients experiencing SCI within the TEVAR cohort all underwent stent coverage from the origin of the left subclavian artery to the diaphragm (p<0.001), and multivariate regression analysis demonstrated chronic renal insufficiency to be independently associated with SCI (p=0.029). At SCI onset, therapeutic interventions increased blood pressure from mean MAP 77mmHg to 99mmHg, and decreased mean lumbar CSF pressure from 10mmHg to 7mmHg, both at time of neurological recovery. There was one mortality within 30 days (1/12, 8%), and 9 of 11 patients experienced complete neurological recovery as a result of the interventions.

Simultaneous closure of two vascular territories A risk model was developed using a prospective 63-patient single-centre cohort [17]. This was then applied to data extracted from the multi-centre European Registry on Endovascular Aortic Repair Complications (EuREC), where 38 of 2235 patients (1.7%) developed SCI (data from 19 centres). In the single-centre cohort direct correlation was seen between the occurrence of symptomatic SCI and both prolonged intraoperative hypotension (p=0.04) and simultaneous closure of at least two independent spinal cord vascular territories (p=0.005), whilst previous closure of a single vascular territory was not associated with an increased risk of symptomatic spinal cord ischemia (p=0.56). The combination of prolonged hypotension and simultaneous closure of at least two territories exhibited the strongest association (p<0.0001). Applying the model to the entire EuREC cohort demonstrated a good correlation between the predicted and observed risk factors (kappa 0.77, 95% CI 0.65-0.90). As a result the study concluded that simultaneous closure of at least two vascular territories supplying the spinal cord is highly relevant, especially in combination with prolonged intraoperative hypotension.

Previous or concomitant abdominal aortic repair Although the putative mechanism of loss of lumbar collateral perfusion in those who had prior aortic repairs appears reasonable, occurrence of SCI in this subset of patients has not been consistent. The outcomes of twenty-eight patients who underwent staged TEVAR following previous or concomitant abdominal aortic repair were reported, of whom twenty-seven had cerebrospinal fluid drainage during and following thoracic repair. SCI developed in four of twenty-eight patients (14.3%); symptoms manifested twelve hours postoperatively in one patient, with delayed onset in the remaining three patients ranging from three days to seven weeks postoperatively [18]. Irreversible cord ischemia occurred in three patients, with full recovery in one patient. This was in comparison to only one of 97 patients (1.0%) who developed SCI following TEVAR only, with no intervention to the abdominal aorta. The study showed that SCI occurred at a markedly higher rate in patients with previous or concomitant abdominal aortic repair, and this risk continued beyond the immediate postoperative period. Another study analysed a case series of 406 patients undergoing thoracic stent-grafting for various aortic pathology [19]. Prophylactic cerebrospinal fluid drainage (CSFD) was used selectively in only four cases. The incidence of paraplegia was 2.7% (n=11), with six patients having major permanent deficit. When analysing conditions influencing SCI, statistical correlation was found for previous conventional or endovascular abdominal aortic aneurysm repair (odds ratio [OR], 4.8) in addition to coverage of the entire descending thoracic aorta (OR, 3.6) and implantation of thoracoabdominal branched and fenestrated stent-grafts (OR, 9.5). Individual analyses revealed other conditions that might have played a role, such as embolization into the segmental arteries, severe visceral ischemia, profound hemorrhagic shock and heparin-induced thrombocytopenia. At our unit we routinely perform CSFD on patients undergoing TEVAR following previous or concomitant abdominal aortic intervention.

1.4. Adjuncts for the prevention of paraplegia

Intercostal artery re-implantation (Figure 5) Acher et al demonstrated an 80% reduction in paraplegia risk using hypothermia, naloxone, steroids, spinal fluid drainage, intercostal ligation and optimizing hemodynamic parameters. The group then demonstrated that intercostal revascularization (either reimplantation or preservation where possible) further reduced their paraplegia risk index by 75% when evaluated using a highly accurate ($R^2 > 0.88$) paraplegia risk index [20]. Intercostal arteries were reimplanted based on magnetic resonance angiography identification of intercostal arteries that supplied radicular arteries feeding the anterior spinal artery, or by patency and location at surgery. The incidence of paralysis after TAAA repair decreased from 4.83% to 0.88% and the paralysis risk index decreased from 0.26 to 0.05 when intercostal artery reimplantation was added to neuroprotective strategies that had already substantially reduced paralysis risk. These findings suggest that factors that affect collateral blood flow and metabolism account for approximately 80% of paraplegia risk and intercostal blood flow accounts for 20% of risk. These figures imply there is a limit in being able to reduce paraplegia risk in patients undergoing endograft treatment for TAAAs.

In the era of endovascular repair, where intercostal artery re-implantation is not possible, physiological factors that affect spinal cord perfusion (MAP, CSFD), metabolism and ischemic tolerance (steroids, naloxone, hypothermia) and oxygen delivery (haemoglobin, MAP, oxygen saturations, temperature, cardiac function) are key tools to prevent paraplegia [14]. There is a range of effectiveness of the applied strategies amongst treatment centres, which tells us that treatment protocols to optimize contributing factors must be established and followed consistently to achieve the best results [14].

Internal iliac revascularization [11] In addition to revascularization of the intercostal vessels, one must also consider the superior and inferior supply to the spinal cord via the subclavian arteries and internal iliac network. Revascularization of the internal iliac arteries should not only be considered in the context of buttock ischemia, but also in an attempt to maintain adequate spinal perfusion. Internal iliac flow should be preserved on at least one side and careful consideration must be given in the context of common and internal iliac aneurysms as well as when a uni-iliac stent-graft is placed.

Left subclavian artery revascularization The left subclavian artery (LSCA) has achieved prominence in discussions regarding case planning for stent-graft insertion. Up to one third of patients undergoing TEVAR require coverage of the LSCA in order to achieve an adequate landing zone and proximal seal [21]. In these situations the stent-graft is placed across the origin of the artery and endovascular embolization of the vessel with percutaneous access via the brachial artery is required to prevent development of a type 2 endoleak (persistent blood flow into the aneurysm sac from collateral vessels). In selected cases LSCA revascularization is undertaken prior to endovascular stent deployment. This can be performed as a single or staged procedure. At our unit this is routinely performed as a single-stage procedure in a hybrid operating suite (surgical operating theatre equipped with advanced medical imaging devices required for endovascular procedures). An open left common carotid to left subclavian artery bypass is performed, commonly with a Dacron graft, prior to endovascular stenting across the origin of the LSCA (Figure 8). The LSCA provides important circulation to the spinal cord, brain, and arm, and therefore coverage is not without clinical consequences. Stroke, SCI and coronary ischemia in the setting of a left internal mammary artery bypass, as well as arm ischemia, have all been described. The left vertebral artery serves as the dominant vessel to the hindbrain in 60% of individuals, and as a result LSCA coverage can lead to a posterior circulation stroke. LSCA coverage can also compromise spinal blood flow with resultant SCI. It contributes to spinal cord perfusion by providing branches to the cephalad portions of the anterior and posterior spinal arteries [22]. Management of patients in whom the LSCA is sacrificed remains a source of considerable debate and controversy. Proponents of routine revascularization cite the increased risk of arm ischemia, stroke and SCI associated with LSCA coverage. Several other studies have shown that intentional coverage of the LSCA without revascularization is not associated with increased morbidity and lend support to those who

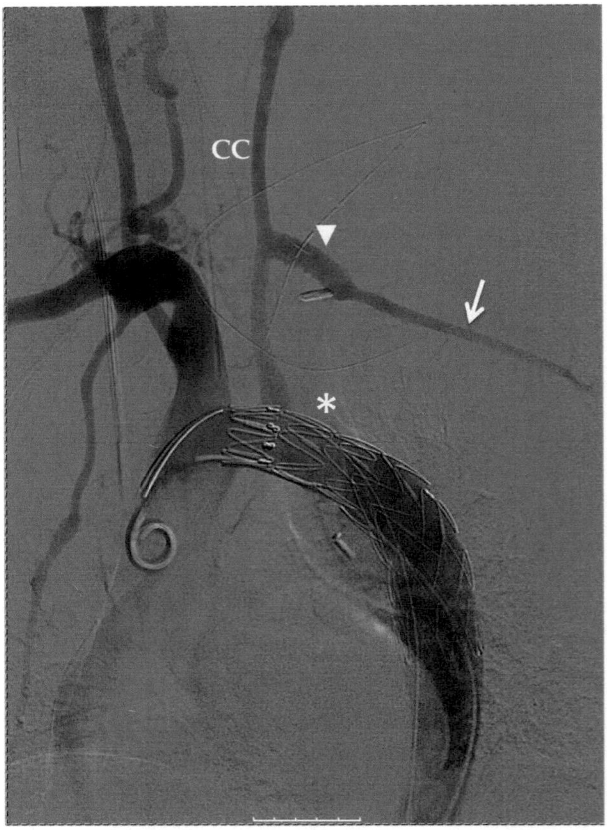

Figure 8. Left subclavian artery revascularization Left common carotid (CC) to left subclavian artery (LSCA, arrow) bypass with Dacron graft (arrow head) performed prior to endovascular stenting across origin of LSCA (star) to create adequate landing zone for exclusion of thoracic aortic aneurysm while maintaining flow to LSCA. Patent LSCA seen (arrow).

advocate more selective revascularization. Despite contributing to critical vascular beds, LSCA coverage is well tolerated in most patients due to collateral blood flow primarily from the right vertebral artery, basilar artery and circle of Willis arcade [22]. In addition, they argue that LSCA bypass and/or transposition is not entirely without risk, and should therefore be stratified according to the individual. Complications include left recurrent laryngeal nerve palsy, left phrenic nerve palsy and neck haematoma necessitating re-exploration. Absolute indications for LSCA revascularization include patent left internal mammary artery coronary bypass graft, dominant left vertebral artery, diminutive or absent right vertebral artery, left arm arterio-venous fistula for dialysis access and patent left axillo-femoral bypass graft. Relative indications include long aortic coverage, previous abdominal aortic surgery and occlusion of the internal iliac or hypogastric arteries.

Two meta-analyses on the subject both reported an increase in SCI when the LSCA is covered. One observed an SCI rate of 2.3 vs. 2.8, p=0.005 for LSCA not covered vs. covered. However there was no protective effect from preoperative revascularization; SCI for the uncovered group 2.7% vs. 0.8% in the revascularized group, p=0.35 [23]. In an effort to establish clinical practice guidelines for management of the LSCA with TEVAR, the Society of Vascular Surgery (SVS) selected a committee of experts within the field and commissioned a systematic review and meta-analysis of the literature. They employed the GRADE method (grading of recommendations assessment, development and evaluation) to develop and present their recommendations. The second study, commissioned by the SVS, demonstrated that coverage of the LSCA is associated with a trend towards increase in paraplegia and anterior circulation stroke and a significant increase in risk of arm ischemia and vertebrobasilar stroke [24]. However there was no association with death, myocardial infarction or transient ischaemic attack. All recommendations listed were made based on level C (low-quality) data, but nonetheless, the proposed SVS guidelines suggest routine preoperative revascularization of the LSA for elective cases requiring coverage of the origin of the vessel [25]. Recommendations include: 1) In patients undergoing elective TEVAR where achievement of a proximal seal necessitates coverage of the LSA, they suggest routine preoperative revascularization (despite the low-quality evidence); 2) In selected patients who have an anatomy that compromises perfusion to critical organs, routine preoperative LSA revascularization is strongly recommended (despite the low-quality evidence); and 3) In patients who need urgent TEVAR for life-threatening acute aortic syndromes where achievement of a proximal seal necessitates coverage of the LSA, they suggest that revascularization should be individualized and addressed expectantly on the basis of anatomy, urgency and availability of surgical expertise.

However, other large single-institution studies with protocols for selective revascularization saw no differences in the rates of SCI. A recent large retrospective multi-centre review was performed on 1189 patients undergoing TEVAR [65]. Subgroup analysis was performed for non-covered LSCA (group A), covered LSCA (group B) and covered and revascularized LSCA (group C) which showed no significant difference between groups B and C (SCI 6.3% vs. 6.1%) and LSCA revascularization was not protective for SCI (7.5% vs. 4.1%, p=0.3). The study concluded that LSCA coverage does not appear to result in an increased incidence of SCI or stroke when a strategy of selective revascularization is adopted, and selective LSCA revascularization results in similar outcomes among the three cohorts studied. Complications from revascularization, understated in most studies, are worth considering. The key to favourable outcomes likely involves careful patient selection when selective revascularization is employed.

Elective sac perfusion via temporary controlled endoleak With endovascular repair, in contrast to open surgical repair, identification and/or direct revascularization of important segmental vessels is not currently possible. SCI therefore remains a major challenge with endovascular repair, and innovations to reduce the occurrence of this complication are necessary. Early experience with a technique for maintaining perfusion of segmental vessels (intercostal and lumbar arteries) in the early postoperative period after endovascular repair of a TAAA with "sac perfusion branches" added to custom-made stent-grafts has been described [27]. The branched stent-graft and bridging stents to the branches are inserted under general anesthesia. The perfusion branches are left open in order to perfuse segmental vessels. The risk of SCI is greatest in the first few days following repair, and so the perfusion branches are left open during this time. Five to ten days postoperatively the branches are then closed with Amplatzer plugs to complete exclusion of the aneurysm. This is performed via a single percutaneous groin puncture under local anesthesia, which allows continuous monitoring of neurological function. Test balloon occlusions of the branches are performed and there is clinical evaluation of the patient's neurological symptoms for approximately 30 minutes. If no symptoms are experienced, the branch is then closed. The choice of five to ten days for closure of the perfusion branch is empiric, as most delayed SCI occurs in the first 72 hours postoperatively. This technique was used in ten patients with type II (the most extensive) TAAAs. One developed monoparesis of the right leg during a period of hypotension secondary to a cardiac event and died within 30 days. Two patients developed lower limb weakness after closure of the perfusion branches, but subsequently recovered full recovery. The concept behind the technique described is that perfusion of the sac by a controlled endoleak may protect spinal cord perfusion in the immediate postoperative period when the risk of hemodynamic instability is greatest. Extensive segmental artery sacrifice can be delayed until the patient has recovered from the first stage of the procedure and some remodeling of the collateral network may have occurred. Two patients in this series developed neurological symptoms after closure of the perfusion branches, thus supporting the hypothesis that perfusion of the sac in the postoperative period does have a protective effect. If any symptoms are experienced the procedure can be abandoned and attempted at a later date when further remodeling of the collateral network is likely to have occurred. This small case series indicates that controlled perfusion of segmental vessels with a temporary controlled endoleak is feasible, and may be a useful adjunct to prevent SCI, providing protection to spinal cord perfusion during the immediate postoperative period when risk of SCI is greatest.

Cerebrospinal fluid drainage (Figure 7) Use of prophylactic cerebrospinal fluid drainage in open surgery has been the subject of two meta-analyses [28, 29]. Although based on a small number of cases, both concluded that prophylactic drainage significantly reduces the risk of perioperative paraplegia or paraparesis. A Cochrane review undertaken to determine the effect of CSFD during thoracic and TAAA surgery on the risk of developing spinal cord injury concluded CSFD may increase the perfusion pressure to the spinal cord and hence reduce the risk of ischemic spinal cord injury [29]. To date, three randomized controlled trials have examined the benefits of lumbar CSFD in open TAAA repairs, which were the three trials included in the Cochrane review with a total of 287 participants operated on for type I or II TAAA. In the first trial of 98 participants (46 patients with CSFD and 52 controls), neurological deficits in the lower extremities occurred in 14 (30%) of the CSFD group and 17 (33%) of the controls [30]. The deficit was observed within 24 hours of the operation in 21 (68%), and from three to 22 days in 10 (32%) participants. CSFD did not have a statistically significant benefit in preventing paraplegia ($p=0.8$), and the only significant predictor of delayed deficits was postoperative hypotension ($p=0.006$). The second trial of 33 participants used a combination of CSFD and intrathecal papaverine (IP, a vasodilator and smooth muscle relaxant); 17 patients randomised to CSFD+IP and 16 to control group [31]. They showed the combined treatment had statistically significant reduction in the rate of postoperative neurological deficit (2/17 developed neurological injury) compared to controls (7/16, $p=0.0392$). Control patients also had lower postoperative motor strength scores (p=0.0340). Multivariate analysis of risk factors for neurological injury included (p<0.05) longer cross-clamp time, failure to actively cool with bypass and postoperative hypotension, whereas CSFD+IP were found to be protective. Logistic regression showed that CSFD+IP and active cooling significantly reduced the risk of injury and that the two combined modalities had a cumulative protective effect. In the third trial, which is the largest and most recent, TAAA repair was performed on 145 participants; 76 with CSFD and 69 without [32]. CSFD was initiated during the operation and continued for 48 hours after surgery. Paraplegia or paraparesis occurred in 9/74 patients (12.2%) in the control group vs. 2/82 (2.7%) receiving CSFD (p=0.03). Overall, CSFD resulted in an 80% reduction in the relative risk of postoperative deficits. The Cochrane meta-analysis showed an odds ratio (OR) of 0.48 (95 % confidence interval (CI) 0.25 to 0.92). For CSFD-only trials, OR was 0.57 (95% CI 0.28 to 1.17) and for intention-to-treat analysis in CSFD-only studies, the OR remained unchanged. The review therefore concluded that there is limited evidence that perioperative CSFD appears to reduce the rate of paraplegia after repair of type I and type II TAAA. CSFD is recommended as a component of the multimodal approach for the prevention of neurological injury, and use of CSFD alone as protection was not established from the available evidence.

The role of prophylactic CSFD in endovascular procedures is more contentious, and level 1 evidence supporting its role is currently lacking. Wong et al undertook a systematic review to determine if preoperative CSFD reduces SCI with TEVAR [33]. Study quality was generally poor to moderate (median Downs and Black score, 9). The systematic review identified 46 eligible studies comprising 4936 patients; overall, SCI affected 3.89% (95% confidence interval, 2.95.05% to 4.95%). Series reporting routine prophylactic drain placement or no prophylactic drain placement reported pooled SCI rates of 3.2% and 3.47% respectively. The pooled SCI rate from 24 series stating that prophylactic drainage was used selectively was 5.6%. However, in all of these series prophylactic CSFDs were placed only in patients deemed at high risk of perioperative SCI. Thus, there is an inherent bias in the analysis in that the CSFD group was at increased risk of SCI. The study concluded that the role of prophylactic CSFD is difficult to establish from the available literature, and high-quality studies are required to determine the role of prophylactic CSF drainage in TEVAR. A single-institution experience of TEVAR using the same proactive spinal cord ischemia protection protocol used in open repair reported proactive spinal cord protective protocols appear to reduce the incidence of spinal ischemia after TEVAR compared with previous series [34]. The spinal cord ischemia protection included routine spinal drainage (spinal fluid pressure <10 mm Hg), endorphin receptor blockade (naloxone infusion), moderate intraoperative hypothermia (<35°C), hypotension avoidance (MAP >90 mmHg) and optimizing cardiac function. From 2005 to 2012, 94 consecutive TEVARs were studied, including 48 for TAA. Mean length of aortic coverage was 161mm, correlating to 59.4% aortic coverage. One patient had delayed paralysis (1.1%) and recovered enough to ambulate easily without assistance. This study recommends that active, as opposed to reactive approaches to spinal ischemia provide a better long-term outcome, and multimodal protection is essential, especially in cases of long segment coverage.

1.5. Adjuncts for the detection of paraplegia

Spinal cord monitoring The priority with thoracic and TAAA repair is the prevention of spinal cord ischemia, followed by the detection and treatment of its occurrence as early as possible to limit injury [35]. These repairs generally require the use of general anesthesia and this is routine practice at our unit. As a result neurological injury is impossible to detect intraoperatively through clinical examination. Neurophysiologic monitoring can therefore be employed in this setting to detect intraoperative injury so that timely interventions can be instigated to improve spinal cord perfusion. In certain institutions TEVAR is performed under loco-regional anaesthesia and if this is the case, routine neuromonitoring or spinal cord protection with CSFD is not required as management such as CSFD can be implemented when clinically required based on examination of the conscious patient.

The two types of intraoperative monitoring used regularly, either alone or in combination, are transcortical motor evoked potentials (MEP) and somatosensory evoked potentials (SSEP) [35]. MEPs are recorded from muscles in the extremities by delivering multi-pulse electrical stimulation to the scalp overlying the motor cortex. The evoked potentials elicited from this stimulation travel from the motor cortex through cortical spinal tracts, anterior horn cell, peripheral nerve, and finally to muscle. An interruption in this pathway will result in loss of the motor evoked potential [36]. Somatosensory evoked potential involves repetitive stimulation of peripheral nerves such as the posterior tibial nerve at the ankle or median nerve at the wrist, followed by the recording of the averaged electrical response in the peripheral nerve, spine, and the cerebral sensory cortex [35]. Most experts in the field believe that intraoperative neuromonitoring is critical in these procedures, although this is largely based on personal clinical experience. These decisions are not based on randomized controlled trials nor do they take into account potential complications and consequences that false positives can have on outcomes in these patients. For example a study examined 97 cases of open (40) and thoracic endovascular stent repairs (57), which were performed with MEP and SSEP monitoring [37]. They used a 50% reduction in amplitude of both cortical SSEPs and transcranial MEP compound motor action potentials as their criteria for potential signs of spinal ischemia. Results included; 63 event-free patients with normal potentials, fourteen patients with accurate correlation between elicited potentials and corresponding neurological outcomes (initial drop and subsequent regeneration in ten patients, six with normal neurological outcomes, four with transient neurological deficit postoperatively and four who suffered paraplegia with no intraoperative evoked potential), three false-positives, one false-negative and sixteen cases with associated with medication (halogenated anesthetic) interaction or technical issues. They observed a sensitivity of 93% and a specificity of 96% for the neurophysiological monitoring.

The choice of whether to use neuromonitoring remains unclear as there still remain difficulties in the successful use of MEPs from the standpoint of safety, technology and experience [35]. In these particular operations there is a significant downside in falsely identifying spinal cord ischemia with MEPs. The maneuvers utilized to treat spinal ischemia such as induced hypertension and arterial reimplantation have potential complications themselves including an increased risk of bleeding, increased length of surgery and even increased mortality [37]. SSEPs may fail to reliably predict all presentations of paralysis and cannot provide evidence as to whether ischemic events are coincidental or isolated peripheral vascular events (clots and emboli causing distal damage) or secondary to a reduction in spinal cord perfusion. Lower extremity perfusion disturbances may occur for a variety of reasons during these procedures and the raw SSEP signals provide ambiguous quantitative correlation to intraoperative events [35]. The use of MEP requires specialized anesthetic protocols such as the use of short-acting paralytics during intubation only and eliminating the use of halogenated agents, which can make the procedure more challenging for the anesthetic team. However, the availability of intravenous anesthetics such as propofol and remifentanyl make MEP monitoring during TAAA repairs feasible when indicated. Patients undergoing these procedures are often sedated in the postoperative period making clinical assessment difficult, and they do not routinely undergo continued neurophysiologic monitoring during this time. The postoperative period is one of great hemodynamic instability and it is quite possible that a number of patients develop SCI at this time. For this reason it is suggested that patients continue to undergo monitoring until they arouse from anesthesia. MEPS cannot be monitored on extubated patients due to the pain involved in delivering the stimulus, but SSEP can be continued postoperatively. Another disadvantage of such neuromonitoring techniques is the need for neurophysiology expertise to interpret the complex waveforms, which is not always available or practical, particularly in the emergency setting. The authors are currently conducting a feasibility study for a technique of physician-interpreted (i.e. anesthetic and surgical teams) MEP monitoring, without the requirement of neurophysiology input.

Monitoring of spinal cord integrity remains challenging and difficult to interpret and further tests for the timely diagnosis of SCI are required. A recent study evaluated the feasibility of non-invasive monitoring of the paraspinal collateral network oxygenation using near-infrared spectroscopy (NIRS) prior to, during and after TAAA repair in a small clinical series [38]. NIRS optrodes were positioned bilaterally over the thoracic and lumbar paraspinous muscles (and thereby the paraspinous vasculature collateral network) to transcutaneously monitor muscle oxygenation in the collateral network to provide real-time non-invasive monitoring potentially indicating pending SCI in 20 patients undergoing repair of type I, II and III TAAAs. Lumbar oxygenation dropped significantly during open repair (n=15) after proximal aortic cross-clamping, but fully recovered after restoration of pulsatile flow to 98.5% of baseline. During TEVAR (n=3), stent-graft deployment did not significantly affect lumbar oxygenation. Three patients developed SCI, and in these patients lumbar oxygenation reduction after aortic cross-clamping was significantly lower compared to those with no neurological deficit (p=0.041). The study demonstrated this technique is feasible, and lumbar collateral network oxygenation levels directly respond to compromise of aortic circulation. Further studies are needed to corroborate these findings.

Biomarkers Although ischemia-related damage with thoracic aortic repair usually occurs intraoperatively, confirmation of neurological injury often does not occur until the postoperative period when anesthetic effects have resolved and the patients can be evaluated clinically [39]. Often patients remain sedated for prolonged periods following their procedure and therefore methods to detect the onset of acute SCI during the intraoperative and immediate postoperative period would be extremely valuable. Biomarkers for the real-time detection of ongoing SCI or prediction of an increased risk for paralysis would potentially provide time to intervene and would be of great benefit in preventing SCI. Tissue ischemia caused by decreased spinal cord or brain perfusion is a potent and powerful stressor that triggers many metabolic and inflammatory pathways [36]. CSF is produced continuously and the total CSF compartment volume is replaced three times a day under normal conditions. The composition of CSF is dependent on metabolite production from the brain, and as CSF bathes the neural tissues of the brain and spinal cord, it should allow detection of the biochemical products of acute central nervous system ischemia more rapidly than in serum, particularly if the blood brain barrier is intact. Specific biochemical markers that have been examined to date include lactate, pCO2, neuron-specific enolase (NSE), glucose, pH and S100β. Existing molecular markers for neurological injury such as S100β have low sensitivity and specificity making them unsuitable for routine clinical use. These markers also increase in serum at other times including during surgical procedures unrelated to acute brain injury, are often slow to increase and hence not useful for rapid 'on-table' detection. The biochemical signs of cerebrospinal injury have been shown to occur in patients without any clinically detectable neurological deficits and it is often difficult to establish a pattern of proportionality between the degree of ischemia and biomarker parameter increases. In addition, the markers can be confounded by conditions such as hemolysis, extra-cerebral sources and resuscitation, thereby not providing a sensitive prognostic tool [39]. As a result, none of the putative markers of injury in blood or CSF reliably detect early brain or spinal cord ischemia or validated surrogate endpoint measures as yet.

Heat shock proteins Heat shock proteins (HSPs) are members of highly conserved families of molecular chaperones that have multiple roles in vivo, and they are rapidly induced by severe stress. The inducible members of the HSP70 and HSP27 families are associated with cellular protection and recovery after a near lethal stress and have also been used as markers for tissues or organs that have been exposed to near-lethal stress [41]. The levels of HSPs in CSF from patients undergoing thoracic aneurysm repair have been analyzed. Blood and CSF samples were collected at regular intervals, and CSF was analyzed by enzyme-linked immunosorbent assay for HSP70 and HSP27. These results were correlated with intraoperative somatosensory-evoked potentials measurements and postoperative paralysis. They found the levels of these proteins in many of these patients are elevated and that the degree of elevation correlates with the risk of permanent paralysis. They hypothesized that sequential intraoperative measurements of heat shock proteins HSP70 and HSP27 levels in CSF could predict those patients who are at greatest risk for paralysis during thoracic aneurysm repair. Further work is in progress by the group to develop these markers to prevent or attenuate this severe complication.

Metabonomics An individual's phenome describes the biochemical expression of genomic and environmental disease risk and is based on the analysis of small molecules and metabolites. Metabonomics is the quantitative measurement of the dynamic multiparametric metabolic response of living systems to pathphysiological stimuli used in patient phenotyping [42]. Emerging techniques enable rapid measurement of large arrays of metabolites, which could greatly enhance the 'on table' decision-making process during surgery. Spectroscopic methods have been applied to generate multivariate profiles of metabolites, mainly using nuclear magnetic resonance (NMR) spectroscopy and mass spectrometry (MS) methods that can measure a wide range of metabolites simultaneously. The data are then analyzed using multivariate statistics [43]. Rapid evaporative ionization mass spectrometry is an emerging technique that allows near real-time characterization of human tissue in vivo by analysis of aerosol smoke released during electrosurgical dissection, and this technique has shown that near real-time spectro-profiling in the clinical environment is a possibility [44]. CSF provides an ideal medium for analysis of biomarkers indicating neurological injury since metabolites of anaesthetic agents and other drugs are restricted by the blood-brain barrier. Patients undergoing TAA and TAAA at our unit routinely have a spinal drain inserted preoperatively if clinically indicated, and this spinal drain remains in situ for approximately 48 to 72 hours postoperatively. This provides a constant source of CSF available for study, and the authors are currently conducting a study to analyse CSF using a metabolic phenotyping approach to identify novel biomarkers for neurological ischemia, with a view to developing a platform for near real-time intraoperative diagnostics.

1.6. Outcomes of paraplegia

In order to define the outcome of patients experiencing SCI after TEVAR and determine the differences in the evolution of long-term functional recovery and the effect on survival, 607 TEVARs performed between 2000 and 2011 were analysed [45]. Fifty-seven patients (9.4%) were noted to have postoperative SCI. SCI developed immediately in twelve patients, had delayed onset in forty and was indeterminate in five patients due to postoperative sedation. Three patients (25%) with immediate SCI had measurable functional improvement based on ambulatory status, whereas twenty-eight (70%) of the delayed-onset patients experienced some degree of neurological recovery (p=0.04). Of the thirty-four patients with complete data available, twenty-six (76%) reported quantifiable functional improvement, but only thirteen (38%) experienced return to their preoperative baseline. Estimated mean survival for patients with and without SCI was 37.2 and 71.6 months respectively (p<0.0006). Patients with functional improvement had a mean survival of 53.9 months compared with 9.6 months for those without improvement (p<0.0001). The study concluded that only a minority of patients experience complete return to baseline function after SCI with TEVAR, and outcomes in patients without early functional recovery are particularly poor. Patients experiencing delayed SCI are more likely to have functional improvement and following neurological recovery may anticipate similar life expectancy compared to patients without SCI.

In addition to the personal consequences to the patient, family and carers, paraplegia is associated with a significant economic burden. Recurring annual costs of caring for patients with chronic spinal cord injury is a large economic burden on health care systems, but information on costs of spinal cord injury care beyond the acute and initial post-acute phase is minimal [46]. The annual direct medical costs associated with healthcare for a sample of 675 patients with chronic spinal cord injury greater than two years after injury were investigated. The total (inpatient and outpatient) annual direct medical cost was $21,450 per patient. Average inpatient cost per patient for complete and incomplete thoracic spinal cord injury was

$30,612 and $24,883 respectively, which included laboratory, nursing, pharmacy, radiology, surgery and inpatient stay costs. Average outpatient costs were $9954 and $8925 respectively. However, community care costs such as nursing home or respite stays, occupational therapy and home adaptations, as well as indirect costs such as carers and sickness benefits also need to be considered. To our knowledge there are no studies to date quantifying the economic burden of paraplegia as a complication of aortic intervention.

1.7. Spinal cord imaging

At our unit magnetic resonance (MR) imaging of the spine is performed if SCI is suspected to confirm the diagnosis and exclude any other cause of myelopathy such as extrinsic compression. MRI is the most sensitive method for verifying cord ischemia or infarction, and current techniques of diffusion-weighted images can be particularly sensitive and diagnostic. Mawad et al conducted a study where magnetic resonance (MR) imaging was obtained on 25 patients developing symptoms of spinal cord ischemia following resection and graft replacement of thoracoabdominal aortic aneurysms [47]. MR studies were abnormal in 17 patients, which correlated well with the somatosensory evoked potential studies, which were abnormal in all 17 patients. All the MRI signal abnormalities were found in the low thoracic cord and conus medullaris, regardless of the severity of the clinical findings. Four patients with mid thoracic aneurysms experienced transient SCI with good clinical outcome where patients were ambulatory following recovery; MR abnormality was in the low thoracic region in one patient and low thoracic region and conus in three, with focal abnormal MR signals limited to grey matter. Twelve patients with mid thoracic and thoracoabdominal aneurysms experienced complete SCI where patients were not ambulatory with 0/5 motor function assessed on the muscle strength scale 0-5; MR abnormality was in the conus in five patients, mid to low thoracic region and conus in five patients, low thoracic region in one and low thoracic region and conus in one, with diffuse abnormal MR signals involving both grey and white matter. Significant advances in MRI modalities and techniques have taken place since the study was published in 1990, but identification of the most common sites for spinal cord ischemia following aneurysm repair remains an important finding.

Abbreviations

TAA-Thoracic aortic aneurysm

TAAA-Thorocoabdominal aortic aneurysm

TAD-Thoracic aortic dissection

TEVAR-Thoracic Endovascular Aortic Repair

MAP-Mean arterial pressure

CSF-Cerebrospinal fluid

SCI-Spinal cord ischemia

http://dx.doi.org/10.5772/57528

CSFD-Cerebrospinal fluid drainage

LSCA-Left subclavian artery

OR-Odds ratio

MEP-Motor evoked potentials

SSEP-Somatosensory evoked potentials

Author details

Anisha H. Perera* and Richard G.J. Gibbs

*Address all correspondence to: r.gibbs@imperial.ac.uk

Department of Vascular Surgery, St Mary's Hospital, Imperial College Healthcare NHS Trust, London, UK

References

[1] Conrad MF, Cambria RP. Contemporary management of descending thoracic and thoracoabdominal aortic aneurysms: endovascular versus open. Circulation. 2008;117(6) 841-52.

[2] Yamauchi T, Takano H, Nishimura M, Matsumiya G, Sawa Y. Paraplegia and paraparesis after descending thoracic aortic aneurysm repair: a risk factor analysis. Ann Thorac Cardiovasc Surg. 2006;12(3) 179-83.

[3] Estrera AL, Rubenstein FS, Miller CC 3rd, Huynh TT, Letsou GV, Safi HJ. Descending thoracic aortic aneurysm: surgical approach and treatment using the adjuncts cerebrospinal fluid drainage and distal aortic perfusion. Ann Thorac Surg. 2001;72(2) 481-6.

[4] Coselli JS, Lemaire SA, Koksoy C, Schmittling ZC, Curling PE. Cerebrospinal fluid drainage reduces paraplegia after thoracoabdominal aortic aneurysm repair: results of a randomized clinical trial. J Vasc Surg. 2002;35(4) 631–9.

[5] Safi HJ, Miller CC 3rd, Huynh TT, Estrera AL, Porat EE, Winnerkvist AN, Allen BS, Hassoun HT, Moore FA. Distal aortic perfusion and cerebrospinal fluid drainage for thoracoabdominal and descending thoracic aortic repair: ten years of organ protection. Ann Surg. 2003;238(3) 372-80.

[6] Svensson LG, Crawford ES, Hess KR, Coselli JS, Safi HJ. Experience with 1509 patients undergoing thoracoabdominal aortic operations. J Vasc Surg. 1993;17(2) 357-70.

[7] Drinkwater SL, Goebells A, Haydar A, Bourke P, Brown L, Hamady M, Gibbs RG; Regional Vascular Unit, St Mary's Hospital, Imperial College NHS Trust. The incidence of spinal cord ischaemia following thoracic and thoracoabdominal aortic endovascular intervention. Eur J Vasc Endovasc Surg. 2010;40(6) 729-35.

[8] Gravereaux EC, Faries PL, Burks JA, Latessa V, Spielvogel D, Hollier LH, Marin ML. Risk of spinal cord ischemia after endograft repair of thoracic aortic aneurysms. J Vasc Surg. 2001;34(6) 997-1003.

[9] von Allmen RS, Anjum A, Powell JT. Incidence of descending aortic pathology and evaluation of the impact of thoracic endovascular aortic repair: a population-based study in England and Wales from 1999 to 2010. Eur J Vasc Endovasc Surg. 2013;45(2): 154-9.

[10] McGarvey ML, Mullen MT, Woo EY, Bavaria JE, Augoustides YG, Messé SR, Cheung AT. The treatment of spinal cord ischemia following thoracic endovascular aortic repair. Neurocrit Care. 2007;6(1) 35-9.

[11] Bicknell CD, Riga CV, Wolfe JH. Prevention of paraplegia during thoracoabdominal aortic aneurysm repair. Eur J Vasc Endovasc Surg. 2009 Jun;37(6) 654-60.

[12] Etz CD, Kari FA, Mueller CS, Silovitz D, Brenner RM, Lin HM, Griepp RB. The collateral network concept: a reassessment of the anatomy of spinal cord perfusion. J Thorac Cardiovasc Surg. 2011;141(4) 1020-8.

[13] Carroccio A, Marin ML, Ellozy S, Hollier LH. Pathophysiology of paraplegia following endovascular thoracic aortic aneurysm repair. J Card Surg. 2003;18(4) 359-66.

[14] Acher C, Wynn M. Paraplegia after thoracoabdominal aortic surgery: not just assisted circulation, hypothermic arrest, clamp and sew, or TEVAR. Ann Cardiothorac Surg. 2012;1(3) 365-72.

[15] Etz CD, Luehr M, Kari FA, Bodian CA, Smego D, Plestis KA, Griepp RB. Paraplegia after extensive thoracic and thoracoabdominal aortic aneurysm repair: does critical spinal cord ischemia occur postoperatively? J Thorac Cardiovasc Surg. 2008;135(2) 324-30.

[16] Ullery BW, Cheung AT, Fairman RM, Jackson BM, Woo EY, Bavaria J, Pochettino A, Wang GJ. Risk factors, outcomes, and clinical manifestations of spinal cord ischemia following thoracic endovascular aortic repair. J Vasc Surg. 2011;54(3) 677-84.

[17] Czerny M, Eggebrecht H, Sodeck G, Verzini F, Cao P, Maritati G, Riambau V, Beyersdorf F, Rylski B, Funovics M, Loewe C, Schmidli J, Tozzi P, Weigang E,Kuratani T, Livi U, Esposito G, Trimarchi S, van den Berg JC, Fu W, Chiesa R, Melissano G, Bertoglio L, Lonn L, Schuster I, Grimm M. Mechanisms of symptomatic spinal cord ischemia after TEVAR: insights from the European Registry of Endovascular Aortic Repair Complications (EuREC). J Endovasc Ther. 2012;19(1) 37-43.

[18] Baril DT, Carroccio A, Ellozy SH, Palchik E, Addis MD, Jacobs TS, Teodorescu V, Marin ML. Endovascular thoracic aortic repair and previous or concomitant abdomi-

nal aortic repair: is the increased risk of spinal cord ischemia real? Ann Vasc Surg. 2006;20(2) 188-94.

[19] Zipfel B, Buz S, Redlin M, Hullmeine D, Hammerschmidt R, Hetzer R. Spinal cord ischemia after thoracic stent-grafting: causes apart from intercostal artery coverage. Ann Thorac Surg. 2013;96(1) 31-8.

[20] Acher CW, Wynn MM, Mell MW, Tefera G, Hoch JR. A quantitative assessment of the impact of intercostal artery reimplantation on paralysis risk in thoracoabdominal aortic aneurysm repair. Ann Surg. 2008 Oct;248(4):529-40.

[21] Peterson BG, Eskandari MK, Gleason TG, Morasch MD. Utility of left subclavian artery revascularization in association with endoluminal repair of acute and chronic thoracic aortic pathology. J Vasc Surg. 2006;43(3) 433-9.

[22] Lee TC, Andersen ND, Williams JB, Bhattacharya SD, McCann RL, Hughes GC. Results with a selective revascularization strategy for left subclavian artery coverage during thoracic endovascular aortic repair. Ann Thorac Surg. 2011;92(1) 97-103.

[23] Cooper DG, Walsh SR, Sadat U, Noorani A, Hayes PD, Boyle JR. Neurological complications after left subclavian artery coverage during thoracic endovascular aortic repair: a systematic review and meta-analysis. J Vasc Surg. 2009;49(6) 1594-601.

[24] Rizvi AZ, Murad MH, Fairman RM, Erwin PJ, Montori VM. The effect of left subclavian artery coverage on morbidity and mortality in patients undergoing endovascular thoracic aortic interventions: a systematic review and meta-analysis. J Vasc Surg. 2009;50(5) 1159-69.

[25] Matsumura JS, Lee WA, Mitchell RS, Farber MA, Murad MH, Lumsden AB, Greenberg RK, Safi HJ, Fairman RM; Society for Vascular Surgery. The Society for Vascular Surgery Practice Guidelines: management of the left subclavian artery with thoracic endovascular aortic repair. J Vasc Surg. 2009;50(5) 1155-8.

[26] Maldonado TS, Dexter D, Rockman CB, Veith FJ, Garg K, Arko F, Bertoni H, Ellozy S, Jordan W, Woo E. Left subclavian artery coverage during thoracic endovascular aortic aneurysm repair does not mandate revascularization. J Vasc Surg. 2013;57(1) 116-24.

[27] Harrison SC, Agu O, Harris PL, Ivancev K. Elective sac perfusion to reduce the risk of neurologic events following endovascular repair of thoracoabdominal aneurysms. J Vasc Surg. 2012;55(4) 1202-5.

[28] Cinà CS, Abouzahr L, Arena GO, Laganà A, Devereaux PJ, Farrokhyar F. Cerebrospinal fluid drainage to prevent paraplegia during thoracic and thoracoabdominal aortic aneurysm surgery: a systematic review and meta-analysis. J Vasc Surg. 2004;40 36-44.

[29] Khan SN, Stansby G.Cerebrospinal fluid drainage for thoracic and thoracoabdominal aortic aneurysm surgery. Cochrane Database Syst Rev. 2012;(10) CD003635.

[30] Crawford ES, Svensson LG, Hess KR, Shenaq SS, Coselli JS, Safi HJ, Mohindra PK, Rivera V. A prospective randomized study of cerebrospinal fluid drainage to prevent paraplegia after high-risk surgery on the thoracoabdominal aorta. J Vasc Surg. 1991;13(1) 36-45.

[31] Svensson LG, Hess KR, D'Agostino RS, Entrup MH, Hreib K, Kimmel WA, Nadolny E, Shahian DM. Reduction of neurologic injury after high-risk thoracoabdominal aortic operation. Ann Thorac Surg. 1998;66(1) 132–8.

[32] Coselli JS, Lemaire SA, Koksoy C, Schmittling ZC, Curling PE. Cerebrospinal fluid drainage reduces paraplegia after thoracoabdominal aortic aneurysm repair: results of a randomized clinical trial. J Vasc Surg. 2002;35(4) 631–9.

[33] Wong CS, Healy D, Canning C, Coffey JC, Boyle JR, Walsh SR. A systematic review of spinal cord injury and cerebrospinal fluid drainage after thoracic aortic endografting. J Vasc Surg. 2012;56(5) 1438-47.

[34] Bobadilla JL, Wynn M, Tefera G, Acher CW. Low incidence of paraplegia after thoracic endovascular aneurysm repair with proactive spinal cord protective protocols. J Vasc Surg. 2013;57(6) 1537-42.

[35] McGarvey ML. Effective tool or necessary evil: intraoperative monitoring during thoracic aneurysm repairs. J Clin Neurophysiol. 2012;29(2) 154-6.

[36] Hecker JG, McGarvey M. Heat shock proteins as biomarkers for the rapid detection of brain and spinal cord ischemia: a review and comparison to other methods of detection in thoracic aneurysm repair. Cell Stress Chaperones. 2011;16(2) 119-31.

[37] ter Wolbeek C, Hartert M, Conzelmann LO, Peivandi AA, Czerny M, Gottardi R, Beyersdorf F, Weigang E. Value and pitfalls of neurophysiological monitoring in thoracic and thoracoabdominal aortic replacement and endovascular repair. Thorac Cardiovasc Surg. 2010;58(5) 260-4.

[38] Coselli JS, Tsai PI. Motor evoked potentials in thoracoabdominal aortic surgery: CON. Cardiol Clin. 2010;28(2) 361-8.

[39] Etz CD, von Aspern K, Gudehus S, Luehr M, Girrbach FF, Ender J, Borger M, Mohr FW. Near-infrared Spectroscopy Monitoring of the Collateral Network Prior to, During, and After Thoracoabdominal Aortic Repair: A Pilot Study. Eur J Vasc Endovasc Surg. 2013;46 (6) 651-6.

[40] Anderson RE, Winnerkvist A, Hansson LO, Nilsson O, Rosengren L, Settergren G, Vaage J. Biochemical markers of cerebrospinal ischemia after repair of aneurysms of the descending and thoracoabdominal aorta. J Cardiothorac Vasc Anesth. 2003;17(5) 598-603.

[41] Hecker JG, Sundram H, Zou S, Praestgaard A, Bavaria JE, Ramchandren S, McGarvey M. Heat shock proteins HSP70 and HSP27 in the cerebral spinal fluid of patients

undergoing thoracic aneurysm repair correlate with the probability of postoperative paralysis. Cell Stress Chaperones. 2008;13(4) 435-46.

[42] Nicholson JK, Lindon JC, Holmes E. 'Metabonomics': understanding the metabolic responses of living systems to pathophysiological stimuli via multivariate statistical analysis of biological NMR spectroscopic data. Xenobiotica. 1999;29(11) 1181-9.

[43] Nicholson JK, Holmes E, Kinross JM, Darzi AW, Takats Z, Lindon JC. Metabolic phenotyping in clinical and surgical environments. Nature. 2012;491(7424) 384-92.

[44] Balog J, Sasi-Szabó L, Kinross J, Lewis MR, Muirhead LJ, Veselkov K, Mirnezami R, Dezső B, Damjanovich L, Darzi A, Nicholson JK, Takáts Z. Intraoperative tissue identification using rapid evaporative ionization mass spectrometry. Sci Transl Med. 2013;5(194) 194ra93.

[45] Desart K, Scali ST, Feezor RJ, Hong M, Hess PJ Jr, Beaver TM, Huber TS, Beck AW. Fate of patients with spinal cord ischemia complicating thoracic endovascular aortic repair. J Vasc Surg. 2013;58(3) 635-42.

[46] French DD, Campbell RR, Sabharwal S, Nelson AL, Palacios PA, Gavin-Dreschnack D. Health care costs for patients with chronic spinal cord injury in the Veterans Health Administration. J Spinal Cord Med. 2007;30(5) 477-81.

[47] Mawad ME, Rivera V, Crawford S, Ramirez A, Breitbach W. Spinal cord ischemia after resection of thoracoabdominal aortic aneurysms: MR findings in 24 patients. AJR Am J Roentgenol. 1990;155(6) 1303-7.

Chapter 3

Spinal Cord Injuries Following Suicide Attempts

Stamatios A. Papadakis, Spyridon Galanakos,
Kleio Apostolaki, Konstantinos Kateros,
Olga Antoniadou, George Macheras and
George Sapkas

Additional information is available at the end of the chapter

http://dx.doi.org/10.5772/57409

1. Introduction

Suicide has become an increasing concern as there are an estimated one million completed suicides per year worldwide. Suicide rates have increased by 60% over the last 50 years, particularly in developing countries. Suicide attempts are up to 20 times more. In 1996 more than 150,000 people committed suicide in 38 countries of the World Health Organization European Region. Suicide is currently one of the most important causes of death in Europe among young and middle-aged people, especially men. In some European Countries, in the age group 15-34, suicide ranks second among the most common causes of death. Nine of the ten countries with the highest suicide rates in the world are in the European Region [1].

In the EUROSAVE (European Review of Suicide and Violence Epidemiology) study, Finland had the highest suicide rate, while Greece had the lowest for the latest available year (1997). Greece also had the lowest undetermined deaths in 1984 and 1997 [2]. According to the Rutz and Wasserman study, increases in male adolescent suicide rates from 1979-1996 that were observed in Sweden, Ireland and Greece can partly be attributed to improved suicide statistics [3]. Botsis [4] suggests that in Greece formal statistics by the National Statistics Office are not representative of reality when they refer to reported suicides. Families avoid reporting suicide as the cause of death for religious reasons. Natural causes are reported instead.

Completed suicide rates for Greece (1960-2009) suggest a fluctuation between 2.8 and 4.0 per 100,000 for the years 1975 and 1985, respectively [1,5]. According to the table of Basic Statistics from Health for All (HFA) for the year 2006 in Greece there is a rate of 3.5 in suicides and self-inflicted injuries at all ages per 100,000. This rate is relatively stable for the years 2000-2009 (3.5-3.6) [1]. Recently, Greece began to experience the effects of the extreme financial crisis, and reports in the mass media and journals support a possible casual link between the economic crisis and suicide rates. However, scientific data concerning this matter is still controversial [5-7].

In many European countries suicidal behavior constitutes a major public and mental health problem. It is also a considerable drain of resources in both primary and secondary health care settings [8]. Furthermore, adolescent suicide and attempted suicide have been recognized as a growing health problem in the rest of the world [9]. Young people of both sexes often make repeated suicide attempts [10-12]. Deliberate self-harm is also associated with increased risk of repetition and suicide [13,14].

Several possible theories have been proposed to explain the increased risk conferred by multiple attempts. One possibility is that multiple attempts reflect persistent risk factors (e.g., a chronic or recurring psychiatric disorder or adverse psychosocial conditions). Esposito et al. [15] studied 74 single attempters (SAs) and 47 multiple attempters (MAs; ages 12-18) seen in an emergency department after a suicide attempt and found higher rates of mood disorder diagnosis among MAs. Joiner [16], suggests that multiple suicide attempts increase the risk for subsequent attempts because practice allows MAs to acquire the ability to engage in more serious suicidal behavior.

In Greece, one study in 76 suicide attempters between the ages of 9-20 years, reported an 18-fold greater frequency of psychiatric disorder, 14-fold greater frequency of other problems (relational), 9.7-fold greater frequency of smoking and 4.7-fold greater frequency of psycho-social and environmental problems [17]. A six year retrospective study of self inflicted burns with ages ranging from 18-90 years concluded that of the 1435 admissions between April 1997-April 2003, 3.69% attempted suicide by self burn. Of these, females 57%, males 43%, with a high mortality rate of 75.4%. In 43.3% there was a preexisting psychiatric disorder [18].

A study in another internal medicine clinic from November 1999 to November 2000 of 146 drug intoxications, of which male 34.2% and female 65.8%, refers that 38.3% had a history of mental illness, 31.5% were in need of psychiatric help and 42.5% had a previous suicide attempt. Mental State Examination diagnoses included depression (20.96%), psychosis (15.32%), dysthymic disorder (16.2%), anxiety disorder (22.58%) and personality disorder (8.8%) [19]. Other studies refer to substance use increasing suicidal ideation or behavior [20], rising trends in male suicides, higher rates among widowed men [21,22], and an unusual peak in the summer [23], or spring and summer [21].

2. Spinal cord injury data

A substantial amount of research indicates that self-harm by falling is a rare phenomenon, accounting for 4–7% of suicidal deaths in the developed world [24,25]. The mostet common mode of attempted suicide is drug ingestion. Completed suicides and violent suicide attempts are less common and include hanging, falls/jumps, and firearms [26]. The incidence of different

http://dx.doi.org/10.5772/57409

methods of suicide may vary from one country to another. In the United States for instance, jumping is among the least common methods of committing suicide (less than 2% of all reported suicides in the United States for 2005), while in Hong Kong, jumping is the most common method of committing suicide, accounting for 52.1% of all reported suicide cases in 2006 and similar rates for the years prior to that [27,28]. Community samples estimate that 8–10% of all those who attempt suicide will eventually die as a result of self-harm, most of these within 5 years of the attempt depending on the diagnosis [29,30].

Patients who attempt suicide by jumping from a height usually suffer from multiple injuries. These may be of two types: deceleration type injuries and direct impact injuries [31]. The former, which are internal organ injuries, result from the tendency to displace the tissue in the direction of motion upon impact, while the movement of the body is arrested by the ground [30]. A number of studies show that most of the patients who attempt suicide by jumping suffer from serious psychiatric disorders. These patients suffer from a broad spectrum of psychiatric symptoms: schizophrenia, depression, drugs or alcohol abuse, personality disorder and manic depression [32,33].

Spinal cord injury (SCI) literature estimates suicide as being responsible for approximately 5% of deaths, though this varies greatly between populations [24-37]. Risk tends to be higher in the years immediately post-injury, but there is an increased life-time risk if an individual has ever attempted suicide or self-harm [24].

Several studies have examined the post-injury predictions for patients who survived after a suicide attempt, and various findings arise. Haenel and Jehle [38], conducted a research in Switzerland, on patients who had become paraplegic after a suicide attempt, and who had to spend a certain time in the Basel and Nottwil (canton of Lucerne) centre for paraplegics. They evaluated the records and catamnestic date of 38 patients with a mean age of 38 years, between the years of 1982-1996 and a follow up study was conducted. Catamnestic investigations performed from one month to 14 years after the suicidal attempt were based on a structured dialogue with a standardized, computerized questionnaire. The results showed that the most frequently encountered suicidal method, leading to the paraplegic lesion, was a fall from a window of a building (89,6 %). In 55% of the cases, a psychiatric disorder had been diagnosed prior to the suicide attempt, with depression, alcohol and drug dependence appearing as the most common diagnoses. Thirty-seven per cent of patients had attempted suicide at least once before and 34 % had been hospitalized for psychiatric reasons prior to the incident. The paraplegic lesions of the patients were equally distributed between thoracic, cervical and lumbar lesions. The most disturbing problem reported by patients after the paralysis was sexual impairment. Despite the limited number of cases and the rather short interval between the suicide attempt and the follow-up investigation, results seem to indicate that such patients are not likely to commit suicide on a later occasion, excluding one single case.

Anderson and Allan [24] conducted a survey in a Scottish spinal rehabilitation unit, on the demographics and patients outcome with vertebral fracture after suicide attempt. Forty-six (44 having detailed data available) patients were identified with 95% of injuries resulting from falls. Thirty-six people had pre-existing mental health problems (82%) with 15 (34%) having this diagnosis established shortly after admission. Seventy-five per cent received follow-up from mental health services. Ninety-five per cent returned to their pre-injury (or similar) residence. Length of stay and functional independence measure for the deliberate self harm group were compared with a non-deliberate self harm group. High levels of mental health and substance abuse problems were detected necessitating formal mental health assessment and follow-up. Deliberate self harm as a mechanism for injury appears to have a significant impact on length of stay in the centre only if the patient has fracture without spinal cord injuries. Immediate rehabilitation outcomes are similar to that of non-deliberate self-harm group. The authors noted in the limitations of the study that the sample size was small and a retrospective methodology concerning an accurate history and outcome was difficult. However, the particular study demonstrates that the patients benefited by their time in rehabilitation and had comparable outcomes to a non-deliberate self harm group in the short term. Despite the fact that substance and mental health problems were significant in this group, these difficulties appear to impact little on immediate rehabilitation and discharge.

Kennedy et al. [34], conducted a retrospective review examining the admission records of 137 individuals, of mean age 32, with SCI as a result of a suicide attempt between the period 1951 to 1992. The research took place in the National Spinal Injuries Centre in Stoke Mandeville Hospital in Bucks, UK. They explored and identified the type of psychiatric condition evident around the time of injury and reviewed outcome information of this sample with specific focus on mortality, especially further evidence of deliberate self harm. The subsequent database comprised among others, cause, level and completeness of injury, height fallen, psychiatric history, psychiatric diagnosis, date of last contact, further suicide attempts, date and cause of death, date and place of discharge. Previous suicide attempts had been made by 23%. The cause of injury in 85% of cases was 'falls'. Thirty-three people are known to have died, of whom eight (24%) committed suicide. During the period between the first and last SCI examined within this study (1951-1992) 1.6% (n=137) of the total sample of patients treated at the rehabilitation centre sustained an SCI as a result of a suicide attempt. Recommendations for further research include an adaptation of the psychological autopsy approach which would provide additional information to that which is normally available in actual suicides.

Stanford et al. [25], conducted a research to State SCI services at New South Wales, Australia to determine the incidence of acute SCI due to suicide attempt from 1970 to 2000. They examined demographics, injuries, mental illness, functional outcomes and nature of subsequent deaths of 2752 acute spinal cord injury admissions. Of these, 56 were attempted suicide (55 falls, one gun-shot wound). The median age was 30 years. Psychiatric diagnoses varied, the most common of which were personality disorder, schizophrenia, depression, chronic alcohol abuse, mood disorder and chronic substance abuse. Follow-up was available in 47 cases (84%) at an average of 8 years. Four subsequent deaths were by suicide. Community placement outcomes for survivors were good, however the subsequent death by suicide was high.

Biering et al. [35], during 1965 to 1987 examined 45 patients who were admitted to the Rehabilitation Hospital in Hornbaek, Denmark because of SCI due to suicide attempts. The median age at injury was 31 years. In 38 instances (84%), SCI was caused by jumps from buildings. 62% had previously been admitted to psychiatric hospitals, and 31% had previously attempted suicide. A follow up study was conducted in 1988-89. At follow up, 11 patients had died, 3 from suicide. Of the 34 alive at follow up, 7 had attempted suicide, and 2 reported suicidal thoughts. A 44% had had a psychiatric admission since the SCI and 56% were taking psychiatric medication.

In another research conducted by Christiansen and Jensen [39] in 2007, the incidence of repetition of suicide attempt, suicide and all deaths was examined, and the influence of psychiatric illness and socio-demographic factors on these was analysed. The study was a Danish register-based survival analysis that retrieved personal data on socio-economic, psychiatric and mortality conditions from various registers. Suicide-attempters (2.614) and non-attempters (39.210) were analysed being matched by gender, age and place of residence. The average follow-up period for suicide-attempters was 3.88 years, during which 271 of them died. By comparison, death occurred four times more often among suicide-attempters than among non-attempters. Suicide was far more common among attempters (61, 2.33%) than among non-attempters (16, 0.04%). A proportion of the attempters (31.33%) repeated their attempt within the follow-up period. The most reliable predictors for suicide and death were repetition, suicide attempt method and treatment for mental illness, while the most reliable predictors for repetition were age, gender and mental illness.

It is clear that the results of the different studies vary, but most of them agree, as Christiansen and Jensen [39] state, that individuals with a history of suicide attempts form a well-defined high-risk group for suicide, and are in need of treatment immediately after the episode. Staff attending to the physical and psychiatric needs of these patients must work together and should inform of the risk of subsequent suicidal behavior, after a first episode of attempted suicide. Furthermore, departments which are in contact with suicidal individuals need action plans to ensure that all such individuals receive proper treatment immediately after the suicide attempt. The injuries and life changing conditions following the suicide attempt, add to the existing problems of the patients, especially those with a psychiatric disorder. Further research could take a closer look at the individual factors that lead to mortality in the spinal cord injuries of the deliberate self-harm patients and perhaps suggest mechanisms to reduce mortality. It may also be profitable to examine the risk to self that all individuals bring with them into rehabilitation by merit of their past deliberate self harm or mental health history, as a way of better focused support for all of those with spinal cord injuries after rehabilitation [24].

3. Sample presentation

3.1. Patients and methods

Thirty-two patients (8 males and 24 females) that were treated for SCIs in the Athens University Orthopaedic Department, as a result of deliberate self harm, are presented. Their ages varied from 18 to 65 years, and the average age was 35 years. There were 16 singles (50%), 14 married (44%) and 2 divorced (6%) patients. Thirteen patients were employed (41%), six housewives (19%), seven unemployed (22%), three students / pupils (9%) and three with various occupations (9%). In terms of religion, 28 were Christian Orthodox (88%), one Roman Catholic (3%), one Jewish (3%), one Muslim (3%) and one (3%) with an unknown religious affiliation.

The cause of injury was a fall from a building in 29 cases (91%), a fall from a window in one case (3%), a fall from a bridge in one case (3%) and a fall inside the house in one case (3%). Concerning the level of injury, in 16 cases (50%) it was at the lumbar level, in 9 cases (28 %) at the cervical, in 5 cases (16%) at thoracic and 2 cases (6%) regarded the sacral vertebrae (Figures 1 and 2). In 20 cases (62.5%) the injury was incomplete and in 12 cases (37.5%) complete. The psychiatric diagnosis was schizophrenia in 12 patients (38%), depression in 8 patients (25%), drugs or alcohol abuse in 3 cases (9%), personality disorder in one patient (3%), bipolar disorder in one patient (3%), other psychiatric reasons in one patient (3%) and in 6 cases (19%) there was no specific diagnosis (generally marital or work related). The height of the falls ranged from 2 to 12 m and all patients landed on solid ground. Operative treatment which included laminectomies, spine instrumentation and fusion was performed in all patients.

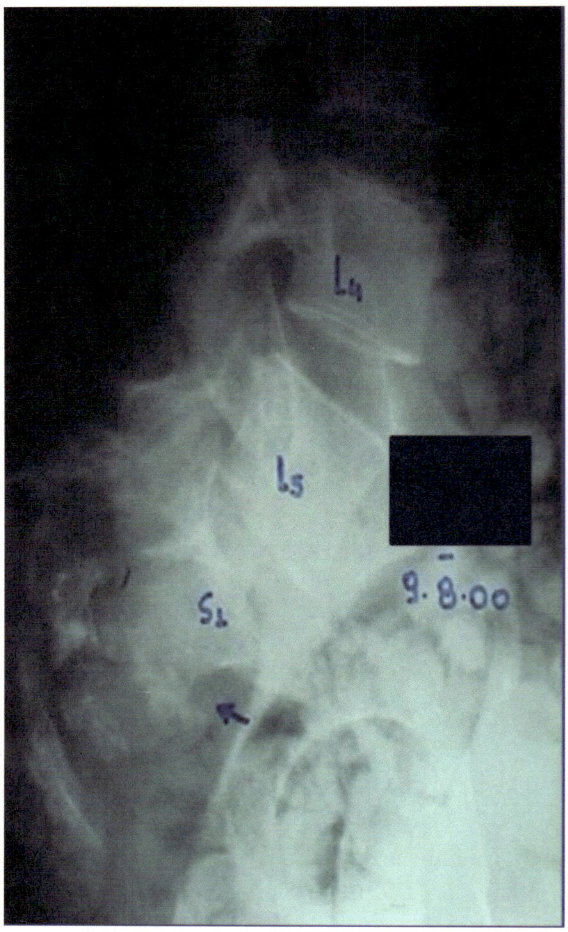

Figure 1. Lateral radiograph showing a fracture of the sacrum.

http://dx.doi.org/10.5772/57409

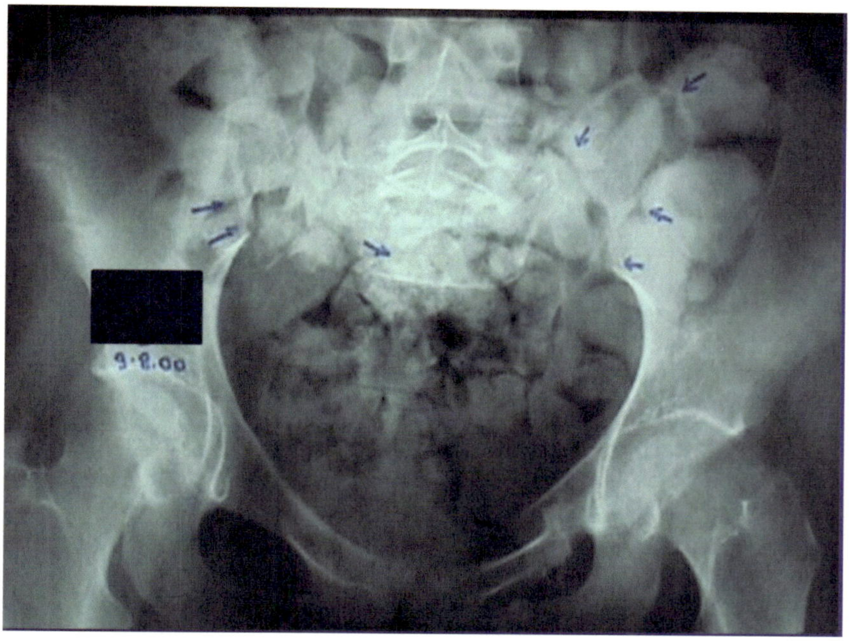

Figure 2. Anteroposterior radiograph of the same case.

3.2. Results

Initial clinical data of the 32 patients included in this study are shown in Table 1. At admission, ATLS guidelines were used for all patients. Associated injuries of the abdomen were present in five patients (patients 1, 4, 10 and 22). In these patients, a laparotomy was necessary for intraperitoneal bleeding, spleen and kidney injury, and mesenteric tear prior to the surgical operation for the spine fracture. Head injuries were revealed with CT scan in six patients (patients 3, 7, 8, 14, 26 and 30). In these cases craniotomy and decompression were performed first, before stabilization of the spinal fractures. Thoracic injuries (ribs fractures or sternum fracture) were present in three patients (patients 3, 5 and 28). Conservative treatment with assisted ventilation was necessary in these cases. Long bone fractures (femoral, tibial, bimalleolar, calcaneal, radial and humeral), including pelvic fractures, were treated by external fixation or closed reduction and immobilization in plaster or temporary splint. Subsequently, reduction and internal fixation, if required, were performed from 8 hours to 5 days later.

Regarding the treatment of the spinal fractures – dislocations, instrumentation devices including titanium rods, transpedicular screws, sacral bars and bone grafting were used on all patients. Patients were evaluated by a consulting psychiatrist as soon as their condition and cooperation permitted. Assessment included an interview and a complete mental status examination.

The only complications encountered were two cases of aspiration pneumonia, one of which resulted in prolonged stay on the intensive therapy unit due to difficulty weaning the patient off the ventilator. All patients were discharged from hospital approximately 6–8 weeks after the operation with a custom-made thermoplastic thoracolumbar or lumbosacral orthosis for another 8 weeks and instructions for physical therapy and rehabilitation programs. After discharge 13 patients returned to their homes and 19 to another hospital or entered residential care.

Patient	Age/ gender	Mechanism of injury	Neurological deficits at admission	Associated Lesion	Surgical treatment	Follow-up	Recovery and outcome
1	23/F	Fall from building	Bowel and bladderdysfunction;saddle anesthesia;incomplete L5-S1 paraplegia	L4 fracture, humeral shaft fracture	Laminectomy; titanium rods and transpedicular screws, humeral external fixation	6 years	Recovery
2	18/M	Fall from building	Incomplete paraplegia	L2 fracture	Laminectomy; titanium rods and transpedicular screws	8 years	Recovery
3	34/F	Fall from building	Completeparaplegia	T9 fracture	Laminectomy; titanium rods and transpedicular screws	2 years	None
4	42/F	Fall from window	Incomplete paraplegia	L3 fracture	Laminectomy; titanium rods and transpedicular screws	18 months	Recovery
5	20/F	Fall from building	Completeparaplegia	T5 - T6 fracture, dislocation	Laminectomies; titanium rods and transpedicular screws	1 year	None
6	48/F	Fall from building	Incomplete paraplegia	L4 fracture	Laminectomy; titanium rods and transpedicular screws	5 years	Recovery
7	65/F	Fall from building	Incompletetetraplegia	C2 - C3 fracture, dislocation	Anterior plating	17 months	Death, second suicide attempt at 2 years

8	56/M	Fall from building	Central cord syndrome	C2 - C3 fracture, dislocation	Anterior plating	2 years	Death (renal failure)
9	41/F	Fall from building	Incomplete paraplegia	L4 fracture	Laminectomy; titanium rods and transpedicular screws	22 months	Recovery
10	27/F	Fall from building	Completeparaplegia	L1 fracture	Laminectomy; titanium rods and transpedicular screws	10 years	None
11	31/F	Fall from building	Bowel and bladderdysfunction;saddle anesthesia;complete L4–S1paraplegia	L4 fracture	Laminectomy; titanium rods and transpedicular screws	9 years	None
12	39/M	Fall from building	Complete tetraplegia	C2 - C3 fracture, dislocation	AnteriorC2 - C3 plating	30 months	None
13	46/F	Fall from building	Complete tetraplegia	C2 - C3 fracture, dislocation	Anterior plating	25 months	None
14	51/F	Fall from building	Complete tetraplegia	C2 - C3 fracture	Anterior plating	3 years	Death (renal failure)
15	36/M	Fall from building	Incomplete tetraplegia	C7 fracture	Anterior plating	1 year	Recovery
16	19/F	Fall from building	Complete tetraplegia	C2 - C3 fracture, dislocation	Anterior plating	14 months	None
17	39/M	Fall from building	Incomplete paraplegia	Sacral fracture, Dennis III	Transiliac sacral bars	34 months	Recovery
18	41/F	Fall from bridge	Complete tetraplegia	C2 - C3 fracture, dislocation	Anterior plating	8 years	None
19	47/F	Fall from building	Incomplete paraplegia	L4 fracture	Laminectomy; titanium rods and transpedicular screws	3 years	Recovery

20	34/F	Fall from building	Incomplete paraplegia	L4 fracture	Laminectomy; titanium rods and transpedicular screws	1 year	Recovery
21	53/M	Fall from building	Complete paraplegia	Transverse fracture of the sacrum with anterior displacement	laminectomies; titanium rods and transpedicular screws; bone grafting	32 months	Death (pneumonia)
22	38/F	Fall from building	Incomplete paraplegia	L1 - L2 fracture, distal radius fracture	Laminectomies; titanium rods and transpedicular screws, cast for the distal radius fracture	23 months	Recovery
23	47/F	Fall from building	Brown - Sequard syndrome	T8 fracture	Laminectomy; titanium rods and transpedicular screws	2 years	Recovery
24	41/F	Fall from building	Incomplete paraplegia	L4 fracture	Laminectomy; titanium rods and transpedicular screws	4 years	Recovery
25	35/M	Fall inside the house	Incomplete paraplegia	L4 fracture	Laminectomy; titanium rods and transpedicular screws	15 months	Recovery
26	36/F	Fall from building	Incomplete tetraplegia	C6 - C7 fracture	Anterior plating	19 months	Recovery
27	27/F	Fall from building	Incomplete paraplegia	L5 fracture	Laminectomy; titanium rods and transpedicular screws	7 years	Recovery
28	33/F	Fall from building	Complete paraplegia	T9 - T10 fracture, dislocation	Laminectomies; titanium rods and	2 years	None

					transpedicular screws		
29	55/F	Fall from building	Incomplete paraplegia	L4 fracture	Laminectomy; titanium rods and transpedicular screws	31 months	Recovery
30	50/F	Fall from building	Complete paraplegia	T8 - T9 fracture, dislocation	Laminectomies; titanium rods and transpedicular screws	13 months	Death (renal failure)
31	44/F	Fall from building	Incomplete paraplegia	L3 fracture, distal radius fracture	Laminectomy; titanium rods and transpedicular screws, cast for the distal radius fracture	4 years	Recovery
32	23/M	Fall from building	Incomplete paraplegia	L4 fracture	Laminectomy; titanium rods and transpedicular screws	8 years	Recovery

Table 1. Clinical data of the patients

The mean follow-up was 6 years (range: 12 months – 10 years). At follow-up, only 27 of the patients were available for evaluation due to the death of 5 patients 1-3 years post injury. Of the five patients one had committed suicide (patient 7) and the other four had presented medical complications [renal failure in 3 patients (patients 8, 14 and 30) and pneumonia in one (patient 21)]. Of the remaining patients, two were involved in further unsuccessful suicide attempts due to psychiatric problems, 1 to 3 years post first injury (patients 10 and 24) (Table 1). All survivors received psychiatric follow-up.

3.3. Discussion

Adolescent suicide and attempted suicide have been recognized as a growing health problem in both Europe and the rest of the world [9]. The highest average person-based ratio of male: female suicide attempt rate was found in the age group 15-24 years (1: 1.9), the next highest in the age group 45-54 years (1: 1.7). This ratio decreases in the age group up to 55 to 1: 1.4 (range: 1:3.4 to 1:0.6) [40].

In the two Greek studies referring to attempted suicide hospitalized in internal medicine wards due to drug intoxication and self poisoning there is a definite precedence of females with the first showing a percentage of male 34.2% and female 65.8% [22], and the second a ratio of male to female of 1:1.97 in an age group of 20-30 years [23]. Other studies also report parasuicide as more common in females and younger ages [41,42]. Contrarily, in the nationwide study of 1980-1995 of suicides a mean age-standardized rate of 5.86/100,000 males to 1.89/100,000 females was demonstrated. In addition, an increase in suicide rates was reported with age for males, with rising trends in the ages of 45-54yrs and decreasing rates for females in the 15-24yrs and 75-84yrs age group. Mostly violent methods are used among men [22]. This male to female trend is confirmed in the Epirus study where a mean age-standardized suicide rate per year 4/100,000 males was reported to 1.29 females/100,000. Once again a significant rising trend was shown for male suicides in the ages 35-44yrs and 65-74yrs, while low female rates were found in the under 35yrs age group [21].

In the current study, the ratio between males to females was 1:3. Females were more likely to make a more dangerous jump that increased their mortality. Others suggest that young males tended to use more lethal methods in attempts and to repeat more often than females [29]. A previous suicide attempt is in itself the strongest predictor of future suicide and local rates of attempted suicide and regional and national suicide rates in young people, especially males, are strongly correlated [43]. There is an association between repeated suicide attempts and completed suicide, particularly in males and when a violent method has been used [44,45].

The underlying psychology of suicide is complex and unique to each individual. However, certain themes emerge from studying individuals who have attempted or completed suicides. In all age groups, depression, alcohol and drug dependence, as well as history of mental illness are known to be risk factors for suicide [46]. Twenty percent of people who attempt suicide will make another attempt within the year, and 10% ultimately succeed [26]. Injuries resulting from direct impact are mostly fractures [47]. The area over which the impact force is applied influences the severity of the fractures [48]. The smaller the area over which the patients land, the greater the load/ unit area. Patients who land on their legs tend to sustain more serious injuries than those who land on their sides.

There were two main combinations of fractures in this series. The patients with spinal fracture combined with pelvic and extremity fractures. Only three of them sustained upper extremity fractures (patients 1, 22 and 31). Twelve patients presented with pelvic or lower extremity fractures associated with upper extremity fractures. The difference between the two groups shows that fractures in the upper extremities usually exclude fractures of the spine. Upon impact, the falling body has a kinetic energy which is converted, in its major part, into fracture energy. In the first group most of the kinetic energy is dissipated to the lower extremities, pelvis and spine, causing fractures at these sites. In the second group, patients use their upper extremities in an attempt to protect themselves, possibly via more flexion at the hip level. This increased flexion converts the remaining energy into forward rotational energy of the trunk exposing the extended upper extremities to fractures. It is probable that this form of energy dissipation protects the spine from fracture.

The initial treatment should be limited to life-saving procedures and short spine and limb stabilization procedures [49]. Fractures should be treated by methods that will allow early mobilization and transfer to the psychiatric ward. Treatment by traction or spica cast is not well tolerated by these patients and interferes with their nursing care. Rigid internal fixation, whenever possible for unstable fractures, is recommended.

The results of our study and others show that most of the patients who attempt suicide by jumping suffer from serious psychiatric disorders [32,33]. These patients suffer from a broad spectrum of psychiatric symptoms: schizophrenia, depression, drugs or alcohol abuse, personality disorder and manic depression. The proportion of patients with schizophrenia is far higher than found in general suicide attempts where it is estimated to range from 5% to 10%. Sometimes they have active suicidal ideation or even a detailed suicidal plan. Thus, the treatment approach for such patients must take into account their psychiatric state. The psychiatric manifestations create subjective distress for the patient and may hinder or even prevent the medical and surgical care of the patient in some instances [50].

In this sample of patients the fact that most individuals appeared to have responded to treatment, indicated that all admissions following self-harm should have access to appropriate psychiatric treatment. The finding that three of the patients within this study, attempted suicide following SCI, suggests that a small number of the people who have attempted suicide will re-attempt. We believe that routine screening for suicide and risk assessments might highlight those who are most at risk of re-attempting suicide, thus allowing healthcare professionals to be aware of these individuals and adopt appropriate strategies to address suicidal ideation and behavior.

The prevalence of psychiatric and mental health problems illustrated in this series highlights the importance of educating staff in the care of patients with mental health problems. In view of the special needs of these individuals, services should ensure regular follow-up to prevent deterioration and monitor progress. Moreover, future clinical research should also evaluate the specific problems of people who have both SCI and a psychiatric diagnosis.

4. Conclusions

Until now it has been difficult to obtain comparable international data on suicide attempts, owing to disparities in definitions, survey designs and study methods. It has been our experience that psychiatric conditions, and especially suicide risk, should be evaluated and treated as early as possible during the orthopaedic or surgical hospitalization. Management requires both psychopharmacological therapy and psychotherapy. It has to be directed towards the achievement of symptomatic relief and, if possible, towards the remission of the primary psychiatric disorder. The management of these patients in the orthopaedic or surgical ward is difficult, because of restlessness, noncooperation of the patient and the problem of staff inexperienced in handling the psychiatric patient. When prolonged orthopaedic and rehabilitation management is necessary, it is suggested that the patient be transferred to the psychiatric hospital while continuing the necessary orthopaedic treatment.

Author details

Stamatios A. Papadakis[1*], Spyridon Galanakos[1], Kleio Apostolaki[2], Konstantinos Kateros[3], Olga Antoniadou[4], George Macheras[1] and George Sapkas[5]

*Address all correspondence to: snapmd@gmail.com

1 D' Department of Orthopaedics, "KAT-EKA" General Hospital, Athens, Greece

2 Private Psychology and Psychotherapy Practice, Athens, Greece

3 A' Department of Orthopaedics, "G. Gennimatas" General Hospital, Athens, Greece

4 Private Psychiatry Practice , Athens, Greece

5 A' Department of Orthopaedics, University of Athens, "Attikon" University Hospital, Haidari, Greece

References

[1] World Health Organisation. Suicide prevention (SUPRE). http://www.who.int/mental_health/prevention/suicide/suicideprevent/en/index.html (accessed 3 November 2013)

[2] Chishti P, Stone DH, Corcoran P, Williamson E, Petridou E; Eurosave Working Group Suicide mortality in the European Union. European Journal of Public Health 2003;13(2): 108-114.

[3] Rutz EM, Wasserman D. Trends in adolescent suicide mortality in the WHO European Region. European Child & Adolescent Psychiatry 2004;13(5):321-331.

[4] Kazalotti E, Xinou A. Suicide. Article, Eleftherotipia, Daily Newspaper 19th January 2008

[5] Fountoulakis KN, Grammatikopoulos IA, Koupidis SA, Siamouli M, Theodorakis PN. Health and the financial crisis in Greece. The Lancet, 2012;379(9820):1001-1002.

[6] Economou M, Madianos M, Peppou LE, Theleritis C, Stefanis CN. Suicidality and the economic crisis in Greece. The Lancet 2012;380(9839):337.

[7] Kentikelenis A, Karanikolos M, Papanicolas I, Basu S, Mckee M, Stuckler D. Health effects of financial crisis: omens of a Greek tragedy. The Lancet 2011;378:1457-1458

[8] Schmidtke A, Bille-Brahe U, Kerkhof A, DeLeo D, Bjerke T, Crepet P, Haring C, Michel K, Salander-Renberg E, Wassermann D, Fricke S, Weinacker B. Results of the WHO/EURO Multicentre Study on Parasuicide: Rates, Trends and Sociodemograph-

ic variables of European parasuicides. Paper presented at the WPA Satellite Symposium"Suicidal Behaviour". Budapest, 1996.

[9] Hultın A., Jiang G.-X., Wasserman D., Hawton K., Hjelmeland H, De Leo D, Ostamo A, Salander-Renberg E, Schmidtke A. Repetition of attempted suicide among teenagers in Europe: frequency, timing and risk factors. European Child & Adolescent Psychiatry 2001;10:161–169.

[10] Brent DA, Kolko DJ,Wartella ME, Boylan M, Moritz G, Baugher M, Zlenak J. Adolescent psychiatric inpatients' risk of suicide attempt at 6-month follow-up. Journal of the American Academy of Child and Adolescent Psychiatry 1993;32:95-105.

[11] Pfeffer CR, Klerman GL, Hurt SW, Kaukuma T, Peskin JR, Siefker CA. Suicidal children grow up: rates and psychosocial risk factors for suicide attempts during follow-up. Journal of the American Academy of Child & Adolescent Psychiatry 1993;32:106–113.

[12] Larsson B,Melin L, Breitholtz E,Andersson M. Short-term stability of depressive symptoms and suicide attempts in Swedish adolescents. Acta Psychiatrica Scandinavica 1991;83:385–390.

[13] Haw C, Bergen H, Casey D, Hawton K. Repetition of deliberate self-harm: a study of characteristics and subsequent deaths in patients presenting to a general hospital according to extent of repetition. Suicide & Life Threatening Behaviour 2007;37(4): 379-396.

[14] Zahl DL, Hawton K. Repetition of DSH and subsequent suicide risk: long-term follow-up study of 11,583 patients. The British Journal of Psychiatry 2004;185:70-75.

[15] Esposito C, Spirito A, Boergers J, Donaldson D. Affective, behavioral, and cognitive functioning in adolescents with multiple suicide attempts. Suicide & Life Threatening Behaviour 2003;33:389-399.

[16] Joiner TE. Why People Die by Suicide. Cambridge, MA: Harvard University Press; 2005;46Y93, 203-222.

[17] Menti E, Lekka NP, Assimakopoulos K, Varvarigou A, Beratis NG, Beratis S. Smoking, psychosocial factor, psychopathologic behaviour and other related conditions in hospitalized youth suicide attempters. Comprehensive Psychiatry 2007;48(6):522-528.

[18] Tsati E, Iconomou T, Tzivaridou D, Keramidas E, Papadopoulos S, Tsoutsos D. Self-inflicted burns in Athens Greece: a six year retrospective study. The Journal of Burn Care & Rehabilitation 2005;26(1):75-78.

[19] Tountas C, Sotiropoulos A, Skliros SA. Kotsini V, Peppas TA, Tamvakos E, Pappas S. Voluntary self-poisoning as a cause of admission to a tertiary hospital internal medicine clinic in Pireaus Greece within a year. BMC Psychiatry 2001;1:4

[20] Giotakos O. Suicidal ideation, substance use, and sense of coherence in Greek male conscripts. Military Medicine 2003;168(6):447-50

[21] Vougiouklakis T, Boumba VA, Mitselou A, Peschos D, Gerontopoulos K. Trends in suicide mortality in the deprived region of Epirus (north-west Greece) during the period 1998-2002. Medicine Science and the Law 2005;45(1):39-46.

[22] Zacharakis CA, Madianos MG, Papadimitriou GN, Stefanis CN. Suicide in Greece 1980-1995:Patterns and Social Factors. Social Psychiatry and Psychiatry Epidemiology 1998;33(10):471-476.

[23] Hatziolis AI, Sion ML, Eleftheriadis NP, Toulis E, Efstratiadis G, Vartzopoulos D, Ziakas AG.Parasuicidal poisoning treated in a Greek medical ward; epidemiology and clinical experience. Human and Experimental Toxicology 2001;20(12):611-617.

[24] Anderson J, Allan DB. Vertebral fracture secondary to suicide attempt: demographics and patient outcome in a Scottish spinal rehabilitation unit. The Journal of Spinal Cord Medicine 2011;34(4):380-387.

[25] Stanford RE, Soden R, Bartrop R, Mikk M, Taylor TKF. Spinal cord and related injuries after attempted suicide: psychiatric diagnosis and long-term follow-up. Spinal Cord 2007;45(6):437-443.

[26] Crandall M, Luchette F, Esposito TJ, West M, Shapiro M, Bulger E. Attempted suicide and the elderly trauma patient: Risk factors and outcomes. Journal of Trauma. 2007; 62(4):1021-1028.

[27] Centre of Suicidal Research and prevention-University of Hong-Kong 2004. http://csrp.hku.hk/WEB/eng/statistics.asp#3.

[28] HKJC Centre for Suicide Research and Prevention, University of Hong Kong 2006. Retrieved 2009-09-10. "Method uses for completing suicide". http://csrp.hku.hk/WEB/eng/statistics.asp#3.

[29] Beautrais AL. Serious suicide attempts in young people: a case control study. American Journal of Psychiatry 1996;153:1009–1014.

[30] Suominen K, Isometsä E, Suokas J, Haukka J, Achte K, Lönnqvist K. Completed suicide after a suicide attempt: a 37-year follow-up study. American Journal of Psychiatry 2004;161(4):563–64.

[31] Maubl KI, Whitley ER, Cardea JA.Vertical deceleration injuries. Surgery Gynecology & Obstetrics 1981;153(2):233-236.

[32] Sims A., O'Brien K. An account of mentally ill people who jump from buildings. Medicine Science and the Law 1979;19:195.

[33] Prasad A., Lloyd GG.Attempted suicide by jumping. Acta Psychiatrica Scandinavica 1983;68:394.

[34] Kennedy P, Rogers B, Speer S, Frankel H. Spinal cord injuries and attempted suicide: a retrospective review. Spinal Cord 1999;37(12):847–852.

[35] Biering-Sorensen F, Pederson W, Giortz Muller P. Spinal cord injury due to suicide attempts. Paraplegia 1992;30(2):139-144.

[36] Hartkopp A, Hansen H, Seidenschnur AM, Biering-Sorensen E. Suicide in a spinal cord injured population: its relation to functional status. Archives of Physical Medicine and Rehabilitation 1998;79(11):1356–1361.

[37] Kewman DG, Tate DG. Suicide in SCI: a psychological autopsy. Rehabilitation Psychology 1998;43(2):143–151.

[38] Haenel T, Jehle O. Paraplegia after suicidal attempt. Psychiatriche Praxis 2003;30(4): 212-215.

[39] Christiansen E., Jensen BF. Risk of repetition of suicide attempt, suicide or all deaths after an episode of attempted suicide: a register-based survival analysis. The Australian and New Zealand Journal of Psychiatry 2007;41(3):257-265.

[40] Petronis KR. Samuels JF, Moscicki EK, Anthony JC. An epidemiologic investigation of potential risk factors for suicide attempts. Social Psqchiatry and Psychiatric Epidemiology. 1990;25:193-199.

[41] Poma SZ, Magno N, Belletti S, Toniolo E (2007) Parasuicide in Rovigo (North of Italy) during the period 2000-2005. J Prev Med Hyg 48(3): 79-82

[42] Prosser JM, Perrone J, Pines JM (2007) The epidemiology of intentional non-fatal self-harm poisoning in the United States: 2001-2004. J Med Toxicol 3 (1): 20-4

[43] Hawton K, Arensman E, Wasserman D, Hultén A, Bille-Brahe U, Bjerke T, Crepet P, Deisenhammer E, Kerkhof A, De Leo D, Michel K, Ostamo A, Philippe A, Querejeta I, Salander-Renberg E, Schmidtke A, Temesváry B. Relation between attempted suicide and suicide rates among young people in Europe. Journal of Epidemiology and Community Health 1998;52(3):191–194.

[44] Granboulan V, Rabain D, Basquin M (1995). The outcome of adolescent suicide attempts.Acta Psychiatrica Scandinavica 91:265-270.

[45] Hawton K, Fagg J, Platt S, Hawkins M. (1993). Factors associated with suicide after parasuicide in young people. British Journal of Psychiatry 306: 1641–1644.

[46] Castle K, Duberstein PR, Meldrum S, Conner KR, Conwell Y. Risk factors for suicide in blacks and whites: an analysis of data from the 1993 National Mortality Followback Survey. American Journal of Psychiatry. 2004; 161:452-458.

[47] Lewis WS, Lee AB, Grantham SA. ``Jumpers syndrome'': the trauma of high free fall as seen at Harlem Hospital. Journal of Trauma 1965;5(6):812-818.

[48] Snyder RG. Human tolerance to extreme impacts in free-fall. Aeroscace Medicine 1963;34: 695-709.

[49] Burri C., Kreuzer U., Limmer J. Principles and practice of fracture treatment in the multiple injured patient. Injury 1982;14(1):44-50.

[50] Katz K, Gonen N, Goldberg I, Mizrahit J Radwan M, Yosipovitch Z..Injuries in attempted suicide by jumping from a height. Injury 1988;19:371-374.

Section 2

Management of Paraplegia

Chapter 4

Role of Decompressive Surgery in Disorders Associated with Spinal Cord Lesions

Ayoub Dakson and Sean D. Christie

Additional information is available at the end of the chapter

http://dx.doi.org/10.5772/58408

1. Introduction

Paraplegia/tetraplegia represents a significant neurologic disability with loss of motor and sensory function in the lower extremities and/or impairment of sexual, urinary and intestinal functions. Involvement of the spinal cord explains most cases of paraplegia/tetraplegia with pathological lesions commonly resulting from trauma or a progressive neoplastic disease of the spine. In such cases, paraplegia/tetraplegia occurs either acutely or results from a chronically progressive spinal pathology, warranting urgent surgical decompression. Surgical decision-making and the rationale for spinal decompression are based on the anticipated increased risk of paraplegia/tetraplegia in cases where there is evidence of progressive functional loss. This chapter aims to review the current state of spinal surgery and to provide an evidence-based approach to the management of common compressive spinal disorders associated with paraplegia/tetraplegia, including degenerative conditions, such as acute traumatic spinal cord injury, cervical spondylotic myelopathy and spinal metastatic disease.The surgical management of each category is discussed separately below.

The anatomical structures maintaining spinal stability and various methods of assessment of spinal instability are discussed. The reminder of the chapter explores up-to-date evidence on the management of compressive myelopathies. In addition, we discuss the most recent evidence and clinical guidelines surrounding the acute management of traumatic cervical spinal cord injury and timing of surgical decompression. Furthermore, this chapter outlines the epidemiology and pathophysiology of cervical spondylotic myelopathy, which is explained in order to provide a foundation to the understanding of prognosis and timing of surgical decompression. Different approaches including anterior and posterior decompression are discussed, explaining the rationale for each approach based on an appraisal of published clinical evidence. The advantages and disadvantages of laminectomy with arthrodesis are reviewed and compared to laminectomy alone and other techniques such as laminoplasty. Finally, management of spinal metastasis as an important etiology for paraplegia is explained. The rationale to surgical decompression is explored on the basis of clinical trials with brief elaboration on the epidemiology and pathophysiology of spinal metastasis.

2. Requirement for spinal stability

Spinal stability constitutes a crucial factor in the surgical management of most spine disorders, serving as a strong indication for surgical intervention in many diseases of the spine. Spinal instability may co-exist with traumatic disorders of the spine as well as non-traumatic disorders such as metastatic and degenerative disease.

Spinal stability has been defined conceptually by Panjabi et al. (1993) as the ability of the spine, under physiologic loads, to limit displacement and deformity in order to prevent neurologic deficits, due to injury to the neural elements (spinal cord and nerve roots), and pain as a result of structural changes. Loss of the ability of the spine to resist displacement is recognized as spinal instability, which increases the risk of neural injury or occurs in association with neural injury. Resistance against such deforming forces stems from passive, active and neural control spinal subsystems, which form the spinal stabilizing system. The skeletal system represents osseous and ligamentous structures including vertebrae, intervertebral discs, spinal ligaments, facet articulations and joint capsules, which all contribute to passive spinal resistance forces. The active subsystem is resembled by muscles and related tendons that surround the spinal column, possessing an active force against spinal deformity and neural injury. Finally, the neural and feedback subsystem is composed of a variety of sensory receptors in ligamentous and muscular structures forming part of the neural feedback system acting reflexively on active and thereby passive subsystems to prevent spinal deformity and neural injury.

The first structural description of spinal stability in the context of a two-column approach was published by Frank Holdsworth et al. (1970). He proposed that spinal instability is sufficiently accounted for by rupture of the posterior ligamentous complex (PLC). However, emerging biomechanical evidence is contradictory in that isolated disruption of the PLC is not necessarily a cause of spinal instability except in cases where evidence of disruption of the posterior longitudinal ligament and tearing of the annulus fibrosis also exists. Therefore, Denis et al. (1983) suggested a three-column approach in assessing the stability of the spine following acute spinal trauma. The anterior longitudinal ligament together with two thirds of the vertebral body form the anterior column, whereas the middle column encompasses the posterior longitudinal ligament, the posterior annulus fibrosis, and the posterior one-third the vertebral body. The posterior column resembles the posterior bony complex (posterior arch) and PLC (supraspinous ligament, interspinous ligament, capsule and ligamentum flavum). This approach will be helpful when describing fractures of the spine and their relation to clinical instability. For instance, one way to differentiate compression fractures from unstable burst fractures is failure of the anterior and middle columns, which is readily visualized on lateral radiographs and CT in burst fractures rendering the spine mechanically unstable (Louis

1985; Denis 1983). This is in contrast to failure of the anterior column only as seen in compression fractures.

More importantly, spinal instability is better represented as a spectrum of instability ranging from stable to unstable spinal injury rather than an all-or-none phenomenon. Two types of spinal instability are described: acute and chronic instability. Acute instability occurs most commonly in the context of trauma, infectious and neoplastic diseases of the spine, whereas chronic instability usually results from a degenerative spinal process or as a consequence of acute instability. In acute spinal instability, two different types occur; overt and limited. The former is defined as loss of the ability of the spine to support the trunk during normal movement, which occurs in the context of loss of the ventral and dorsal integrities of the spinal column. For instance, compromise of the vertebral body integrity is seen in compression and burst fractures resulting in ventral column disruption, which can be assessed with plain radiographs or CT. Compromise of the dorsal integrity of the spinal column often results from disruption of the ligamentous structures or fractures of the dorsal elements. Assessment of ligamentous injury is aided by MRI imaging with the addition of fat suppression or short T1 inversion recovery (STIR) sequences for better visual distinction of the ligamentous structures. Isolated MRI signal change indicates increased water content within the ligamentous structures and does not necessarily confirm complete disruption of the disco-ligamentous structures unless accompanied by evidence of locked facets or facet dislocation, which is considered an absolute indication of posterior ligamentous disruption (Vaccaro 2007). The presence of overt instability requires definite surgical stabilization.

On the other hand, limited instability is represented by disruption of either the anterior or posterior integrity of the spine with preservation of the other. For instance, wedge or burst fractures of the vertebral body with no evidence of disruption of the posterior integrity resemble limited instability, which allows for non-operative management, and may include external orthoses such as a brace. Having said that, overt instability can be missed and misjudged as limited instability especially when in the context of overlooking disruption of the posterior ligamentous structures.

In current practice, few scoring systems exist to aid assessment of spinal instability in cervical and thoracolumbar spinal injury. As discussed above, the Spine Trauma Study Group published a classification system for subaxial cervical spine injuries, named the Subaxial Injury Classification (SLIC) and Severity Scale, describing the morphological, discoligamentous complex (DLC) and clinical neurological parameters associated with cervical spine injury (Anderson 2007; Vaccaro 2007). In terms of describing the morphology of the fracture, the greater instability associated with the spinal fracture, the higher the number of points given (Table 1). For instance, facet dislocation and fracture-dislocation injuries are considered highly unstable with failure of three columns (4 points), compared to simple compression fractures, which are associated with single column failure (1 point). In addition, the SLIC severity scoring system sheds further light on the importance of disruption of the posterior column, which requires evidence of perched or dislocated facet and facet diastasis > 2mm, as well as MRI signal change at the entire disc (2 points). The presence of T2-weighted STIR MRI signal change at the ligamentous structures or isolated widening of the interspinous space on plain radiographs is considered intermediate evidence of ligamentous disruption (1 point). SLIC score of ≥ 5 points is highly suggestive of spinal instability and requirement for surgical stabilization, with or without spinal cord or nerve root decompression (Arabi 2013).

Sub-Axial Injury Classfication Scale	Points
Morphology	
No abnormality	0
Compression	1
Burst	2
Distraction (facet perch, hyperextension)	3
Rotation/translation (facet dislocation, unstbale teardrop fracture)	4
Disco-ligamentous Complex (DLC)	
Intact	0
Intermediate (isolated interspinous widening, MRI signal change only)	1
Disrupted (widening of disc space, facet perch or dislocation)	2
Neurological status	
Intact	0
Root injury	1
Complete cord injury	2
Incomplete cord injury	3
Continous cord compression (in setting of neurological deficit)	+1

Table 1. Subaxial Injury Classification (SLIC) and severity scale

3. Traumatic cervical spinal cord injury

Trauma to the spinal cord is commonly associated with considerable disability and is manifested by loss of function, including tetra-/paraplegia as well as genitourinary and gastrointestinal dysfunction, and chronic pain. Acute SCI affects about 250,000 individuals in North America, and has been estimated to account for a lifetime cost of $500,000 to $2 millions per case, with an overall annual cost of $7 billion in the USA (DeVivo 1997; Sadowsky 1999). The annual incidence of traumatic SCI ranges from 28 and 55 cases per million people with about 10,000 cases reported annually in the USA (McDonald 2002). Patients sustain considerable deficits and disabilities that require multidisciplinary approach to treatment and an intensive neurorehabilitation program. Much research has been published in an effort to establish what factors alter the neurologic and functional outcomes after SCI in order to optimize targeted management of acute SCI. The management of acute SCI, particularly cervical SCI includes a multifaceted and stepwise approach starting with pre-hospital care, leading to emergency medical or physiological strategies as well as decompressive spinal surgery with large emphasis on timely diagnosis of acute SCI. The main role of surgical interventions is to restore spinal stability and prevent further neurologic deterioration.

The most commonly injured part of the spinal cord is the cervical cord, accounting for more than two-thirds of all SCI and commonly associated with tetraplegia more so than paraplegia. This is important since patients with cervical traumatic SCI are prone to developing hemodynamic instability and respiratory failure in the acute setting, which are thought to worsen their end outcome. In this chapter, the scope is limited to cervical spine injuries, and their management, highlighting recent evidence and guidelines publications.

3.1. Epidemiology

Young males are most commonly affected by spinal cord injury. Males are 3 to 20 times more likely to suffer SCI than females. Bimodal age preference is observed in SCI patients with the second peak occurring in elderly patients following a fall (Hall 1978; DeVivo 1980). The prevalence of SCI in the USA is estimated to reach up to 400,000, with estimated hospital occupancy of about 2000 beds annually. Although about a third of spinal fractures occur in the cervical region, only 10-20% of these are associated with spinal cord injuries (Hu 1996). SCI co-exists with traumatic brain injuries in up to 8% of cases and up to 10% of patients with SCI demonstrate other spinal fractures (Holly 2002). The most common cause of traumatic SCI is traffic collisions including motor vehicle collisions, or other traumas involving a motorcycle or a pedestrian. Elderly patients over the age of 65 are at risk of SCI following a fall, which often occurs at home. Pre-existing cervical canal stenosis or degenerative spondylosis in this age group are associated with certain clinical types of incomplete SCI, specifically central cord syndrome.

3.2. Pathophysiology and types of cervical SCI

Timely and careful pre-hospital and initial in-hospital acute management should optimize the role of surgery in helping patients with SCI. Understanding the pathophysiology of cervical SCI is a pre-requisite to explaining the rationale and research basis of acute prompt management of cervical SCI. Respiratory compromise and hypoventilation are common in cervical cord injuries, resulting from paralysis of the intercostal muscles. Residual diaphragmatic function allows for independent breathing unless the injury is above the outflow of the phrenic nerves at the spinal nerve roots C3-C5. Furthermore, patients with cervical SCI can present frequently with hypothermia due to disruption of the connections to the sympathetic chain, which has a substantial outflow within the thoracic spinal cord segments T8-10. Hypotension in the context of cervical spine injury may result from loss of the sympathetic tone and reduced peripheral vascular resistance. This is commonly associated with bradycardia and hypothermia.

Injury to the spinal cord occurs because of stretching, crushing, vascular compromise or compression. Incomplete cervical SCI encompasses three different subtypes with potentially different pathophysiological mechanisms. These include central cord syndrome, anterior cord syndrome and spinal cord hemisection or Brown-Sequard syndrome. Traumatic central cord syndrome (TCCS) is the most common incomplete cervical cord injury accounting for up to half of SCI clinical syndromes and about 9% of all SCIs in one series (McKinley 2007; Bosch 1971). It occurs more frequently in elderly patients with spinal canal stenosis associated with cervical spondylosis in the form of bony spurs anteriorly and thickened ligamentum flavum posteriorly (Schneider 1954). The pathophysiology of TCCS is poorly understood, however, the proposed mechanism of injury is thought to be secondary to a hyperextension injury during a fall resulting in inward buckling of the ligamentum flavum and compression of the cord dorsoventrally, occasionally with central cord hemorrhage and venous infarction (Quencer 1992). The spinal segments C3-4 and C4-5 are commonly affected in more than two thirds of TCCS cases (Aarabi 2011). In post-mortem reports of patients deceased following TCCS, spinal cord damage adopts tubular and central orientation, which may or may not extend several cervical segments rostrocaudally (Schneider 1954). Histological examination suggests a predominant white matter injury with axonal damage associated with myelin loss affecting the lateral columns (Quencer 1992). Clinically, patients with TCCS exhibit motor weakness in the upper extremities out of proportion to weakness in the lower extremities. One systematic review of the literature searching a common diagnostic criterion of TCCS found an average 11 ASIA motor points difference between upper and lower extremities motor scores, suggesting it can be utilized to aid diagnosis (Pouw 2010). Some sensory disturbance occurs variably and includes allodynia as well as sphincter dysfunction in the form of urinary retention. The prognosis in more than two thirds of cases is favorable with recovery of lower extremities motor function permitting independent ambulation and recovery of bladder function (Schneider 1958; Roth 1990; Dvorak 2005). However, some residual fine motor deficits in the hands frequently persist.

Patients with traumatic anterior cord syndrome present with immediate or delayed bilateral paralysis associated with dissociated sensory loss manifesting as loss of pain and temperature consistent with the level of the lesion and preservation of dorsal column function including discriminatory touch, proprioception and vibratory sense. The incidence is very rarely and found to be less than 1% in one series by McKinley et al. (2007). Pollock et al. (1953) first described these neurologic deficits in a series of 27 patients, with a proposition that anterior spinal artery occlusion is the mechanism for the injury following traumatic vertical and anterior compression. However, acute traumatic injury to the anterior portion of the cervical cord by structural disruption and dislocated bone fragments or herniated disc or actual direct destruction of the ventral aspect of the cord was also described in the central cord syndrome (Schneider 1954). These patients unfortunately have the poorest prognosis especially if no improvement is observed within the first 24 hours post-injury (Schneider 1954; Foo 1981; Stuaffer 1975).

The Brown-Sequard syndrome is associated with a rare incidence of 3.6% and usually results from a penetrating injury, such as gunshot or knife wounds, although its development in the context of blunt injury and extra-dural cord compression was also described (McKinley 2007; Roth 1991). Patient manifest with ipsilateral motor and proprioceptive, touch and vibratory sense loss associated with contralateral pain sensation loss. The majority of patients with Brown-Sequard syndrome are able to ambulate independently and recover their bladder control (Roth 1991).

3.3. Initial evaluation and acute management of SCI

An initial rapid approach for assessment of the airway, circulation and breathing is employed in acute prompt management of cervical spine injuries. Pre-hospital safe immobilization of the cervical spine and maintenance of normal axial alignment of the body is required in order to avoid iatrogenic spinal cord injury or worsening of an existing injury. Cervical spinal cord injury is associated with respiratory failure manifesting as hypoventilation secondary to paralysis of chest wall musculature. Unilateral or bilateral paralysis of the diaphragm may result in injuries with tetraplegia when the C3-C5 spinal segmental outflow to the phrenic nerves is disrupted. The laryngeal mask airway has been used increasingly in the setting of acute trauma and respiratory insufficiency with satisfactory outcomes (Moller 2000). In addition to respiratory compromise, loss of sympathetic tone occurs in cervical SCI, resulting in decreased cardiac preload secondary to venous pooling and loss of compensatory sympathetic reflex tachycardia (Troll 1975), thereby causing hemodynamic instability and hypotension. According to clinical guidelines, admission of cervical SCI to the intensive care unit is recommended on the basis of class III evidence in order to ensure cardiac monitoring of respiratory and cardiovascular parameters and prompt treatment of respiratory and cardiovascular compromise (Hadley 2013; Casha and Christie 2011). Furthermore, data from retrospective investigations found significant association between mean arterial pressure of 85 – 90 mmHg post-operatively for 7 days and clinical recovery, necessitating adequate augmentation of blood pressure in an intermediate or intensive care unit (Casha and Christie 2011; Ryken 2013).

According to early retrospective studies, intravenous glucocorticoid administraiton in the early stage of traumatic SCI was thought to harbor some beneficial effect in halting secondary neuronal injury and improving neurologic outcome (Short 2000). However, prospective randomized studies provided class I, II and III evidence demonstrating increased risk of adverse effects such as wound infection, acute steroid myelopathy, respiratory failure, sepsis and death in SCI patients treated with steroids. A number of landmark studies have been published in the field including the National Acute Spinal Cord Injury Study (NASCIS) I, II and III trials. In NASCIS I, investigators conducted a multicenter, double-blinded randomized trial comparing low-dose methylprednisone (MP) to high-dose regimen in patients with acute SCI treated for 10 days (Bracken 1984 and 1985). The study failed to demonstrate a difference in outcome at 6 weeks, 6 months and 12 months follow-up periods. Although the study was limited due to lack of a control group and absent power analysis, the authors noted significantly higher rate of infections at the surgical site with mortality being three-folds higher in the high-dose MP treatment group. The second NASCIS trial was published in 1990 with 487 patients with acute SCI randomized into to MP, naloxone and placebo groups (Bracken 1990, 1991 and 1992). No difference in primary neurologic utcomes was observed. However, post-hoc subanalysis demonstrated mean improvement of 5 points in the ASIA motor score and mean improvement of 4 points in the ASIA sensory score in the MP group compared to controls at 6 months. However, this treatment effect was only realized when treatment was administered within 8 hours of injury, excluding 291 patients who were treated outside this time window. Furthermore, complications such as gastrointestinal hemorrhage, wound infections and pulmonary embolism occured more frequently in patients treated with MP. NASCIS II has been downgraded by some to level III evidence indicating weak positive evidence supporting MP use. This is due to the inconsistency of claimed benefits, lack of functional outcome assessments, the arbitary nature of the eight-hour cut-off time and the high rate of patient exclusion in the subanalysis. NASCIS II provided class I evidence demonstrating harmful adverse effects of steroid use. In NASCIS III, 16 centers in the United States and Canada were enrolled in a prospective double-blinded study including 499 patients presenting with acute SCI within 8 hours randomized into treatment with MP IV infusion for 24 hours (n=166), MP IV infusion for 48 hours (n=166) and tirilazad treatment for 48 hours (n=167) which is a chemically engineered "super-steroid" (Bracken 1997 and 1998). Because of the reported positive effect of steroids in NASCIS II, all three groups patients received a loading dose of MP prior to randomization and no placebo-controlled group was included. The study failed to demonstrate a significant difference in neurologic outcome between the three treatment groups at one year (P=0.053), providing class I evidence lacking positive effect of steroid use in acute SCI even when initiated within 8 hours of injury. Of note, there was a transient 5 and 6 ASIA motor score improvements in the 48-hour MP treatment group compared to the 24-hour MP group at 6 weeks (P=0.04) and 6 months (p=0.01), respectively. Similar to NASCIS I and II, there was a trend towards serious complications associated with steroid use in NASCIS III reporting a consistent pattern of adverse effects. Furthermore, a French investigator group published the fourth prospective randomized trial investigating the use of steroids in acute SCI (Pointillart 2000). In this study, 106 patients were randomized into treatment with MP, nimodipine, MP+nimodipine and no pharmacological treatment. The authors demonstrated no significant difference in neurologic recovery between the treatment groups. Therefore, current clinical practice guidelines are not in favor of administering IV steroids even during the early stage of acute SCI due to the higher incidence of adverse effects and lack of clear clinical benefit (Hurlbert 2013). As a result a number of professional organizations in North America have relegated steroid use following spinal cord injury to a weak treatment option only.

3.4. Surgical indications

The goals of surgery in the context of cervical spinal cord injury are to facilitate neurologic recovery and prevent further injury to the neural elements and to restore spinal stability. This is achieved via anterior, posterior or combined surgical approaches focused at decompression of the neural elements and surgical arthrodesis in patients with a mechanically unstable spine in order to provide immediate stabilization and early mobilization as well as preventing further spinal deformity and pain. Therefore, the presence of clinical evidence of cervical cord injury as well as spinal instability represents surgical indications for decompressive and stabilization surgery. In patients with complete cervical cord injury, the primary goal of surgery is to restore spinal stability due to the low likelihood of neurologic recovery given the severity of cord injury. On the other hand, patients with incomplete cervical cord injury and evidence of compromise of the spinal canal should undergo surgical decompression and stabilization in order to aid neurologic recovery. Class II evidence based on the Surgical Timing in Acute Spinal Cord Injury Study (STASCIS) suggests improvement of neurologic function particularly when early surgery (within 24 hours) was instituted. In this prospective, multi-centre cohort study of 313 patients with acute cervical SCI, the authors found that about 20% of patients treated early showed 2 or more AIS grade improvements, compared to 9% in the late surgery group at 6 months follow-up (OR=2.6, 95% CI:1.1-6.0). However, in the context of other subgroups of incomplete cervical SCI, such as traumatic central cord syndrome, there is only class III evidence based on retrospective studies suggesting superiority of surgical decompression over conservative management (Dahdaleh 2013). There is no class I or II evidence examining the efficacy or timing of surgical decompression in TCCS. Therefore, early clinical diagnosis of spinal cord injury and characterization of its severity is crucial when considering surgical management to optimize the potential for neurologic recovery.

Furthermore, classification of cervical spine fractures may assist in surgical-decision making. Cervical spinal fractures or dislocations may or may not be accompanied by spinal cord injury or neurologic deficits such as paraplegia. In either case, reduction of these injuries can be achieved by closed reduction techniques including tong and halo traction, followed by restoration of spinal stability (if compromised). The latter is accomplished via surgical stabilization or external orthosis, such as various cervical collars, cervicothoracic braces and halo orthoses.

Cervical spine fractures are generally classified into fractures of the atlas, axis and fractures of the subaxial cervical vertebrae. Fractures of the atlas and axis rarely present with neurologic deficits (Sonntag 1988;Crockard 1993; Sonntag 1988), and therefore their discussion is out of the scope of this chapter. On the other hand, fractures of cervical spine below the level of the atlas and axis are relatively common and more frequently involved in decompressive spinal surgery; they affect C5 and C6 vertebrae accounting, respectively, for 40% and 36% of cervical spine fractures in one review (Benzel 1987). The morphology of these fractures is crucial in determining the course of management and likelihood of neurologic compromise, and includes compression, burst, teardrop fractures and facet dislocation injuries. The Subaxial Injury Classification (SLIC) and Severity Scale is recommended as a valid and useful tool to guide surgical management. It describes the morphological, ligamentous and clinical neuro-logical parameters associated with cervical spine injury (Table 1) (Anderson 2007; Vaccaro 2007). The overall inter-rater reliability has a correlation coefficient of 0.71. Clinical guidelines for acute cervical spine injuries published recommendations based on class I evidence to utilize

SLIC as a clinical and radiographic tool to assess and communicate information regarding spinal cord injury (Arabi 2013). SLIC scores of 1 to 3 suggest non-operative management, whereas scores 5 and above are suggestive of surgical management. A SLIC score of 4 represents indeterminate management when clinical judgment of the surgeon plays an important rule in deciding between operative and non-operative managements.

3.4.1. Surgical approaches

The determination of the surgical approach (anterior, posterior or combined) is influenced by the type of spinal cord injury, the mechanism of injury and the location of spinal cord compression in the anterior-posterior dimension of the cervical canal.

3.4.2. Posterior surgical approaches

In patients with flexion-type injuries to the subaxial cervical spine, the preferred surgical approach is posterior decompression and fusion. The rationale behind this surgical plan is restoring spinal stability and decompressing the spinal cord at the direction of main tissue disruption. The indications for posterior approaches include the presence of posterior ligamentous injury, facet dislocation and traumatic subluxation (Dvorak 2007). The integrity of the anterior column has to be preserved and there should be no evidence of anterior spinal cord compression, otherwise, a combined anterior-posterior approach should be considered.

Facet dislocation may occur unilaterally in association with flexion-rotation injury, or bilaterally in the context of hyperflexion injury indicating increased instability due to the disruption of the posterior ligamentous complex. A quarter of patients with unilateral dislocated facet are neurologically intact, with more than one-third manifesting with nerve root injuries and one-third with either complete or incomplete injuries (Andreshak 1997). On the other hand, bilateral facet dislocation is associated with a high rate of spinal cord injury and, hence, surgical reduction and stabilization with or without decompression may be indicated. For instance, in a retrospective review of 68 patients with facet fracture-dislocation injuries 68% of patients with bilateral facet dislocation were found to have complete spinal cord injuries, with ≤ 10 patients being neurologically intact (Hadley 1992). Since more than two-third of patients with unilateral or bilateral facet dislocations demonstrate evidence of poor anatomic alignment, surgical stabilization is indicated (Sears 1990). Despite that facet injuries result from flexion-type trauma, up to at least 50% of patients with facet dislocation injuries demonstrate evidence of disco-ligamentous injury with traumatic disc herniation in pre-reduction MRI. Although class I prospective, randomized evidence has demonstrated that surgical stabilization with anterior discectomy and fusion compared to posterior fixation is equally viable treatment option for unilateral facet dislocation injuries (Kwon 2007), the presence of traumatic disc herniation influences the choice of surgical approach. An anterior approach is favored in this context because of direct decompression of the anterior aspect of spinal canal and subsequent restoration of spinal stability by closed reduction and anterior bone graft placement and plate fixation (Lanuzzi 2006; Razack 2000). The risk profile of this approach in this clinical situation includes incomplete reduction intra-operatively and possible posterior ligament in folding. Therefore, tight and full reduction must be ensured prior to anterior fixation in cases with facet dislocation associated with traumatic disc herniation. On the other hand, patients sustaining spinal cord injury in the context of unilateral or bilateral facet dislocation and no evidence of traumatic disc herniation, there is no evidence favoring one approach over another. However, an informed decision could be made based on patient's preferences in terms of the different risk profiles of both surgical approaches which include mainly dysphagia and hoarseness of voice and risk of injury to visceral organs such as the trachea and esophagus in anteriorly treated patients, versus local wound infection and post-operative pain with posterior approaches. The advantage of a posterior approach is increased surgeon's familiarity (Dvorak 2007). Should a posterior approach be employed, open reduction with complete resection of ligamentum flavum and lateral mass fixation and fusion are achieved. Of note, some degrees of post-surgical kyphosis are identified in patients treated with posterior fixation, which is thought to result from intervertebral disc injury and progressive collapse. Although the long-term clinical effects of this finding is yet to be evaluated, pre-operative sagittal alignment of the spinal column in patients with facet injuries should be noted prior to undergoing anterior or posterior stabilization (Lifeso 2000; Elgafy 2006).

3.4.3. Anterior surgical approaches

Anterior surgical decompression and stabilization can be utilized even in cases with posterior spinal instability as demonstrated above in the context of unilateral facet injury. Furthermore, burst fractures are associated with disruption of two columns and retropulsion of bone fragments into the cervical canal, rendering spinal cord injury common. The mechanism of injury is largely the result of axial compression forces. Post-traumatic syringomyelia may ensue in patients with persistent canal compression and impairment of CSF circulation. The presence of posterior column failure and neurologic deficits specific to neurologic injury at the level of the burst fracture necessitates surgical decompression and stabilization. An anterior surgical approach with corpectomy or cage fitting and plate fixation is suggested by one retrospective investigation favoring anterior rather than posterior approaches with better decompression and better neurologic recovery and mechanical reconstitution of the motion segments (Toh 2006; Lanuzzi 2006).

Teardrop fractures represent about 5% of cervical spine fractures and result from flexion compression injury, which is commonly seen in injuries associated with diving into shallow waters (Gehweiler 1979; Torg 1991). They represent chip fractures commonly affecting the anterior-inferior aspect of the vertebral body. The severity of injury varies considerably with the most severe injuries seen in the context of a coronal split through the anterior aspect of the vertebral body with dislocation of the other part of the vertebral body posteriorly into the spinal canal (Schneider 1956). Surgical management is indicated in these fractures due to their high likelihood of spinal instability and neurologic injury. Other surgical indications include posterior column failure suggested by distraction and dislocation of the facet joint(s) with or without increased interlaminar distance (Allen 1982). Fisher and Leith et al. (2002) published retrospective data showing greater degrees of improved sagittal alignment with lower rate of treatment failures when patients are treated surgically via anterior cervical plating. However, a combined anterior and posterior approach has been recommended in cases with severe bony and ligamentous injury (Toh 2006; Cybulski 1992).

4. Cervical spondylotic myelopathy

Cervical spondylosis refers to a chronic degenerative process that affects the disco-ligamentous structures of the cervical spine leading to symptoms related to compression of the spinal cord (myelopathy) or nerve roots (radiculopathy). The progressive nature of the disease process warrants timely operative intervention in order to prevent motor paralysis and autonomic dysfunction related to severe myeloradiculopathy. Cervical spondylotic myelopathy (CSM) is the most common cause of myelopathy in elderly patients, and is associated with significant morbidity in its moderate and severe forms. Although some of the surgical approaches for the treatment of both is similar, the goal of surgery for cervical myelopathy differs in that it aims to provide decompression of the spinal cord to halt the progression of myelopathy, and to stabilize the spine and reinstate its alignment. In addition, the natural history of both disorders is different, with myelopathy being largely a progressive disease, interrupted by long periods of plateauing (Lees 1963; Nurick 1972). On the other hand, a certain degree of myelopathy and radiculopathy may co-exist warranting treatment of both.

4.1. Pathophysiology

Cervical spondylopathy results in loss of the intervertebral disc height secondary to non-inflammatory disc degeneration associated with a "wear-and-tear" process and, in some cases, repetitive trauma. Other accompanying changes include hypertrophy of the facet/zygopophyseal joint and hypertrophy of the posterior longitudinal ligament and ligamentum flavum causing ligamentous laxity and buckling into the cervical canal. Loss of the hydrophilic proteoglycan content of the intervertebral disc occurs as aging advances. This results in loss of the disc height and reduces its ability as a shock absorber, which in turn shifts axial loading force into the annulus fibrosis at the outer periphery of the disc. Eventually, the annulus undergoes wear and tear associated with thinning and weakening of the outer fibers of the annulus that provide anchoring to the bony matrix of the outer periphery of the vertebral body. This part of the annulus is named Sharpey's fibers. Their weakness is associated with formation of osteophytes due to reactive bony growth. Protrusion of the nucleus content of the disc through the strained and weakened annulus occurs, acutely. The process of disc herniation and osteophyte formation has a knock-on effect on the posterior longitudinal ligament causing ligamentous hypertrophy and ossification.

Mechanical pain symptoms have been postulated to originate from degenerative cervical disc and facet joints, based on the finding of rich innervations occurring in these structures (Ahn 2007; Dwyer 1990; Bogduk 2003). It is thought that a tear through the annulus fibrosis is sufficient to cause axial neck pain through afferent sensory fibers.

Pain related to acute or chronic radiculopathy is distinctively different from axial neck pain in that it follows the dermatomal distribution of the affected nerve root. Acute radiculopathy usually occurs in a younger group of patients and results from acute cervical disc herniation in association with cytokine-mediated inflammatory demyelinating effect on the large-fiber axons leading to motor deficits in the first week (Yoshizawa 1995). In contrast, chronic radiculopathy is associated with osteophyte formation, annulus wear and tear, laxity and peeling of the ligamentous structures with facet hypertrophy.

Spinal cord injury or myelopathy in the context of degenerative cervical disease occurs in relation to static, dynamic and ischemic factors (Dadashev 2011). Static factors include the spondylotic process through which narrowing of the cervical canal occurs, as described above. The normal diameter of the cervical canal is about 17-18 mm wide, with significant cervical canal stenosis considered to be less than 13 mm (Yue 2001). Dynamic factors result in episodic compression of the spinal cord with flexion being association with ventral cord compression against osteophytes and with extension causing dorsal cord compression secondary to ligamentous hypertrophy. Finally, an ischemic process ensues as being evidenced from pathological changes within both gray and white mater undergoing ischemic changes. It is postulated that spinal cord compression secondary to cervical stenosis restricts pial and intramedullary arterioles as well as causing venous engorgement leading to infarction. In severe and chronic cases, formation of a syringomyelia can also occur.

4.2. Surgical management

The natural history of CSM is variable and differs across cases, making prediction of the clinical course very challenging. On the other hand, selection of cases and the indication for surgery can be guided by the extent of clinical severity (Matz 2009). Kadanka and colleagues et al. (2000) conducted a prospective trial of 48 patients with mild CSM (mJOA scale score >12), randomized to surgery (n=21) or non-operative treatment (n=27). The modified Japanese Orthopedic Association (mJOA) scale score is a grading system used for myelopathy, with mJOA scale score > 12 used to define mild CSM. Both groups in that study improved equally on the mJOA scale score, 10-minute walk test and activity-dependent livings at 2 years follow-up. Similarly, the same authors randomized a larger sample of 64 patients to surgical or conservative treatment groups, demonstrating no significant difference in neurologic recovery at a longer follow-up period of 3 years (Kadanka 2005). At much longer follow-up of 10 years, the authors presented results on 25 patients treated conservatively, compared to 22 patients treated surgically with no difference in improvement (Kadanka 2011). However, this study is limited with a small sample size and its power analysis showed reduced statistical capacity to detect smaller differences between the two groups. Based on these findings (Class II evidence), clinical guidelines and a systematic review of the literature suggested that both operative and non-operative management options may be offered in the treatment of mild CSM (defined as mJAO scale score > 12) in the short term (3 years) (Mummaneni 2009). Non-operative strategies include prolonged immobilization in a stiff cervical collar, "low-risk" activity modification or bed rest, and anti-inflammatory analgesia. Furthermore, Bednarik et al. (1999) and Wada et al. (2001) prospectively followed patients with moderate to severe CSM (mJOA scale score < 12) postoperatively at 2 years and 5-15 years, respectively, demonstrating neurologic improvement. However, a non-operative comparison group was lacking, thereby conferring Class III evidence for the operative management of moderate to severe CSM (Matz 2009). On the other hand, patients with severely progressive CSM were observed to demonstrate low likelihood of spontaneous partial remission or cessation of progression of CSM (Clarke and Robinson 1956).

In addition to the severity of CSM, surgical treatment < 1 year from the onset of CSM is associated with improved neurologic outcome, compared to patients treated within 1-2 years or > 3 years (Phillips 1973). Early treatment within one year was found to be a predictor of good prognosis in one systematic review (Tetreault 2013). Similarly, the severity of baseline myelopathic changes correlates with the prognosis postoperatively suggesting reduced likelihood of reversibility of myelopathy in its severe stage. It is not entirely clear whether the progression of severe disease could be significantly halted by surgical decompression.

4.3. Surgical approaches

The surgical approach for the treatment of CSM is broadly categorized into anterior and posterior approaches. The superiority of any one approach over another in terms of the rate of neurologic recovery has been the subject of debate for a few decades. Furthermore, all up-to-date evidence demonstrated comparable neurologic recovery between the different anterior and posterior surgical approaches, although the risk profiles of these approaches are different as being shown by two systematic reviews of the literature (Mummaneni 2009; Cunningham 2010). Unfortunately, current studies suffer many methodological flaws associated with bias and the presence of confounding factors. Nonetheless, in order to select the optimal approach for the patient with CSM, knowledge of the advantages and disadvantages of each technique is pre-requisite for informed and rationale surgical decision-making (Table 2).

	Advantages	*Disadvantages*
Anterior approach	Direct decompression Stabilization with arthrodesis Correction of deformity Good axial pain relief	Technically challenging Graft complications Loss of motion Adjacent segment disease
Posterior approach	Less loss of motion No graft complications Less technically demanding	Indirect decompression Postoperative kyphosis Instability limitations Late instability Inconsistent axial pain relief

Table 2. Summary of the advantages and disadvantages of anterior and posterior approaches for CSM. Adapted from Dadashev et al. (2011)

Options for posterior surgical approaches for the treatment of CSM encompass laminectomy without fusion, laminectomy with lateral mass fusion and laminoplasty. In comparing laminectomy alone with laminectomy with fusion, the retrospective review by Perez-Lopez et al. (2001) revealed similar rates of neurologic improvement as represented by improved Nurick scores of 0.84 in the laminectomy group compared to 1.24 in the group treated with laminectomy and fusion, at 3.3 years follow-up. However, the authors also noted increased incidence of postoperative kyphotic deformity in the laminectomy alone group (24%), compared to 7% in the fusion group. This holds true in reviews of cases with CSM treated with laminectomy and fusion demonstrating very low or zero rate of swan neck deformity post-operatively (Kumar 1999;Houten 2003), whereas cases treated with laminectomy are predisposed to develop late deformity as well as destabilization which requires repeat surgery (Guigui 1998; Sim 1974; Mastunagna 1999). Therefore, laminectomy with fusion is recommended over laminectomy alone especially in young patients, or in cases associated with risk of spinal instability (Class III; strength of recommendation D) (Mummaneni 2009).

Laminoplasty has been used with comparable results to laminectomy with fusion in terms of improved neurologic recovery in the treatment of CSM (Class III; recommendation D) (Mummaneni 2009). In patients with CSM or ossification of the posterior longitudinal ligament, Heller et al. (2001) retrospectively compared laminectomy with fusion (13 patients) and laminoplasty (13 patients). The authors noted statistically non-significant greater improvement in Nurick scores in the laminoplasty group (from 2.2 to 1.1) compared to the laminectomy with fusion group (from 2.2 to 1.5). However, the range of cervical movement was retained in the laminoplasty group compared to laminectomy with fusion ($P<0.002$). In addition, a significantly greater complication rate was reported in the latter group with development of hardware failure in 2, neurologic deterioration in 2, pseudoarthrosis in 5 and deep infection in one case. No complications were noted in the laminoplasty group. The difference in complication rate is subject to criticism in relation to probable selection bias associated with selection of matched controls in whom fusion is more likely due to kyphosis, thereby rendering this study Class III evidence (Mummaneni 2009). In addition, two retrospective reviews of laminectomy with fusion found favorable neurologic recovery (improved neurologic outcome or no deterioration) and zero or low rate of complication associated with this approach (Houten 2003; Huang 2003). Therefore, no recommendation was made of laminoplasty over laminectomy with fusion in terms of improved neurologic recovery in evidence-based published guidelines.

Anterior surgical approaches for decompression of the cervical spine in CSM include anterior cervical discectomy with fusion (ACDF) and anterior cervical corpectomy with fusion (ACCF). Based on class III evidence, patients with CSM have been shown to respond to multilevel anterior cervical spine decompression, however, with varying proportions of complications associated with each technique (Mummaneni 2009; Cunningham 2011). In a retrospective study by Nirala et al. (2004), 201 patients underwent multilevel anterior cervical spine decompression with fusion (autograft) and without anterior plate fixation. Patients were subdivided into ACDF (n=69) and ACCF (n=132), with the functional outcome was assessed using Odom's criteria, whereas dynamic plain films were used to assess radiographic outcomes. Patients wore a hard cervical collar for 3 months postoperatively. After 10 years, the fusion rate was higher in the ACCF group (94%) compared to the ACDF group (69.6%) ($P< 0.001$). There was no statistically significant difference in the functional outcome between the two groups. This study presents class III evidence favoring ACCF over ACDF when plate fixation is not used (Grade D recommendation). In contrast, anterior plate fixation in ACDF and ACCF is associated with equal fusion rates reported in one systematic review to reach greater than 90% (Fraser and Hartl 2007). However, in three-level disc disease, the fusion rate was significantly lower in the ACDF group (82.5%) compared to cases treated with ACCF (96%) (P=0.03). This systematic review represents class III evidence due to the lack of application of a standardized methodology for systematic reviews and to violating the inclusion and exclusion criteria. Therefore, a grade D recommendation underlies the utilization of either ACDF or ACCF with plate fixation in the treatment of multilevel anterior CSM.

Furthermore, the use of anterior plate fixation in ACDF and ACCF is associated with non-union rates of 42% and 31%, respectively at about 3.3-year follow-up (Swank 1997). Of note, a major confounding factor is the increased use of dynamic plates in ACDF compared to constrained plates in ACCF with the latter being associated with higher fusion rates. Another study by Wang et al. (2001) failed to find a statistically significant difference in fusion rates between the two groups.

Early complications in ACDF include dysphagia (9.5%), neck hematoma (5.6%) with 2.4% of patients requiring surgery, recurrent laryngeal nerve palsy (3.1%), dural laceration (0.5%) and esophageal perforation (0.3%). The latter was associated with death in one patient (1 about 1000 patients). Less common complications include wound infection and Horner's syndrome. Late complications of ACDF include non-union and adjacent-segment disease. The presence for adjacent-segment disease was found to be associated with a plate-to-disc distance of < 5 mm. This complication is thought to occur at an annual rate up to 3% over 10 years. Further studies are required to elucidate the clinical nature of these changes. Furthermore, other factors that can affect the fusion rate include plate fixation and smoking (Bolesta 2000; Fraser and Hartl 2007).

To summarize, the location of spinal cord compression in relation to the anterior-posterior diameter of the cervical canal is a crucial factor influencing the direction of the surgical approach. In cases with predominantly anterior multilevel disease affecting more three levels, ACCF with plate fixation could be considered over ACDF due to a suggestion of lower rates of fusion in the latter group. However, patients with CSM resulting from less than three-level disease, ACDF and ACCF with plate fixation are equally indicated. On the other hand, patients with features of CSM resulting from multi-level disease affecting more than three levels may benefit from a posterior approach. Laminoplasty is associated with significantly increased incidence of neck pain, but fewer complications and possibly greater range of cervical motion range as well as comparable neurologic improvement rate when compared to laminectomy with fusion and even to anterior approaches including ACDF and multilevel ACCF. Therefore, laminoplasty maybe utilized in patients who are able to tolerate some post-operative neck pain with the benefit of retained cervical mobility. Furthermore, laminectomy without fusion is discouraged in patients with a kyphotic deformity or straight spine due to a significant risk of development of postoperative swan-neck deformity of the cervical spine (Rao 2006; Benzel 1991;Anderson 2009; Kaptain 2009). In younger and healthier patients with significant anterior and posterior compression of the cord resulting in significant progressive myelopathy, a combined anterior-posterior approach is recommended to ensure complete decompression.

5. Metastatic spinal diseases

5.1. Epidemiology

Cancer-related complications led to about half a million deaths in 2008, with annual newly detected cancer rate of about 1.4 million new cases (Sciubba 2010). Up to 70% of all cancer patients will develop metastasis, most commonly to the lungs and liver, followed by skeletal structures. The most common osseous site for metastasis is the spine, which occurs in 40% of all cancer patients (Aaron 1994;Black 1979; Zerick 1994). Of these patients with spinal metastatic disease, up to 20% will develop symptomatic epidural spinal cord compression, which accounts for 20,000 to 30,000 cases per year in the USA (Kwok 2006). Post-mortem studies showed that up to 90% of patients deceased with cancer were found to have evidence of spinal metastatic disease (Wong 1990; Cobb 1977). Up to half patients with spinal metastasis require treatment, with 5-10% being surgically treated (Bell 1997;Bilsky 2005; Walsh 1997; York 1999).

The incidence of metastatic spinal disease peaks at the age groups between 40-65 years (Perrin 1982). The most common primary tumors that metastasize to the spine are breast, lung, melanoma or prostate cancers, which correspond to the common occurrence of these primary malignancies (Constans 1983; Helweg-Larsen 1994). The rates of spinal metastases in prostate, breast, melanoma and lung cancers correspond to about 90%, 74%, 55% and 45%, respectively (Wong 1990). Of note, 10% of cases present clinically with spinal metastatic disease without previous history of known primary malignancy (Gerszten 2000), with 50% of these cases found to have primary lung malignancy (Stark 1982).

5.2. Characteristics of spinal metastasis

The most common region of the spine affected by metastatic disease is the thoracic spine, which corresponds to 70%, followed by the lumbar spine (20%) and cervical (10%) spine, (Gerszten 2000, Byme 1992; Gilbert 1978). Metastases occur extra-durally, with the intra-dural and intra-medullary spaces being very rare metastatic targets representing up to about 8% of cases (Schijns 2000). The vertebral body is involved in more than 80% of cases with the posterior half being the initial site of invasive disease (Gerszten 2000). The reminder of cases often manifest with paravertebral metastasis.

The routes of metastatic spread include hematogenous spread, which is the most common mechanism, manifest by metastases to the vertebral body occurring through hematogenous spread secondary to their rich blood supply (Arguello 1990), followed by direct invasion and spread through shedding of tumor cells in the CSF. Direct invasion to the sacral and lumbar spine were reported in the context of prostate cancer (Ross 2005). CSF seeding of tumor cells occurs following mobilization of intra-axial cranial malignancies, and may result in drop metastasis (Perrin 1982).

5.3. Clinical manifestation

Patients with spinal metastatic disease may present with pain symptoms and/or neurologic deficits, associated with constitutional or systematic symptoms including weight loss and anorexia.

Pain is the initial complaint in up to 95% of patients with spinal metastases, preceding any neurologic deficits by weeks to months (Bach 1990; Helweg-Larsen 1994; Weinstein 1987). In contrast, about 10% of patients with undiagnosed extra-spinal primary malignancy present with pain as their initial complaint (Livingston 1978). Patients with spinal metastases describe three different categories of pain; tumor-related, mechanical and radicular pain. Tumor-related or local pain is often progressive and characterized as dull constant ache localized to the metastatic region of the spine, and responsive to nonsteroidal antiinflammatory drugs (Gokaslan 1996). It may worsen in the morning or nocturnally. It's postulated to result from dilatation and engorgement of spinal venous channels secondary to tumor growth leading to mass effect on pain-sensitive structures, such as the dura, periosteum and spinal cord. Pain radiating to the sacro-iliac region and to the interscapular area occur in association with lumbar and thoracic metastatic disease, respectively. On the other hand, mechanical pain results from vertebral body destruction and collapse, associated with some degree of spinal instability leading to increased physiological stress on spinal support structures including ligamentous and muscular structures. Mechanical pain manifests as pain provoked by movement and standing, as well as coughing, and relieved by resting. Radicular pain is caused by invasion of the intervertebral foramina leading to compression of nerve roots and pain radiating across the dermatome subserved by the affected nerve root.

Neurological symptoms result from either compression of the spinal cord or nerve roots, causing myelopathy or radiculopathy, respectively, or both. Myelopathy related to spinal metastasis usually presents with gait difficulty associated with spasticity and motor weakness, which is the most common presenting symptom second to pain in up to 85% of patients (Greenberg 1980; Posner 1995). Myelopathic motor weakness is often followed by bladder and bowel dysfunction (Schiff 1996). Urinary retention and increased frequency of urinary tract infection in males suggest a diagnosis of neurogenic bladder. Isolated autonomic or bladder dysfunction rarely occurs in isolation and is usually accompanied by other symptoms, except in cases with conus medullaris compression. Without treatment, patients with motor deficits progress to complete paraplegia (Botterell 1959). The initial neurological status of the patient correlates with prognosis, thereby necessitating a thorough neurologic examination. Certain scales can be used for neurological and functional assessments, including the American Spinal Injury Association (ASIA) Impairment Scale (AIS), the Frankel scale and the Eastern Cooperative Oncology Group (ECOG) Performance Score.

5.4. Rationale for selection of cases for surgical management

The management of spinal metastatic disease can be challenging and requires a multidisciplinary approach involving neurosurgical expertise as well as radiation and medical oncology and patient's input. Surgical interventions in most cases are palliative, aimed at relieving pain symptoms refractory to medical treatment, obtaining a tissue diagnosis and preserving ambulation and autonomic function by decompressing the neural elements.

Surgical intervention is considered in tumors relatively resistant to radiation treatment including sarcoma, lung and colon cancers, renal cell carcinoma, and breast cancer (Cole 2008). Other indications for surgery include evidence of spinal instability, compression of the cord or nerve roots, pain refractory to medical treatment and deterioration of neurologic function during radiation therapy indicating treatment failure. The three-column involvement, discussed above, has been used by Tomita et al. (Tomita 2001) as evidence of increased spinal instability and therefore an indication for surgical management. The authors discussed other features suggesting spinal instability including vertebral body collapse > 50%, transitional deformity and involvement of the same column in more than one level. Other investigators regarded bone fragments repulsion into the spinal canal as evidence of spinal instability (Cybulski 1989). Although spinal instability has been discussed as a strong indication for surgery in different conditions related to spinal injury, a clear unifying definition of spinal instability is still debated.

On the other hand, patient's life expectancy represents a crucial factor in surgical decision-making, with an estimated life expectancy greater than 3 or 6 months considered favorable in the context of surgical management of spinal metastatic disease (Sciubba 2010). Different prognostic systems have been devised in order to help stratify patients into different groups according to prognosis to help guide surgical treatment.

Tokuhashi and colleagues et al (Tokuhashi 2005; Tokuhashi 1990) established a scoring system based on the general medical condition as described by the Karnofsky performance status, number of extra-spinal metastases, number of vertebral metastases, the treatment status of major internal organ metastases, primary tumor type and the presence of neurologic dysfunction (Table 4). Non-operative or radiation treatment is indicated in cases with scores ranging from 0 to 8, with an estimated life expectancy less than 6 months. Patients with scores ranging from 12 to 15 were found to have a life expectancy of one year or more, and were treated with circumferential excisional surgery with reconstruction and stabilization. Palliative decompression surgery utilizing a posterior approach with or without instrumentation is offered to patients with a score of 9 to 11. Stratification of cases according to the Tokuhashi scoring system has been validated and used in other studies (Ulmar 2005; Enkaoua 1997).

Furthermore, Tomita and colleagues et al. (2001) devised a scoring system based on the advances of surgical techniques taking into account the grade of malignancy (slow, moderate or rapid growth), visceral metastases and bone metastases. Patients with scores of up to 3 points, wide marginal excision is recommended for local long-term control, whereas scores of 4 or 5 indicate marginal or intralesional excision for intermediate-term control. Scores of 6 or 7 suggest short-term palliation with palliative surgery, and scores of 8 to 10 indicates non-operative supportive care. These scoring systems represent useful tools to communicate a host of important prognostic factors rather than absolute conclusions for surgical decision-making, which relies on other factors such as spinal instability and patient's factors including co-morbidities.

The Spinal Instability Neoplastic Score (SINS) is a useful tool for the assessment of spinal instability in patients with spinal metastatic disease. It utilises clinical and radiographic data in order to facilitate the classification and assessment of spinal instability (Table 3). SINS was formulated by the Spine Oncology Study Group (Fisher and colleagues et. al.,2010) on the basis of a systematic review and modified Delphi criteria evaluating factors crucial for the assessment of spinal stability. With a sensitivity and specificity of 95.7% and 79.5%, respectively, and confirmed near-perfect inter-and intra-rater reliability (Fourney 2011; Fisher 2010), SINS stratifies patients with spinal metastatic disease into three categories; those with stable spine (0-6 points), potentially unstable spine (7-12 points) and unstable spine (13-15points).

Location	Rigid (S2-5)	0
Semi-rigid (T3-T10)	1	
Mobile spine (C3-C6,L2-L4)	2	
Junctional (Occiput-C2,C7-T2,T11-L1,L5-S1)	3	
Pain	Pain-free lesion	0
	Occasional pain but not mechanical	1
	Yes – mechanical pain	3
Bone lesion	Blastic	0
	Mixed (lytic/blastic)	1
	Lytic	2
Radiographic spinal alignment	Normal alignment	0
	De novo deformity (kyphosis/scoliosis)	2
	Sublaxation/translation present	4
Vertebral body collapse	None	0
	No collapse with "/> 50% body involvement	1
	< 50%	2
	"/> 50% collapse	3
Posterolateral involvement of spinal elements	None	0
	Unilateral	1
	Bilateral	3

Table 3. The Spinal Instability Neoplastic Score (SINS) system.

General condition	Poor PS <40%	0
Moderate 50-70%	1	
Good > 80%	2	
No. Of extraspinal bone metastases foci	3 or more	0
	1-2	1
	0	2
No of metastases in the vertebral body	3 or more	0
	1-2	1
	0	2
Metastases to the major organs	Unremovable	0
	Removable	1
	No mets	2
Primary cancer	Lung, osteosarcoma, stomach, bladder, pancreas, esophagus	0
	Liver, gallbladder, unknown	1
	Others	2
	Kidney, uterus	3
	Rectum	4
	Thyroid, prostate, breast, carcinoid tumor	5
Spinal cord palsy	Complete (Frankel A, B)	0
	Incomplete (Frankel C, D)	1
	None (Frankel E)	2

Table 4. Tokuhashi prognostic scoring system for spinal metastatic disease

5.5. Surgical management

Substantial development in the surgical techniques and approach for spinal stabilization over the past three decades have been associated with longer survival and improved neurologic outcomes in patients with spinal metastatic disease (Scuibba 2010). Historically, the mainstay of surgical intervention was based on simple laminectomy, representing the only surgical intervention at the time. The aim of the procedure was to obtain tissue diagnosis or relief of pain. However, a high rate of complications reaching up to 11% was associated with this approach, including spinal instability, wound infection and dehiscence (Findlay 1984). In addition, a retrospective study of 235 patients treated with posterior decompressive laminectomy with or without radiation demonstrated no difference in the rate of neurologic recovery between the two groups (Gilbert 1978). The association of simple laminectomy with morbidity such as increased risk of spinal instability and its susceptibility to failure rendered surgical management of spinal metastatic disease less efficacious with little value. In addition, simple laminectomy did not also address anterior compression of the spinal cord or thecal sac resulting from a metastatic lesion at the vertebral body.

Therefore, radiation alone was the only effective treatment available until the evolution of spinal stabilization and instrumentation techniques. Some early reports of internal fixation in addition to laminectomy suggested improved surgical outcomes, which re-introduced surgical management as an effective and safe intervention in spinal metastatic disease. For instance, more than 90% of patients treated with internal fixation demonstrated increased ambulation and improved pain control postoperatively, compared to 57% treated with laminectomy alone (Sherman 1986). Results from the first prospective randomized controlled trial were presented in 2005 by Patchell et al. comparing the efficacy of radiation treatment alone and combined surgical circumferential decompression of the spinal cord with tumor resection and stabilization, followed by adjuvant radiation therapy. There was a statistically significant higher rate of post-treatment ambulation in the surgery group reaching 84% compared to 57% in the radiation treatment group (P=0.001) (Table 5). The median duration of ambulation in the surgery group was found to be 122 days, compared to 13 days in the radiation group (P=0.003). About 60% of patients regained the ability to walk post-surgically compared to 19% receiving radiation alone (P=0.012). Other secondary outcomes associated with surgery included improved continence rates, muscle strength (ASIA scores) and improved functional ability (Frankel scores).

	Ambulation				
	Posttreatment ambulatory rate (%)	**Retained (days)**	**Maintained ambulation (%)**	**Re-gained (%)**	**Mean survival (days)**
Surgery and XRT	84	122	94	62	126
XRT alone	57	13	74	19	100

Table 5. Outcomes following treatment with radiation alone versus surgery with radiation (Patchell 2005).

Furthermore, Witham et al. (2006) performed a systematic review assessing the literature on the treatment of spinal metastatic disease between 1964 and 2005. The author found a mean 64% improvement in motor function associated with mean 88% improvement of pain control when laminectomy with posterior stabilization is utilized, compared to a mean 42% improvement in motor function in laminectomy with or without radiation treatment. Importantly, patients with anterior decompression and stabilization demonstrated the highest rate of neurologic improvement with 75% of cases exhibiting improvement. The role of anterior decompression of the spinal cord has become more apparent since the majority of the tumour burden in metastatic disease is often found anterior or antero-lateral to the spinal cord. This finding was highlighted by Siegal and colleagues et al. (1982), illustrating 91% rate of regaining ambulation in patients with ventral metastatic compression of the cord following anterior decompression. Multiple studies demonstrated similar results, thereby underlining circumferential spinal cord decompression as one of the principles of surgical management of spinal metastatic diseases beside reconstruction and stabilization (Klimo 2011).

5.6. Surgical approach

Posterior approaches to surgical management of spinal metastatic disease have become more popular especially with the introduction of the transpedicular approach, which allows for circumferential decompression of the spinal cord and reconstruction of the vertebral body. This approach has been found effective in the lumbar and thoracolumbar spine according to a review of 140 patients in whom this approach was utilized leading to 75% rate of regain of the ability to walk post-operatively and more than 95% improvement of pain. Alternatively, single-stage posterolateral vertebrectomy (SPLV) with costotransversectomies provide wider exposure compared to direct posterior approaches in the surgical management of thoraco-lumbar spinal metastases. Street and colleagues et al. (2007) provide data on 42 patients treated with this approach demonstrating that all patients remained neurologically stable or improved after surgery. The complication rate was 26% (n=11) with nine patients requiring early reoperation including seven patients for wound failures. The approach involves performing laminectomy at the metastatic level with pedicle screw insertion prior to bilateral total facetectomies and complete pedicle resection to the base of the vertebral body. Circumferential decompression of the neural elements is achieved with resection of the posterior rib, rib head and costrotransverse joint to facilitate wide resection. Reconstruction of the vertebrectomy defect is achieved by introducing cement. Placing bilateral rods to ensure spinal stabilization completes the procedure. The authors favor this approach over the combined anteroposterior approach due to the increased risk of respiratory adverse effects and prolonged anesthetic time in the combined approach. In addition, the wide exposure and improved working angle offered by SPLV provide greater advantage compared to the conventional posterolateral transpedicular approach.

The utilization of minimally invasive spine surgery has been extrapolated to thoracolumbar spinal metastatic disease (Deutsch 2008; Huang 2006; Singh 2006). Deutsch and colleagues et al. (2008) described the results of a minimally invasive transpedicular vertebrectomy in 8 patients with spinal thoracic metastatic disease in whom an anterior approach via thoracotomy was deemed unsuitable due to significant co-morbidities and limited life expectancy. For patients presenting with metastases affecting thoracic spinal levels T4 to T11, in whom minimally invasive surgery was performed, the authors described resection of the pedicles though a 22-mm diameter tubular retractor, followed by dorsal decompression of the neural elements with partial vertebrectomy and ventral decompression. A bilateral approach with transpedicular resection was used in order to ensure total decompression of the ventral canal. No instrumentation was used in this approach and all patients received postoperative radiation treatment. The average length of the procedure is 2.2 hours. The authors noted neurologic improvement in 5 out of 8 patients (62.5%) post-surgically with a similar rate of improvement in pain. In addition, two patients with paraparesis preoperatively were able to ambulate unassisted post-surgery. The one-year survival was 37.5% and no evidence of tumor recurrence and spinal instability at one-year follow-up in survivors. The authors recommended this approach as a palliative measure in selected cases in order to provide pain relief and improved ambulation without significant tissue trauma and increased risk of adverse effects otherwise noted in open anterior approaches. A major disadvantage of this approach is limited visualization and risk of incomplete decompression. On the other hand, the role of minimally invasive technique is greatly employed in percutaneous vertebroplasty and kyphoplasty in the treatment of painful pathological fractures secondary to underlying metastases (Fourney 2003; Binning 2004). Vertebroplasty is performed by injecting cement percutaneously into the vertebral body. This technique is used in patients with a painful osteolytic metastatic lesion without evidence of disruption of the posterior aspect of the body cortex and without severe loss of the body height (Jensen 2002; Weill 1996). Vertebroplasty is particularly helpful in this group of patients since radiation treatment may not provide pain relief for up to two weeks post-treatment (Binning 2004). Kyphoplasty differs from vertebroplasty in that an expandable balloon is placed into the vertebral body to create space hosting the cement. This technique has been shown to reduce the risk of kyphotic deformity and provides effective and sustained pain relief (Pflugmacher 2007; Fourney 2003.

Author details

Ayoub Dakson and Sean D. Christie

Dalhousie University, Dept. Surgery (Neurosurgery), Dept. Medical Neurosciences, Halifax, Nova Scotia, Canada

References

[1] Aarabi, B. *et al.* Predictors of outcome in acute traumatic central cord syndrome due to spinal stenosis. *Journal of neurosurgery. Spine* 14, 122-130, doi: 10.3171/2010.9.SPINE09922 (2011).

[2] Aarabi, B. *et al.* Subaxial cervical spine injury classification systems. *Neurosurgery* 72 Suppl 2, 170-186, doi:10.1227/NEU.0b013e31828341c5 (2013).

[3] Aaron, A. D. The management of cancer metastatic to bone. *JAMA : the journal of the American Medical Association* 272, 1206-1209 (1994).

[4] Ahn, N. U., Ahn, U. M., Ipsen, B. & An, H. S. Mechanical neck pain and cervicogenic headache. *Neurosurgery* 60, S21-27, doi:10.1227/01.NEU.0000249258.94041.C6 (2007).

[5] Allen, B. L., Jr., Ferguson, R. L., Lehmann, T. R. & O'Brien, R. P. A mechanistic classification of closed, indirect fractures and dislocations of the lower cervical spine. *Spine* 7, 1-27 (1982).

[6] Anderson, P. A. *et al.* Laminectomy and fusion for the treatment of cervical degenerative myelopathy. *Journal of neurosurgery. Spine* 11, 150-156, doi: 10.3171/2009.2.SPINE08727 (2009).

[7] Anderson, P. A. *et al.* Cervical spine injury severity score. Assessment of reliability. *The Journal of bone and joint surgery. American volume* 89, 1057-1065, doi:10.2106/JBJS.F.00684 (2007).

[8] Andreshak, J. L. & Dekutoski, M. B. Management of unilateral facet dislocations: a review of the literature. *Orthopedics* 20, 917-926 (1997).

[9] Arguello, F. *et al.* Pathogenesis of vertebral metastasis and epidural spinal cord compression. *Cancer* 65, 98-106 (1990).

[10] Bach, F. *et al.* Metastatic spinal cord compression. Occurrence, symptoms, clinical presentations and prognosis in 398 patients with spinal cord compression. *Acta neurochirurgica* 107, 37-43 (1990).

[11] Baptiste, D. C. & Fehlings, M. G. Pathophysiology of cervical myelopathy. *The spine journal : official journal of the North American Spine Society* 6, 190S-197S, doi:10.1016/j.spinee.2006.04.024 (2006).

[12] Bednarik, J. *et al.* The value of somatosensory- and motor-evoked potentials in predicting and monitoring the effect of therapy in spondylotic cervical myelopathy. Prospective randomized study. *Spine* 24, 1593-1598 (1999).

[13] Bell, G. R. Surgical treatment of spinal tumors. *Clinical orthopaedics and related research*, 54-63 (1997).

[14] Benzel, E. C., Lancon, J., Kesterson, L. & Hadden, T. Cervical laminectomy and dentate ligament section for cervical spondylotic myelopathy. *Journal of spinal disorders* 4, 286-295 (1991).

[15] Benzel, E. C. & Larson, S. J. Functional recovery after decompressive spine operation for cervical spine fractures. *Neurosurgery* 20, 742-746 (1987).

[16] Bilsky, M. H., Boakye, M., Collignon, F., Kraus, D. & Boland, P. Operative management of metastatic and malignant primary subaxial cervical tumors. *Journal of neurosurgery. Spine* 2, 256-264, doi:10.3171/spi.2005.2.3.0256 (2005).

[17] Binning, M. J., Gottfried, O. N., Klimo, P., Jr. & Schmidt, M. H. Minimally invasive treatments for metastatic tumors of the spine. *Neurosurgery clinics of North America* 15, 459-465, doi:10.1016/j.nec.2004.04.010 (2004).

[18] Black, P. Spinal metastasis: current status and recommended guidelines for management. *Neurosurgery* 5, 726-746 (1979).

[19] Bogduk, N. The anatomy and pathophysiology of neck pain. *Physical medicine and rehabilitation clinics of North America* 14, 455-472, v (2003).

[20] Bolesta, M. J., Rechtine, G. R., 2nd & Chrin, A. M. Three- and four-level anterior cervical discectomy and fusion with plate fixation: a prospective study. *Spine* 25, 2040-2044; discussion 2045-2046 (2000).

[21] Bosch, A., Stauffer, E. S. & Nickel, V. L. Incomplete traumatic quadriplegia. A ten-year review. *JAMA : the journal of the American Medical Association* 216, 473-478 (1971).

[22] Botterell, E. H. & Fitzgerald, G. W. Spinal cord compression produced by extradural malignant tumours; early recognition, treatment and results. *Canadian Medical Association journal* 80, 791-796 (1959).

[23] Bracken, M. B. Treatment of acute spinal cord injury with methylprednisolone: results of a multicenter, randomized clinical trial. *Journal of neurotrauma* 8 Suppl 1, S47-50; discussion S51-42 (1991).

[24] Bracken, M. B. *et al.* Efficacy of methylprednisolone in acute spinal cord injury. *JAMA : the journal of the American Medical Association* 251, 45-52 (1984).

[25] Bracken, M. B. *et al.* Methylprednisolone or naloxone treatment after acute spinal cord injury: 1-year follow-up data. Results of the second National Acute Spinal Cord Injury Study. *Journal of neurosurgery* 76, 23-31, doi:10.3171/jns.1992.76.1.0023 (1992).

[26] Bracken, M. B. *et al.* A randomized, controlled trial of methylprednisolone or naloxone in the treatment of acute spinal-cord injury. Results of the Second National Acute Spinal Cord Injury Study. *The New England journal of medicine* 322, 1405-1411, doi: 10.1056/NEJM199005173222001 (1990).

[27] Bracken, M. B. *et al.* Methylprednisolone and neurological function 1 year after spinal cord injury. Results of the National Acute Spinal Cord Injury Study. *Journal of neurosurgery* 63, 704-713, doi:10.3171/jns.1985.63.5.0704 (1985).

[28] Bracken, M. B. *et al.* Administration of methylprednisolone for 24 or 48 hours or tirilazad mesylate for 48 hours in the treatment of acute spinal cord injury. Results of the Third National Acute Spinal Cord Injury Randomized Controlled Trial. National Acute Spinal Cord Injury Study. *JAMA : the journal of the American Medical Association* 277, 1597-1604 (1997).

[29] Bracken, M. B. *et al.* Methylprednisolone or tirilazad mesylate administration after acute spinal cord injury: 1-year follow up. Results of the third National Acute Spinal Cord Injury randomized controlled trial. *Journal of neurosurgery* 89, 699-706, doi: 10.3171/jns.1998.89.5.0699 (1998).

[30] Byrne, T. N. Spinal cord compression from epidural metastases. *The New England journal of medicine* 327, 614-619, doi:10.1056/NEJM199208273270907 (1992).

[31] Casha, S. & Christie, S. A systematic review of intensive cardiopulmonary management after spinal cord injury. *Journal of neurotrauma* 28, 1479-1495, doi:10.1089/neu.2009.1156 (2011).

[32] Clarke, E. & Robinson, P. K. Cervical myelopathy: a complication of cervical spondylosis. *Brain : a journal of neurology* 79, 483-510 (1956).

[33] Cobb, C. A., 3rd, Leavens, M. E. & Eckles, N. Indications for nonoperative treatment of spinal cord compression due to breast cancer. *Journal of neurosurgery* 47, 653-658, doi:10.3171/jns.1977.47.5.0653 (1977).

[34] Cole, J. S. & Patchell, R. A. Metastatic epidural spinal cord compression. *Lancet neurology* 7, 459-466, doi:10.1016/S1474-4422(08)70089-9 (2008).

[35] Constans, J. P. *et al.* Spinal metastases with neurological manifestations. Review of 600 cases. *Journal of neurosurgery* 59, 111-118, doi:10.3171/jns.1983.59.1.0111 (1983).

[36] Crockard, H. A., Heilman, A. E. & Stevens, J. M. Progressive myelopathy secondary to odontoid fractures: clinical, radiological, and surgical features. *Journal of neurosurgery* 78, 579-586, doi:10.3171/jns.1993.78.4.0579 (1993).

[37] Cunningham, M. R., Hershman, S. & Bendo, J. Systematic review of cohort studies comparing surgical treatments for cervical spondylotic myelopathy. *Spine* 35, 537-543, doi:10.1097/BRS.0b013e3181b204cc (2010).

[38] Cybulski, G. R., Douglas, R. A., Meyer, P. R., Jr. & Rovin, R. A. Complications in three-column cervical spine injuries requiring anterior-posterior stabilization. *Spine* 17, 253-256 (1992).

[39] Dahdaleh, N. S. & Hitchon, P. W. Thoracolumbar spinal extradural arachnoid cysts. *Neurosurgery* 72, E318-319, doi:10.1227/NEU.0b013e31827bc093 (2013).

[40] Denis, F. The three column spine and its significance in the classification of acute thoracolumbar spinal injuries. *Spine* 8, 817-831 (1983).

[41] Deutsch, H., Boco, T. & Lobel, J. Minimally invasive transpedicular vertebrectomy for metastatic disease to the thoracic spine. *Journal of spinal disorders & techniques* 21, 101-105, doi:10.1097/BSD.0b013e31805fea01 (2008).

[42] DeVivo, M. J. Causes and costs of spinal cord injury in the United States. *Spinal cord* 35, 809-813 (1997).

[43] Dvorak, M. F. *et al.* The surgical approach to subaxial cervical spine injuries: an evidence-based algorithm based on the SLIC classification system. *Spine* 32, 2620-2629, doi:10.1097/BRS.0b013e318158ce16 (2007).

[44] Dvorak, M. F. *et al.* Factors predicting motor recovery and functional outcome after traumatic central cord syndrome: a long-term follow-up. *Spine* 30, 2303-2311 (2005).

[45] Dwyer, A., Aprill, C. & Bogduk, N. Cervical zygapophyseal joint pain patterns. I: A study in normal volunteers. *Spine* 15, 453-457 (1990).

[46] Elgafy, H. *et al.* The radiographic failure of single segment posterior cervical instrumentation in traumatic cervical flexion distraction injuries. *Topics in spinal cord injury rehabilitation* 12, 20-29 (2006).

[47] Enkaoua, E. A. *et al.* Vertebral metastases: a critical appreciation of the preoperative prognostic tokuhashi score in a series of 71 cases. *Spine* 22, 2293-2298 (1997).

[48] Fehlings, M. G. & Wilson, J. R. Multicenter clinical research networks for traumatic spinal cord injury: a critical pathway to discovery. *Journal of neurosurgery. Spine* 17, 4-5; discussion 5, doi:10.3171/2012.5.AOSPINE12416 (2012).

[49] Findlay, G. F. Adverse effects of the management of malignant spinal cord compression. *Journal of neurology, neurosurgery, and psychiatry* 47, 761-768 (1984).

[50] Fisher, C. G. *et al.* A novel classification system for spinal instability in neoplastic disease: an evidence-based approach and expert consensus from the Spine Oncology Study Group. *Spine* 35, E1221-1229, doi:10.1097/BRS.0b013e3181e16ae2 (2010).

[51] Fisher, C. G. *et al.* A novel classification system for spinal instability in neoplastic disease: an evidence-based approach and expert consensus from the Spine Oncology Study Group. *Spine* 35, E1221-1229, doi:10.1097/BRS.0b013e3181e16ae2 (2010).

[52] Fisher, C. G., Dvorak, M. F., Leith, J. & Wing, P. C. Comparison of outcomes for unstable lower cervical flexion teardrop fractures managed with halo thoracic vest versus anterior corpectomy and plating. *Spine* 27, 160-166 (2002).

[53] Foo, D., Subrahmanyan, T. S. & Rossier, A. B. Post-traumatic acute anterior spinal cord syndrome. *Paraplegia* 19, 201-205, doi:10.1038/sc.1981.42 (1981).

[54] Fourney, D. R. *et al.* Spinal instability neoplastic score: an analysis of reliability and validity from the spine oncology study group. *Journal of clinical oncology : official journal of the American Society of Clinical Oncology* 29, 3072-3077, doi:10.1200/JCO.2010.34.3897 (2011).

[55] Fourney, D. R. *et al.* Percutaneous vertebroplasty and kyphoplasty for painful vertebral body fractures in cancer patients. *Journal of neurosurgery* 98, 21-30 (2003).

[56] Fraser, J. F. & Härtl, R. Anterior approaches to fusion of the cervical spine: a metaanalysis of fusion rates. *Journal of Neurosurgery: Spine* 6, 298-303 (2007).

[57] Gehweiler, J. A., Jr., Clark, W. M., Schaaf, R. E., Powers, B. & Miller, M. D. Cervical spine trauma: the common combined conditions. *Radiology* 130, 77-86, doi:10.1148/130.1.77 (1979).

[58] Gerszten, P. C. & Welch, W. C. Current surgical management of metastatic spinal disease. *Oncology* 14, 1013-1024; discussion 1024, 1029-1030 (2000).

[59] Gilbert, R. W., Kim, J. H. & Posner, J. B. Epidural spinal cord compression from metastatic tumor: diagnosis and treatment. *Annals of neurology* 3, 40-51, doi:10.1002/ana.410030107 (1978).

[60] Gokaslan, Z. L. Spine surgery for cancer. *Current opinion in oncology* 8, 178-181 (1996).

[61] Greenberg, H. S., Kim, J. H. & Posner, J. B. Epidural spinal cord compression from metastatic tumor: results with a new treatment protocol. *Annals of neurology* 8, 361-366, doi:10.1002/ana.410080404 (1980).

[62] Guigui, P., Benoist, M. & Deburge, A. Spinal deformity and instability after multilevel cervical laminectomy for spondylotic myelopathy. *Spine* 23, 440-447 (1998).

[63] Hadley, M. N., Fitzpatrick, B. C., Sonntag, V. K. & Browner, C. M. Facet fracture-dislocation injuries of the cervical spine. *Neurosurgery* 30, 661-666 (1992).

[64] Hadley, M. N. & Walters, B. C. Introduction to the Guidelines for the Management of Acute Cervical Spine and Spinal Cord Injuries. *Neurosurgery* 72 Suppl 2, 5-16, doi: 10.1227/NEU.0b013e3182773549 (2013).

[65] Hall, F. M. Radiographs in cervical spine trauma. *AJR. American journal of roentgenology* 131, 555-556, doi:10.2214/ajr.131.3.555 (1978).

[66] Helweg-Larsen, S. & Sorensen, P. S. Symptoms and signs in metastatic spinal cord compression: a study of progression from first symptom until diagnosis in 153 patients. *Eur J Cancer* 30A, 396-398 (1994).

[67] Holdsworth, F. Fractures, dislocations, and fracture-dislocations of the spine. *The Journal of bone and joint surgery. American volume* 52, 1534-1551 (1970).

[68] Holly, L. T. *et al.* Cervical spine trauma associated with moderate and severe head injury: incidence, risk factors, and injury characteristics. *Journal of neurosurgery* 96, 285-291 (2002).

[69] Houten, J. K. & Cooper, P. R. Laminectomy and posterior cervical plating for multilevel cervical spondylotic myelopathy and ossification of the posterior longitudinal ligament: effects on cervical alignment, spinal cord compression, and neurological outcome. *Neurosurgery* 52, 1081-1087; discussion 1087-1088 (2003).

[70] Houten, J. K. & Cooper, P. R. Laminectomy and posterior cervical plating for multilevel cervical spondylotic myelopathy and ossification of the posterior longitudinal ligament: effects on cervical alignment, spinal cord compression, and neurological outcome. *Neurosurgery* 52, 1081-1087; discussion 1087-1088 (2003).

[71] Hu, R., Mustard, C. A. & Burns, C. Epidemiology of incident spinal fracture in a complete population. *Spine* 21, 492-499 (1996).

[72] Huang, P., Gupta, M. C., Sarigul-Klijn, N. & Hazelwood, S. Two in vivo surgical approaches for lumbar corpectomy using allograft and a metallic implant: a controlled clinical and biomechanical study. *The spine journal : official journal of the North American Spine Society* 6, 648-658, doi:10.1016/j.spinee.2006.04.028 (2006).

[73] Huang, R. C., Girardi, F. P., Poynton, A. R. & Cammisa Jr, F. P. Treatment of multilevel cervical spondylotic myeloradiculopathy with posterior decompression and fu-

sion with lateral mass plate fixation and local bone graft. *Journal of spinal disorders & techniques* 16, 123-129 (2003).

[74] Hurlbert, R. J. *et al.* Pharmacological therapy for acute spinal cord injury. *Neurosurgery* 72 Suppl 2, 93-105, doi:10.1227/NEU.0b013e31827765c6 (2013).

[75] Ianuzzi, A. *et al.* Biomechanical evaluation of surgical constructs for stabilization of cervical teardrop fractures. *The spine journal : official journal of the North American Spine Society* 6, 514-523, doi:10.1016/j.spinee.2005.12.001 (2006).

[76] Jensen, M. E. & Kallmes, D. E. Percutaneous vertebroplasty in the treatment of malignant spine disease. *Cancer journal* 8, 194-206 (2002).

[77] Kadanka, Z., Bednarik, J., Novotny, O., Urbanek, I. & Dusek, L. Cervical spondylotic myelopathy: conservative versus surgical treatment after 10 years. *European spine journal : official publication of the European Spine Society, the European Spinal Deformity Society, and the European Section of the Cervical Spine Research Society* 20, 1533-1538, doi: 10.1007/s00586-011-1811-9 (2011).

[78] Kadanka, Z. *et al.* Conservative treatment versus surgery in spondylotic cervical myelopathy: a prospective randomised study. *European spine journal : official publication of the European Spine Society, the European Spinal Deformity Society, and the European Section of the Cervical Spine Research Society* 9, 538-544 (2000).

[79] Kadanka, Z. *et al.* Predictive factors for spondylotic cervical myelopathy treated conservatively or surgically. *European journal of neurology : the official journal of the European Federation of Neurological Societies* 12, 55-63, doi:10.1111/j.1468-1331.2004.00896.x (2005).

[80] Kaptain, G. J., Simmons, N. E., Replogle, R. E. & Pobereskin, L. Incidence and outcome of kyphotic deformity following laminectomy for cervical spondylotic myelopathy. *Journal of Neurosurgery: Spine* 93, 199-204 (2000).

[81] Klimo, P., Jr., Thompson, C. J., Kestle, J. R. & Schmidt, M. H. A meta-analysis of surgery versus conventional radiotherapy for the treatment of metastatic spinal epidural disease. *Neuro-oncology* 7, 64-76, doi:10.1215/S1152851704000262 (2005).

[82] Kumar, V. G., Rea, G. L., Mervis, L. J. & McGregor, J. M. Cervical spondylotic myelopathy: functional and radiographic long-term outcome after laminectomy and posterior fusion. *Neurosurgery* 44, 771-777; discussion 777-778 (1999).

[83] Kwok, Y., Tibbs, P. A. & Patchell, R. A. Clinical approach to metastatic epidural spinal cord compression. *Hematology/oncology clinics of North America* 20, 1297-1305, doi: 10.1016/j.hoc.2006.09.008 (2006).

[84] Kwok, Y., Tibbs, P. A. & Patchell, R. A. Clinical approach to metastatic epidural spinal cord compression. *Hematology/oncology clinics of North America* 20, 1297-1305, doi: 10.1016/j.hoc.2006.09.008 (2006).

[85] Kwon, B. K. *et al.* A prospective randomized controlled trial of anterior compared with posterior stabilization for unilateral facet injuries of the cervical spine. *Journal of neurosurgery. Spine* 7, 1-12, doi:10.3171/SPI-07/07/001 (2007).

[86] Lees, F. & Turner, J. W. Natural History and Prognosis of Cervical Spondylosis. *British medical journal* 2, 1607-1610 (1963).

[87] Lifeso, R. M. & Colucci, M. A. Anterior fusion for rotationally unstable cervical spine fractures. *Spine* 25, 2028-2034 (2000).

[88] Livingston, K. E. & Perrin, R. G. The neurosurgical management of spinal metastases causing cord and cauda equina compression. *Journal of neurosurgery* 49, 839-843, doi: 10.3171/jns.1978.49.6.0839 (1978).

[89] Louis, R. Spinal stability as defined by the three-column spine concept. *Anatomia clinica* 7, 33-42 (1985).

[90] Matsunaga, S., Sakou, T. & Nakanisi, K. Analysis of the cervical spine alignment following laminoplasty and laminectomy. *Spinal cord* 37, 20-24 (1999).

[91] Matz, P. G. *et al.* The natural history of cervical spondylotic myelopathy. *Journal of neurosurgery. Spine* 11, 104-111, doi:10.3171/2009.1.SPINE08716 (2009).

[92] McDonald, J. W. & Sadowsky, C. Spinal-cord injury. *Lancet* 359, 417-425, doi:10.1016/S0140-6736(02)07603-1 (2002).

[93] McKinley, W., Santos, K., Meade, M. & Brooke, K. Incidence and outcomes of spinal cord injury clinical syndromes. *The journal of spinal cord medicine* 30, 215-224 (2007).

[94] Moller, F., Andres, A. H. & Langenstein, H. Intubating laryngeal mask airway (ILMA) seems to be an ideal device for blind intubation in case of immobile spine. *British journal of anaesthesia* 85, 493-495 (2000).

[95] Mummaneni, P. V. *et al.* Cervical surgical techniques for the treatment of cervical spondylotic myelopathy. *Journal of neurosurgery. Spine* 11, 130-141, doi: 10.3171/2009.3.SPINE08728 (2009).

[96] Nirala, A. P., Husain, M. & Vatsal, D. K. A retrospective study of multiple interbody grafting and long segment strut grafting following multilevel anterior cervical decompression. *British journal of neurosurgery* 18, 227-232 (2004).

[97] Nurick, S. The natural history and the results of surgical treatment of the spinal cord disorder associated with cervical spondylosis. *Brain : a journal of neurology* 95, 101-108 (1972).

[98] Panjabi, M. M. *et al.* Articular facets of the human spine. Quantitative three-dimensional anatomy. *Spine* 18, 1298-1310 (1993).

[99] Patchell, R. A. *et al.* Direct decompressive surgical resection in the treatment of spinal cord compression caused by metastatic cancer: a randomised trial. *Lancet* 366, 643-648, doi:10.1016/S0140-6736(05)66954-1 (2005).

[100] Perez-Lopez, C. *et al.* [Efficacy of arthrodesis in the posterior approach of cervical myelopathy: comparative study of a series of 36 cases]. *Neurocirugia* 12, 316-323; discussion 323-314 (2001).

[101] Perrin, R. G., Livingston, K. E. & Aarabi, B. Intradural extramedullary spinal metastasis. A report of 10 cases. *Journal of neurosurgery* 56, 835-837, doi:10.3171/jns.1982.56.6.0835 (1982).

[102] Pflugmacher, R., Beth, P., Schroeder, R. J., Schaser, K. D. & Melcher, I. Balloon kyphoplasty for the treatment of pathological fractures in the thoracic and lumbar spine caused by metastasis: one-year follow-up. *Acta radiologica* 48, 89-95, doi: 10.1080/02841850601026427 (2007).

[103] Phillips, D. G. Surgical treatment of myelopathy with cervical spondylosis. *Journal of neurology, neurosurgery, and psychiatry* 36, 879-884 (1973).

[104] Pollock, L. J. *et al.* Relation of recovery of sensation to intraspinal pathways in injuries of the spinal cord. *A.M.A. archives of neurology and psychiatry* 70, 137-150 (1953).

[105] Pouw, M. H. *et al.* Diagnostic criteria of traumatic central cord syndrome. Part 1: a systematic review of clinical descriptors and scores. *Spinal cord* 48, 652-656, doi: 10.1038/sc.2009.155 (2010).

[106] Quencer, R. M. *et al.* Acute traumatic central cord syndrome: MRI-pathological correlations. *Neuroradiology* 34, 85-94 (1992).

[107] Rao, R. D., Gourab, K. & David, K. S. Operative treatment of cervical spondylotic myelopathy. *The Journal of bone and joint surgery. American volume* 88, 1619-1640, doi: 10.2106/JBJS.F.00014 (2006).

[108] Razack, N., Green, B. A. & Levi, A. D. The management of traumatic cervical bilateral facet fracture-dislocations with unicortical anterior plates. *Journal of spinal disorders* 13, 374-381 (2000).

[109] Roth, E. J., Lawler, M. H. & Yarkony, G. M. Traumatic central cord syndrome: clinical features and functional outcomes. *Archives of physical medicine and rehabilitation* 71, 18-23 (1990).

[110] Ryken, T. C. *et al.* The acute cardiopulmonary management of patients with cervical spinal cord injuries. *Neurosurgery* 72 Suppl 2, 84-92, doi:10.1227/NEU.0b013e318276ee16 (2013).

[111] Schijns, O. E., Kurt, E., Wessels, P., Luijckx, G. J. & Beuls, E. A. Intramedullary spinal cord metastasis as a first manifestation of a renal cell carcinoma: report of a case and review of the literature. *Clinical neurology and neurosurgery* 102, 249-254 (2000).

[112] Schneider, R. C. The diagnosis and treatment of trauma to the central nervous system. *The Medical clinics of North America* 40, 1369-1384 (1956).

[113] Schneider, R. C., Cherry, G. & Pantek, H. The syndrome of acute central cervical spinal cord injury; with special reference to the mechanisms involved in hyperextension injuries of cervical spine. *Journal of neurosurgery* 11, 546-577, doi:10.3171/jns.1954.11.6.0546 (1954).

[114] Schneider, R. C., Thompson, J. M. & Bebin, J. The syndrome of acute central cervical spinal cord injury. *Journal of neurology, neurosurgery, and psychiatry* 21, 216-227 (1958).

[115] Sciubba, D. M. & Gokaslan, Z. L. Are patients satisfied after surgery for metastatic spine disease? *The spine journal : official journal of the North American Spine Society* 10, 63-65, doi:10.1016/j.spinee.2009.10.004 (2010).

[116] Sciubba, D. M. *et al.* Diagnosis and management of metastatic spine disease. A review. *Journal of neurosurgery. Spine* 13, 94-108, doi:10.3171/2010.3.SPINE09202 (2010).

[117] Siegal, T., Siegal, T., Robin, G., Lubetzki-Korn, I. & Fuks, Z. Anterior decompression of the spine for metastatic epidural cord compression: a promising avenue of therapy? *Annals of neurology* 11, 28-34, doi:10.1002/ana.410110106 (1982).

[118] Sim, F. H., Svien, H. J., Bickel, W. H. & Janes, J. M. Swan-neck deformity following extensive cervical laminectomy. A review of twenty-one cases. *The Journal of bone and joint surgery. American volume* 56, 564-580 (1974).

[119] Singh, K. *et al.* Current concepts in the management of metastatic spinal disease. The role of minimally-invasive approaches. *The Journal of bone and joint surgery. British volume* 88, 434-442, doi:10.1302/0301-620X.88B4.17282 (2006).

[120] Sonntag, V. K., Hadley, M. N., Dickman, C. A. & Browner, C. M. Atlas fractures: treatment and long-term results. *Acta neurochirurgica. Supplementum* 43, 63-68 (1988).

[121] Stark, R. J., Henson, R. A. & Evans, S. J. Spinal metastases. A retrospective survey from a general hospital. *Brain : a journal of neurology* 105, 189-213 (1982).

[122] Stauffer, E. S. Diagnosis and prognosis of acute cervical spinal cord injury. *Clinical orthopaedics and related research*, 9-15 (1975).

[123] Street, J. *et al.* Single-stage posterolateral vertebrectomy for the management of metastatic disease of the thoracic and lumbar spine: a prospective study of an evolving surgical technique. *Journal of spinal disorders & techniques* 20, 509-520, doi:10.1097/BSD.0b013e3180335bf7 (2007).

[124] Swank, M. L., Lowery, G. L., Bhat, A. L. & McDonough, R. F. Anterior cervical allograft arthrodesis and instrumentation: multilevel interbody grafting or strut graft reconstruction. *European spine journal : official publication of the European Spine Society, the European Spinal Deformity Society, and the European Section of the Cervical Spine Research Society* 6, 138-143 (1997).

[125] Tetreault, L. A., Karpova, A. & Fehlings, M. G. Predictors of outcome in patients with degenerative cervical spondylotic myelopathy undergoing surgical treatment: results of a systematic review. *European spine journal : official publication of the European Spine Society, the European Spinal Deformity Society, and the European Section of the Cervical Spine Research Society*, doi:10.1007/s00586-013-2658-z (2013).

[126] Toh, E., Nomura, T., Watanabe, M. & Mochida, J. Surgical treatment for injuries of the middle and lower cervical spine. *International orthopaedics* 30, 54-58, doi:10.1007/s00264-005-0016-4 (2006).

[127] Tokuhashi, Y., Matsuzaki, H., Oda, H., Oshima, M. & Ryu, J. A revised scoring system for preoperative evaluation of metastatic spine tumor prognosis. *Spine* 30, 2186-2191 (2005).

[128] Tokuhashi, Y., Matsuzaki, H., Toriyama, S., Kawano, H. & Ohsaka, S. Scoring system for the preoperative evaluation of metastatic spine tumor prognosis. *Spine* 15, 1110-1113 (1990).

[129] Tomita, K. *et al.* Surgical strategy for spinal metastases. *Spine* 26, 298-306 (2001).

[130] Torg, J. S., Pavlov, H., O'Neill, M. J., Nichols, C. E., Jr. & Sennett, B. The axial load teardrop fracture. A biomechanical, clinical and roentgenographic analysis. *The American journal of sports medicine* 19, 355-364 (1991).

[131] Troll, G. F. & Dohrmann, G. J. Anaesthesia of the spinal cord-injured patient: cardiovascular problems and their management. *Paraplegia* 13, 162-171, doi:10.1038/sc.1975.27 (1975).

[132] Ulmar, B. *et al.* The Tokuhashi score: significant predictive value for the life expectancy of patients with breast cancer with spinal metastases. *Spine* 30, 2222-2226 (2005).

[133] Vaccaro, A. R. *et al.* The subaxial cervical spine injury classification system: a novel approach to recognize the importance of morphology, neurology, and integrity of the disco-ligamentous complex. *Spine* 32, 2365-2374, doi:10.1097/BRS.0b013e3181557b92 (2007).

[134] Wada, E. *et al.* Subtotal corpectomy versus laminoplasty for multilevel cervical spondylotic myelopathy: a long-term follow-up study over 10 years. *Spine* 26, 1443-1447; discussion 1448 (2001).

[135] Walsh, G. L. *et al.* Anterior approaches to the thoracic spine in patients with cancer: indications and results. *The Annals of thoracic surgery* 64, 1611-1618 (1997).

[136] Wang, J. C. *et al.* Single-stage posterolateral transpedicular approach for resection of epidural metastatic spine tumors involving the vertebral body with circumferential reconstruction: results in 140 patients. Invited submission from the Joint Section Meeting on Disorders of the Spine and Peripheral Nerves, March 2004. *Journal of neurosurgery. Spine* 1, 287-298, doi:10.3171/spi.2004.1.3.0287 (2004).

[137] Wang, J. C., McDonough, P. W., Kanim, L. E., Endow, K. K. & Delamarter, R. B. Increased fusion rates with cervical plating for three-level anterior cervical discectomy and fusion. *Spine* 26, 643-646; discussion 646-647 (2001).

[138] Weill, A. *et al.* Spinal metastases: indications for and results of percutaneous injection of acrylic surgical cement. *Radiology* 199, 241-247, doi:10.1148/radiology.199.1.8633152 (1996).

[139] Weinstein, S. M. & Walton, O. Management of pain associated with spinal tumor. *Neurosurgery clinics of North America* 15, 511-527, doi:10.1016/j.nec.2004.04.017 (2004).

[140] Witham, T. F., Khavkin, Y. A., Gallia, G. L., Wolinsky, J. P. & Gokaslan, Z. L. Surgery insight: current management of epidural spinal cord compression from metastatic spine disease. *Nature clinical practice. Neurology* 2, 87-94; quiz 116, doi:10.1038/ncpneuro0116 (2006).

[141] Wong, D. A., Fornasier, V. L. & MacNab, I. Spinal metastases: the obvious, the occult, and the impostors. *Spine* 15, 1-4 (1990).

[142] York, J. E. *et al.* Combined chest wall resection with vertebrectomy and spinal reconstruction for the treatment of Pancoast tumors. *Journal of neurosurgery* 91, 74-80 (1999).

[143] Yoshizawa, H., Kobayashi, S. & Morita, T. Chronic nerve root compression. Pathophysiologic mechanism of nerve root dysfunction. *Spine* 20, 397-407 (1995).

[144] Yue, W. M., Tan, S. B., Tan, M. H., Koh, D. C. & Tan, C. T. The Torg--Pavlov ratio in cervical spondylotic myelopathy: a comparative study between patients with cervical spondylotic myelopathy and a nonspondylotic, nonmyelopathic population. *Spine* 26, 1760-1764 (2001).

[145]

Chapter 5

Functional Electrical Stimulation in Paraplegia

Aris Papachristos

Additional information is available at the end of the chapter

http://dx.doi.org/10.5772/58625

1. Introduction

Functional Electrical Stimulation (FES) is a technique of eliciting controlled neural activation through the application of low levels of electrical current. FES was initially referred to as Functional Electrotherapy by Liberson [1] and it was not until 1967 that the term Functional Electrical Stimulation was established by Moe and Post [2]. In 1965 Offner patented a system used to treat foot drop with the title "Electrical stimulation of muscle deprived of nervous control with a view of providing muscular contraction and producing a functionally useful moment" [3]. Another term often used equally to FES is Functional Neuromusclular Stimulation (FNS or FNMS).

The first commercially available FES devices treated foot drop in hemiplegic patients by stimulating the peroneal nerve during gait. In this case, a switch, located in the heel end of a user's shoe, would activate a stimulator worn by the user.

Structural discontinuity in the spinal cord after injury results in a disruption in the impulse conduction resulting in loss of various bodily functions depending upon the level of injury. The initial goal of FES technology was to provide greater mobility to the patients after SCI. However, with the advances in biomedical engineering within the last 2 decades, FES is no more limited to locomotion alone. Therefore, the definition of FES has changed considerably and is now considered to be the technique of applying safe levels of electric current to stimulate various organs of the body rendered disabled due to SCI. Electrical stimulation in the form of functional electrical stimulation (FES) can help facilitate and improve limb mobility along with other body functions lost due to injury e.g. sexual, bladder or bowel functions.

2. Mechanism of FES operation

Both nerves and muscle fibres respond to electric current. However, for practical purposes FES is mostly used to directly stimulate nerve fibres, as a much lower amount of current is required to generate an action potential in a nerve than the one required for muscular depolarisation.

The main component of a FES system is the microprocessor-based electronic stimulator which determines when and how the stimulation is provided, with channels for delivery of individual pulses through a set of electrodes connected to the neuromuscular system. The microprocessor contains programs for sitting, standing, walking etc. It serves to generate a train of impulses that grossly imitate the neural triggers that would have normally passed through the spinal cord to the appropriate peripheral nerves below spinal cord lesion for these different programs. These stimuli thus trigger action potentials in the peripheral nerves which in turn activate muscle contractions in the associated muscles fibers [11]. When properly applied, the energy transfer is both safe and efficient. Low levels of current can be safely injected to neural tissue with a minimal but biologically acceptable response. Furthermore, the energy amplification is substantial, since a small stimulus can generate a considerable action. For example, an electrical stimulus of a few milliwatts generates as much as a hundred newton-meters of torque in the lower limb.

It is proven nowadays that FES exersice is improving cardiovascular fitness, and decreasing the risk of diabetes, as well as reducing osteoporosis [12, 54-59]. FES exercise and weight bearing also reduce the risk of pressure sores by improving tissue oxygen levels, increasing muscle bulk, and altering seated pressure distribution [12]

Another use of electrical signals is to use afferent signals from intact structures whose communication links with other body systems have been destroyed or diminished by an injury or disease to provide feedback to guide motor activity.

It is conceptually possible, therefore, to obtain "artificial" control with electrical stimulation over virtually all structures which rely upon neural communication for their activation. This encompasses virtually all of the critical motor and sensory pathways involved in paralysis of the central nervous system.

The frequency, pulse width/duration, duty cycle, intensity/amplitude, ramp time, pulse pattern, program duration, program frequency, and muscle groups activated are parameters taken into account. Frequency refers to the pulses produced per second during stimulation and is stated in units of Hertz (Hz, e.g., 40 Hz=40 pulses per second). The frequencies of electrical stimulation used can vary widely depending on the goals of the task or intervention, but most clinical regimens use 20-50Hz patterns for optimal results [20]. In order to avoid fatigue or discomfort, constant low frequency stimulation is typically used, which produces a smooth contraction at low force levels. In a study comparing several different frequencies and stimulation patterns, frequencies under 16Hz were not sufficient to elicit a strong enough contraction to allow the quadriceps to extend to a target of 40º. Commercial stimulators provide many different waveforms and pulse settings capable of producing contractions at therapeutic

http://dx.doi.org/10.5772/58625

levels. The source should be flexible to generate complex electrical waveforms, such as triangular or quasitrapezoidal waveforms [60].

The numbers of channels, which can range from one to several, govern the sophistication required for complex outputs like FES assisted standing. The programmable microprocessor activates the various channels sequentially or in unison to synchronize the complex output of the stimulator. Electrodes provide the interface between the electrical stimulator and the nervous system. Various types of electrodes have been developed and are available ranging from non-invasive surface electrodes to invasive implantable ones. Implantable electrodes provide more specific and selective stimulation to the desired muscle group than the surface electrodes. The feedback control of the FES system can be either open-looped or closed-looped. Open-looped control is used for simple tasks such as for muscle strengthening alone, and requires a constant electrical output from the stimulator. In a closed-looped system, the parameters for electrical stimulation are constantly modified by a computer via feedback information on muscle force and joint position thus stimulating various muscle groups simultaneously leading to a combination of muscular contraction needed for a complex sophisticated functional activity such as walking.

3. Standing and walking

The efforts to develop a suitable human functional stimulator which can achieve synergistic activity of various muscles accelerated in the late 1980s and early 1990s. In 1987, Davis proposed the development of a FES system based on multi-cochlear implant technology to restore function in paraplegic patients [9]. Kralj proposed the use of FES for restoring standing and walking in spinal cord injured (SCI) patients [4]. Other parallel studies at that time also concluded that FES assisted walking is feasible in patients with incomplete SCI even with severe motor loss [7, 10]. In all lower limb applications the general method for restoration of standing is the application of electrical stimulation to the quadriceps. The restoration and/or improvement of gait has typically involved the stimulation of two sites. These have been the quadriceps, during the stance phase of gait and the peroneal nerve, producing a patterned flexion response during the swing phase of the ipsilateral limb [6]. FES has greater potential for functional use in incomplete spinal cord injury (ISCI) patients due to the preservation of some motor and sensory function [7,8]. Paraplegic patients using FES for ambulation still require the use of walker or other orthotic devices for stabilising the ankle, knees and hips. Several gait programs for the ISCI subjects have been established. Applications of FES can be divided into two classes: (A) neuroprostheses for use as permanent assistive devices, and (B) FES to facilitate exercise and be used in temporary therapeutic interventions to improve voluntary function. This latter class of applications has been termed functional electrical therapy (FET). Therapeutic applications include cardiovascular conditioning and the prevention of muscular atrophy through exercise. Functional applications assist with vital body functions lost due to SCI. The FES devices were initially designed in an attempt to provide assistance with standing or walking, provided the paraplegic patient had adequate upper body motor control and strength [13,32].

The use of these FES devices designed to permit or improve ambulation is not simple or without risks. Paraplegic patients require extensive training to build muscle strength in the upper body in order to achieve FES assisted ambulation. The amount of energy spent with FES walking is almost twice than that for normal walking, although the achievable speed is slower than that of normal walking [18,19]. The risk of injury with FES assisted ambulation is more likely to be higher due to fatigue of the stimulated muscle causing an increase incidence of fall and fractures. These factors limit the true functional utilisation of these systems. Another major practical problem associated with the current FES locomotive models is mainly related to feedback control. In spite of these associated limitations for everyday mobility in daily life, there are potential functional, medical and psychological benefits of FES assisted standing and walking. These devices can help increase their level of independence by providing some assistance with standing while transferring from the wheelchair to a car, climbing a few steps or reaching for a higher object.

3.1. Non-invasive FES systems

Parastep I is a FDA approved FES system for short distance ambulation that uses a walker support for balance [14,15]. The Parastep is a non-invasive system and consists of the following components:

- a microcomputer controlled neuromuscular stimulation unit
- a battery
- a unit for pre-testing main system operation and electrode cables
- surface applied skin electrodes
- power and electrode cables
- a control and stability walker with finger activated control switches.

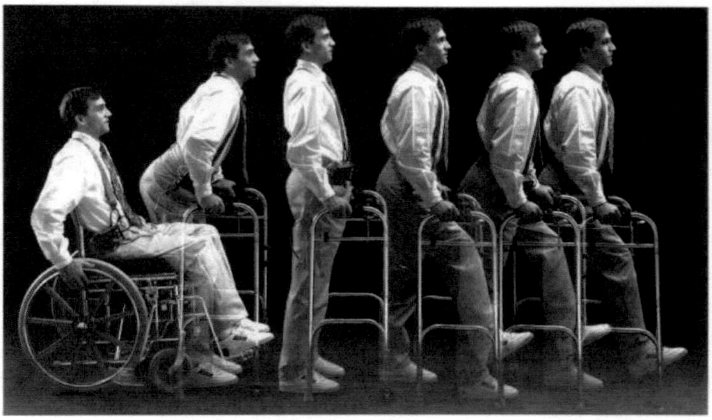

Figure 1. Advertisement of the Parastep System

The system provides stimulation output to 12 surface electrodes that are attached to the skin at appropriate placements. These stimulation pulses trigger action potentials in the intact peripheral nerves to generate muscle contraction. Another noninvasive, transcutaneous FES system is the six-channel stimulator from the Ljubljana University but it was not commercialized and not FDA approved. In opposite the Parastep system received FDA approval in 1994 is nowadays widely available. It has been evaluated for its ambulation performance and medical/psychological effects.[14,16,17]. Factors considered to be a candidate for ambulation with the Parastep system include the presence of neurologically stable and complete SCI, level of injury (preferably between T4 and T12), patient motivation, degree of spasticity, muscle contractile response to electrical stimulation, cardio-respiratory capacity, and musculoskeletal integrity.

3.2. Implanted FES systems

Current technology using surface and percutaneous electrodes has distinct disadvantages. Systems using percutaneous electrodes are prone to infection if poorly maintained, and systems using surface electrodes make donning and doffing difficult. Moreover, as the number of channels increases, surface electrodes become impractical and inconvenient, making them generally best suited for short-term therapeutic applications. In addition, selectively activating individual muscles deep to the skin (such as the hip flexors) with surface stimulation or obtaining repeatable stimulated responses from day to day is difficult or impossible. Neural prostheses or Neuroprosthetics are implantable devices which use electrical current that can substitute a motor, sensory or cognitive modality that might have been damaged as a result of an injury or a disease. Familiar examples include cochlear implants and cardiac pacemakers. The Freehand system was the first motor-system neuroprosthesis to receive marketing approval. These devices have been safely and effectively installed worldwide in the upper limbs in patients with cervical SCI to provide active handgrasp after paralysis without major complications. External system components included a custom rechargeable wearable external control unit, command hand switch, transmitting coil, charger, and clinical programming station.

Fully implanted pacemaker-like systems offer numerous advantages over surface and percutaneous stimulation for long-term clinical use, including improved convenience, cosmesis, reliability, and repeatability. In these systems, muscle or nerve-based electrodes are installed surgically and connected to an implanted stimulation device, so no material crosses the skin.

FES systems using implanted intramuscular electrodes with percutaneous leads have provided up to 48 channels of stimulation for improved stability and forward progression and finer control of movement during walking. Multichannel implanted FES systems for walking after motor complete paraplegia have provided a swing-through and reciprocal gait [29,30]. They reduced donning time and improved day-to-day repeatability compared with surface FES systems and eliminated site care of percutaneous systems.

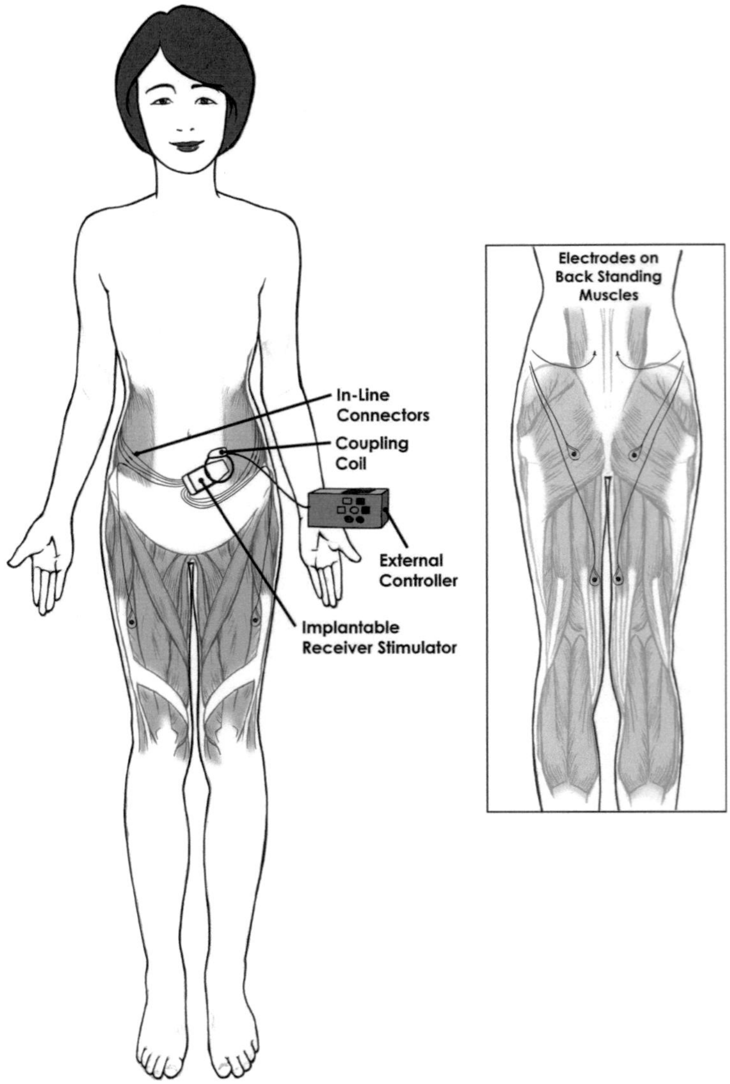

Figure 2. Cleveland FES Standing/Transfer System.

3.3. Hybrid FES-Orthosis ambulation systems

A variety of mechanical orthoses have been designed and tested for lower-limb function after SCI. The reciprocal gait orthosis (RGOs) stabilize ankles, knees, hips, and trunk to provide upright posture and couple hip flexion with contralateral hip extension to facilitate walking. The long leg braces only fix the ankle and knee joints to provide stability and prevent collapse. In some configurations, the addition of a pelvic band provides extra stability. Most orthoses provide good postural stability, especially when the hip joints are reciprocally coupled to prevent bilateral hip flexion. With all mechanical braces, upper-body strength is required for standing up and for forward progression during walking. Clinical reviews also indicate that brace users are consistently unable to achieve significant functional ambulation without some sort of pelvic control and that adequate hip flexion is an essential component of walking with braces. In conclusion only few individuals with paraplegia choose to use their orthosis for activities other than therapeutic exercise [34].

First in 1973, a hybrid actuator was described for orthotic systems in which the anatomical joint could be controlled internally by means of FES or externally by means of a hypothetical three-state joint actuator incorporated onto an exoskeletal brace [33]. This work initiated the field of hybrid orthotics and, specifically, defined the concept of a hybrid neuroprosthesis (HNP), in which FES is combined with external mechanical components.

Hybrid neuroprosthesis (HNP) potentially can combine the best features of mechanical bracing and FES into new systems for walking after SCI that offer more advantages than the individual components acting alone. The exoskeletal mechanical components of hybrid systems have been generally passive devices to minimize size, weight, and energy consumption, while the FES component serves as an active mechanism for limb propulsion.

Surface and intramuscular FES systems have been combined with a conventional trunk-hip-knee-ankle-foot orthosis (THKAFO) for reciprocal gait in individuals with complete thoracic level SCI. The addition of FES to the glutei for example during stance when individuals used lower-limb bracing reduced crutch forces [51,52] and provided forward propulsion by driving the stance leg into extension. Users with paraplegia (complete T4-T12 SCI) required 70 percent of their maximum upper-limb aerobic capacity when walking with an RGO alone, while walking with an RGO combined with FES required 32 percent of the upper-limb and 25 percent of the lower-limb aerobic capacity, effectively shifting the metabolic burden from the muscles of the arms, shoulders and trunk to the large, otherwise paralyzed, muscles of the legs [53].

The RGO Generation II is a reciprocating gait orthosis combined with FES which was developed by Louisiana State University Medical Center and Durr-Fillauer Medical, Inc. It employs concurrent electrostimulation of the rectus femoris and hamstrings to assist in rising and balancing and a ratchet-type latching device to improve safety and stability in standing. Alternating stimulation of the rectus femoris and contralateral hamstrings are used for locomotion [42].

In summary, an HNP combining bracing and FES has been shown to significantly improve walking distance and reduce energy consumption. A reciprocal coupling of the hips provides good trunk stability, and flexion-to-extension coupling ratios favoring flexion improve step length and energy cost. Unlocking the orthotic knee joints during the swing phase of gait improves foot-to-floor clearance and reduces energy cost, while locking them during stance postpones muscle fatigue from stimulation.

3.4. Hybrid FES – External Powered Orthosis Ambulation systems

To date only a few ambulatory external powered exoskeletons have been built. An ambulatory system named HAL that combines a powered exoskeleton with a customized walker was designed at the Sogang University [43-45]. A walker ensures complete balance and reduces the weight of the device by housing the battery, DC motors, and control unit, with cables transmitting power to the joints.

ReWalk developed by Argo Medical Technologies Ltd. enables paraplegics, with the aid of crutches for balance, to stand up, sit

down, walk about including slopes, and even climb stairs.[46]. ReWalk features servomotors located at the hip and knee joints, rechargeable batteries, and a wrist remote control that commands the type of desired motion. Since ambulatory exoskeletons are meant to be used by paraplegics and people with severely impaired locomotion capabilities, two crucial problems must be considered – ensuring full balance and determining the intention of the motion of the user. To overcome these problems, external balancing aids have been considered – crutches, canes, or walkers are used to ensured balance, whereas joysticks or keypads are used to command the desired motion.

In 2010 Berkeley Bionics unveiled eLEGS, which stands for "Exoskeleton Lower Extremity Gait System". eLEGS is another hydraulically powered exoskeleton system, and allows paraplegics to stand and walk with crutches or a walker. In 2011 eLEGS was renamed Ekso. Ekso weighs 20 kg, it has a maximum speed of 3.2 km/h and a battery life of 6 hour [47].

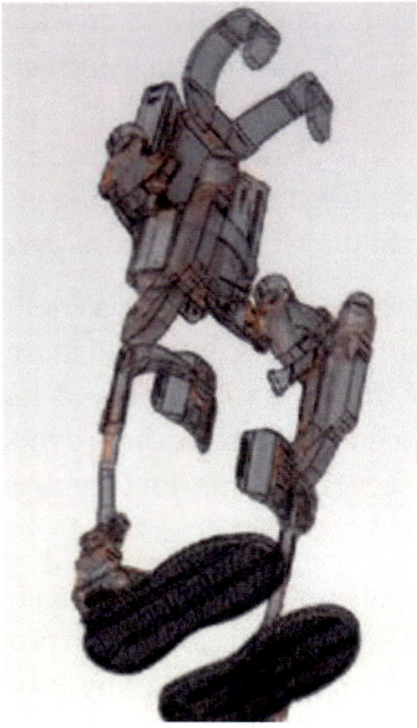

Figure 3. "eLegs" exoskeleton by Berkeley Bionics

A new promising exoskeleton named Indego is seeking for FDA approval in 2015 developed in Vanderbilt University [49,50].

All of these devices can be coupled with FES. Compared to using FES alone, the powered exoskeleton provides joint motions that are otherwise difficult to achieve consistently (e.g. hip flexion). Even for motions that can be achieved using FES, the exoskeleton ensures that the joint trajectories stay consistent in the presence of time-varying muscle behavior, providing consistent and repeatable gait. Compared to using a powered exoskeleton alone, the addition of FES reduces electrical power consumption while providing additional joint torques. Certain therapeutic effects of the use of FES have been studied. The medical advantages of short distance ambulation include increased blood flow to lower limbs, increase in lower limb muscle mass, reduced spasticity, lower heart rate at sub peak work intensities and beneficial effects on digestion, bowel and bladder. Psychological benefits achieved through FES assisted walking such as the associated increase in self esteem and reduction in depression are all well documented. Most of the studies conducted which have evaluated the role of FES assisted walking have a very small sample size and a short follow up time [48,51].

4. Bladder, bowel and sexual function

Other functional applications of FES which help to restore useful functions and thus improve the quality of life include bladder and bowel voiding and electro-ejaculation. Voluntary control of bowel and bladder function is either lost or considerably impaired depending upon the level and severity of SCI and can lead to multiple complications. The Vocare bladder system (Finetech-Brindley bladder system) is a surgically implantable sacral anterior root stimulator that allows individuals with complete spinal cord injury to urinate on demand [60].

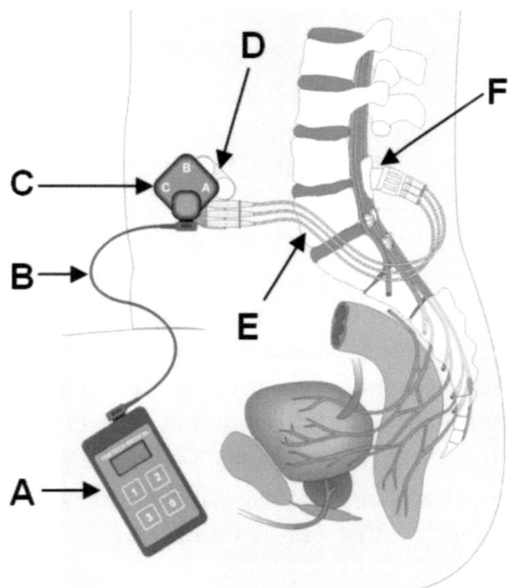

Figure 4. The Finetech-Brindley Bladder Control System

Secondary use of the device is to aid in bowel evacuation. It was approved by FDA in 1998. It consists of an external controller and transmitter and an implantable receiver-stimulator and electrodes. This system is operated by radio frequency signals transmitted to electrodes placed on the sacral spinal nerves (S2-S4) and leads to bladder/large bowel and urethral/ anal sphincter contraction. At the time of implantation, a posterior rhizotomy through laminectomy at sacral level is performed to abolish the uninhibited reflex bladder contractions. This eliminates the reflex incontinence caused by the activation of the sensory reflex pathway. However it also causes a loss of perineal sensations and reflex erection and ejaculation if present. Patient selection criteria for Vocare implantation include neurologically stable and clinically complete supra-sacral SCI and intact parasympathetic innervation to detrusor musculature. The major disadvantage of this system is the need for major surgery for implantation and posterior rhizotomy. However, this device offers an improved quality of life, social ease, as well as a reduction and prevention of urinary tract infections and their associated complication (61,62,65li) Another added benefit of this system is enhanced bowel evacuation with most patients reporting a reduction in the time required for bowel evacuation along with a reduction in constipation and faecal impaction. A slower stimulation time sequence is required for defeacation than for micturation. Approximately 60% of men can also produce penile erection using this device. Electroejaculation is one of the several techniques now available to harvest viable sperm for the purposes of artificial insemination or in vitro fertilization. An electric probe is inserted into the rectum near the prostate to stimulate the nerves and contract the pelvis muscles, causing ejaculation [63,64]. The ejaculate is collected from the urethra and prepared for use in artificial insemination. Caution need to be taken in men with SCI who have a history of autonomic dysreflexia as electroejaculation can cause a significant increase in blood pressure and heart rate.

4.1. FES cycling and rowing

A safe and economic alternative to FES-induced gait training is the employment of FES synchronized to the cycling movement, which entails a coordinated activation of the lower limb muscles, approximating the cyclic movements of locomotion. In contrast to FES standing and walking systems, an FES-cycling system uses stimulator cycling software to control sequential stimulation of the large leg-actuating muscles of paralyzed leg muscles to produce cyclical leg motion. Currently, FES cycling exercise (FESCE) is often used in rehabilitation therapy. There are a number of subsequent investigations reporting physiological adaptations after regular cycling exercise training, which demonstrated that cycling exercise increases muscle strength and endurance and bone density [66-71] suppresses spasticity [72,73], improves cardiopulmonary function, and provides many other physiological and psychological benefits for subjects with an SCI [74-78]. Typically, the quadriceps,hamstrings, and gluteus groups are activated in an appropriate sequence which is out of phase bilaterally to maintain a forward driving torque. The level of stimulation applied to the muscles (which, in turn, determines the amount of torque and cadence produced at the pedals) is controlled by the stimulation software. The advantage of FES-cycling over FES-walking and standing exercise is that individuals with paralysis can perform the exercise, and it can also enhance an individual's suitability for FES standing and walking. Presently, there are many commercial FES cycling ergometers available, such as the BerkelBike (BerkelBike BV, AV's-Hertogenbosch, the Netherlands), Ergys and Regys (Therapeutic Alliances, Fairborn, Ohio, USA), and Motomed (Reck, Betzenweiler, Germany).

http://dx.doi.org/10.5772/58625

In general, FES cycling ergometers can be divided into two major types, mobile and stationary types. The mobile type, a locomotion device, focuses on muscle training as well as giving some mobility to subjects whose muscles can still be excited. Several research groups have developed a mobile cycling system using standard or recumbent tricycles for SCI subjects. Usually, the mobile type of cycling ergometer is an open-loop system, which is not only a rehabilitation modality but also a recreational activity.

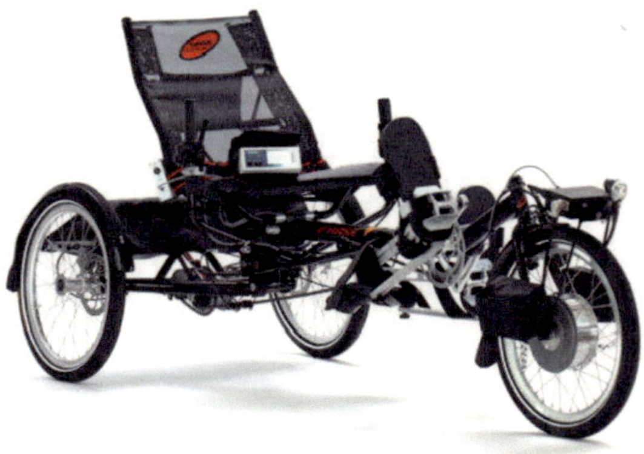

Figure 5. The"RehaBike"by Hasomed (outdoor bike)

The stationary type of cycling ergometer is usually used for aerobic exercise training in subjects with an SCI to condition their muscle strength and enhance cardiopulmonary function.

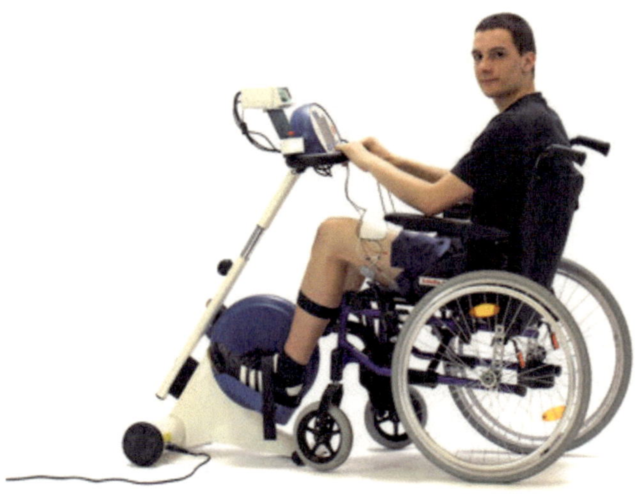

Figure 6. "RehaMove" FES System coupled with Motomed stationary bike

The time course and training frequency are major factors that determine the therapeutic effects of cycling exercise. It is commonly recommended that subjects with an SCI receive at least 2-3 times per week and 30 min per time in a cycling rehabilitation program. In addition, it was reported that detraining from cycling exercise can soon induce a quick reversal of physical fitness within 1 week. The selection of electrical stimulation parameters is also an important issue considered in FESCE studies. Commonly, the FES cycling stimulation current is delivered to the large paralyzed leg muscles via surface electrodes. The stimulation output can either be regulated current or regulated voltage, which depends on the control design of the FES cycling stimulator. Commonly, the stimulation frequency is selected in the range of 10~50 Hz. However, a relatively higher stimulation frequency (> 50 Hz) can produce higher forces and therefore higher power for pedaling the ergometer compared to lower stimulation frequencies (10~50 Hz). But higher stimulation frequencies may rapidly result in ATP depletion at neuromuscular junctions and cause muscle fatigue.

In conclusion FES cycling plays an important role for each individual. It enables – in addition to the described beneficial physiological effects – the implementation of a physical activity and thereby, in terms of an improved participation, leads to a better quality of live.

Author details

Aris Papachristos*

Address all correspondence to: arispapa76@gmail.com

Rehabilitation Center "Kentavros", Volos, Greece

References

[1] Liberson, W. T.; Holmquest, H. J.; Scot, D.; Dow, M. (1961). "Functional electrotherapy: Stimulation of the peroneal nerve synchronized with the swing phase of the gait of hemiplegic patients". *Archives of physical medicine and rehabilitation* 42: 101–105.

[2] J. H. Moe and H. W. Post, "Functional electrical stimulation for ambulation in hemiplegia," The Lancet, vol. 82, pp. 285–288, July 1962

[3] Offner et al. (1965), Patent 3,344,792

[4] Kralj A, Orobelnik S (1973) Functional electrical stimulation-A new hope for paraplegic patients? Bull Prosthet Res 10(20): 75-102

[5] Bajd T, Kralj A, Turk R, Benko H, Sega J (1983) The use of a four channel stimulator as an ambulatory aid for paraplegic patients. Phys Ther 63: 1116-1120.

[6] Bajd T, Andrews BJ, Kralj A, Katakis J (1986) Restoration of walking in patients with incomplete spinal cord injuries by use of electrical stimulation-preliminary results. Clin Prosthet Orthot 10: 111-114.

[7] Bajd T, Kralj A, Turk R, Benko H, Sega J (1989) Use of functional electrical stimulation in the rehabilitation of patients with incomplete spinal cord injuries. J Biomed Eng 11: 96-102 doi: 10.1016/0141-5425(89)90115-5.

[8] Kralj A, Bajd T (1989) Functional Electrical Stimulation: Standing and Walking After Spinal Cord Injury. CRC Press, Inc, Boca Raton, Florida, USA.

[9] Davis R, Eckhouse J, Patrick J, et al. Computerised 22 channel stimulator for limb movement. Appl Neurophysiol. 1987;50:444–448. doi: 10.1159/000100760

[10] Graupe D, Kohn KH. Functional neuromuscular stimulator for short distance ambulation by certain thoracic level spinal cord injured paraplegics. Surg Neurol. 1998;50(3):202–207. doi: 10.1016/S0090-3019(98)00074-3

[11] Rattay F, Resatz S, Dimitrijevic MR, et al. Mechanisms of electrical stimulations with neural prosthesis. Neuromodulation.2003;6(1):42–56. doi: 10.1046/j.1525-1403.2003.03006

[12] Samar Hamid and Ray Hayek. Role of electrical stimulation for rehabilitation and regeneration after spinal cord injury: an overview. Eur Spine J. 2008 Sep;17(9):1256-69. doi: 10.1007/s00586-008-0729-3.

[13] Gorman PH. An update on functional electrical stimulation after spinal cord injury.Neurorehabil Neural Repair. 2000;14:251–263.

[14] Graupe D. An overview of the state of the art of noninvasive FES for independent ambulation by thoracic level paraplegics.Neurol Res. 2002;24(5):431–442. doi: 10.1179/016164102101200302

[15] SIGMEDICS, INC. http://www.sigmedics.com

[16] Brissot R, Gallien P, Le Bot MP, et al. Clinical experience wit functional electrical stimulation-assisted gait with parastep in spinal cord injured patients. Spine. 2000;25(4):501–508. doi: 10.1097/00007632-200002150-00018.

[17] Gallien P, Brissot R, Eyssette M, et al. Restoration of gait by functional electrical stimulation for spinal cord injured patients. Paraplegia. 1995;33(11):660–664

[18] Jacobs PL, Johnson B, Mahoney ET. Physiologic responses to electrically assisted and frame-supported standing in persons with paraplegia. J Spinal Cord Med.2003;26(4): 384–389.

[19] Spadone R, Merati G, Bertocchi E, Mevio E, Veicsteinas A, Pedotti A. et al. Energy consumption of locomotion with orthosis versus Parastep-assisted gait: a single case study. Spinal Cord. 2003;41(2):97–104 (x) Sadowsky CL. Electrical stimulation in spinal cord injury. Neurorehabilitation.2001;16:165–169

[20] Baker LL, Bowman BR, McNeal DR. Effects of waveform on comfort during neuromuscular electrical stimulation. Clin Orthop.1988;233:75–85.

[21] Scheiner A, Polando G, Marsolais EB. Design and clinical application of a double helix electrode for functional electrical stimulation. IEEE Trans Biomed Eng. 1994;41(5): 425-31.DOI:10.1109/10.293216

[22] Marsolais EB, Kobetic R. Implantation techniques and experience with percutaneous intramuscular electrodes in the lower extremities. J Rehabil Res Dev. 1986;23(3):1-8.

[23] Nandurkar S, Marsolais EB, Kobetic R. Percutaneous implantation of iliopsoas for functional neuromuscular stimulation. Clin Orthop Relat Res. 2001 Aug;(389): 210-17.DOI:10.1097/00003086-200108000-00030

[24] Shimada Y, Sato K, Abe E, Kagaya H, Ebata K, Oba M, Sata M. Clinical experience of functional electrical stimulation in complete paraplegia. Spinal Cord. 1996;34(10): 615-19

[25] Kobetic R, Marsolais EB. Synthesis of paraplegic gait with multichannel functional neuromuscular stimulation. IEEE Trans Rehabil Eng. 1994;2(2):66-79. DOI: 10.1109/86.313148

[26] Kobetic R, Triolo RJ, Marsolais EB. Muscle selection and walking performance of multichannel FES systems for ambulation in paraplegia. IEEE Trans Rehabil Eng. 1997; 5(1):23-29. DOI:10.1109/86.559346

[27] Holle J, Frey M, Gruber H, Kern H, Stohr H, Thoma H. Functional electrostimulation of paraplegics: Experimental investigations and first clinical experience with an implantable stimulation device. Orthopedics. 1984;7(7):1145-60

[28] Brindley GS, Polkey CE, Rushton DN. Electrical splinting of the knee in paraplegia. Paraplegia. 1979;16(4):428-37

[29] Kobetic R, Triolo RJ, Uhlir JP, Bieri C, Wibowo M, Polando G, Marsolais EB, Davis JA Jr, Ferguson KA. Implanted functional electrical stimulation system for mobility in paraplegia: A follow-up case report. IEEE Trans Rehabil Eng. 1999;7(4):390-98. DOI: 10.1109/86.808942

[30] Von Wild K, Rabischong P, Brunelli G, Benichou M, Krishnan K. Computer added locomotion by implanted electric stimulation in paraplegic patients (SUAW). Acta Neurochir Suppl. 2001;79:99-104.

[31] Guiraud D, Stieglitz T, Koch KP, Divoux JL, Rabischong P. An implantable neuroprosthesis for standing and walking in paraplegia: 5-year patient follow-up. J Neural Eng. 2006; 3(4):268-75. DOI:10.1088/1741-2560/3/4/003

[32] Kobetic R, To CS, Schnellenberger JR, Audu ML, Bulea TC, Gaudio R, Pinault G, Tashman S, Triolo RJ. Development of hybrid orthosis for standing, walking, and stair climbing after spinal cord injury. J Rehabil Res Dev. 2009;46:447–62.

[33] Christopher and Dana Reeve Foundation's(32) Paralysis Resource Center http://www.christopherreeve.org/

[34] Tomovic R, Vukobratovic M, Vodovnik L. Hybrid actuators for orthotic systems: Hybrid assistive systems. In: Popovic D, editor. Advances in external control on human extremities. proceedings I-X of the Fourth International Symposium on External Control of Human Extremities; 1972 Aug 28-Sep 2: Dubrovnik, Yugoslavia. Aalborg (Denmark): Center for Sensory-Motion Interaction; 1972.

[35] Moore P, Stallard JS. A clinical review of adult paraplegic patients with complete lesion using the ORLAU Parawalker. Paraplegia. 1991;29:191-96.

[36] Isakov E, Douglas R, Berns P. Ambulation using the reciprocating gait orthosis and functional electrical stimulation. Paraplegia. 1992;30(4):239-45.

[37] Yang L, Granat MH, Paul JP, Condie DN, Rowley DI. Further development of hybrid functional electrical stimulation orthoses. Spinal Cord. 1996;34(10):611-14.

[38] Solomonow M, Aguilar E, Reisin E, Baratta RV, Best R, Coetzee T, D'Ambrosia R. Reciprocating gait orthosis powered with electrical muscle stimulation (RGO II). Part I: Performance evaluation of 70 paraplegic patients. Orthopedics. 1997;20(4):315-24

[39] Nene AV, Jennings SJ. Hybrid paraplegic locomotion with the ParaWalker using intramuscular stimulation: A single subject study. Paraplegia. 1989;27(2):125-32.

[40] Marsolais EB, Kobetic R, Polando G, Ferguson K, Tashman S, Gaudio R, Nandurkar S, Lehneis HR. The Case Western Reserve University hybrid gait orthosis. J Spinal Cord Med. 2000;23(2):100-108.

[41] Kobetic R, Marsolais EB, Triolo RJ, Davy DT, Gaudio R, Tashman S. Development of a hybrid gait orthosis: A case report. J Spinal Cord Med. 2003;26(3):254-58.

[42] Solomonow M, Baratta R, Hirokawa S, Rightor N, Walker W, Beaudette P, Shoji H, D'Ambrosia R. The RGO Generation II: muscle stimulation powered orthosis as a practical walking system for thoracic paraplegics.Orthopedics (1989, 12(10): 1309-1315)

[43] Suzuki K, Mito G, Kawamoto H, Hasegawa Y, Sankai Y. Intention-based walking support for paraplegia patients with Robot Suit HAL. Advanced Robotics. 2007 Dec; 21:1441–1469.

[44] Tsukahara A, Kawanishi R, Hasegawa Y, Sankai Y. Sit-to-Stand and Stand-to-Sit Transfer Support for Complete Paraplegic Patients with Robot Suit HAL. Advanced Robotics. 2010;24:1615–1638.

[45] Neuhaus PD, Noorden JH, Craig TJ, Torres T, Kirschbaum J, Pratt JE. Design and evaluation of Mina: A robotic orthosis for paraplegics. Rehabilitation Robotics (ICORR), 2011 IEEE International Conference; 2011. pp. 1–8

[46] Baker, B., ''Walk of Life,'' The Engineer, Vol. 293, No. 7750, pp. 30–31, June 16, 2008.

[47] Ekso Bionics, Berkeley, California. http://eksobionics.com/

[48] Ragnarsson KT. Functional electrical stimulation after spinal cord injury: current use, therapeutic effects and future directions. Spinal Cord. 2008 Apr;46:255–74

[49] Quintero HA, Farris RJ, Goldfarb M. Control and implementation of a powered lower limb orthosis to aid walking in paraplegic individuals. IEEE Int Conf Rehabil Robot. 2011 Jun;2011:1–6.

[50] Farris RJ, Quintero HA, Goldfarb M. Preliminary Evaluation of a Powered Lower Limb Orthosis to Aid Walking in Paraplegic Individuals. Neural Systems and Rehabilitation Engineering, IEEE Transactions 2011;19:652–659

[51] R. Jailani, M.O. Tokhi and S. Gharooni, 2010. Hybrid Orthosis: The Technology for Spinal Cord Injury. *Journal of Applied Sciences, 10: 2785-2792.*

[52] McClelland M, Andrews BJ, Patrick JH, Freeman PA, El Masri WS. Augmentation of the Oswestry Parawalker orthosis by means of surface electrical stimulation: Gait analysis of three patients. Paraplegia. 1987;25(1):32-38.

[53] Stallard J, Major RE. The influence of orthosis stiffness on paraplegic ambulation and its implications for functional electrical stimulation (FES) walking systems. Prosthet Orthot Int. 1995;19(2):108-14

[54] Petrofsky JS, Smith JB. Physiologic costs of computer-controller walking in persons with paraplegia using a reciprocating-gait orthosis. Arch Phys Med Rehabil. 1991; 72(11):890-96

[55] Edwards BG, Marsolais EB. Metabolic responses to arm ergometry and functional neuromuscular stimulation. J Rehabil Res Dev. 1990;27(2):107-14

[56] Mahoney ET, Bickel CS, Elder C, Black C, Slade JM, Apple D Jr, Dudley GA. Changes in skeletal muscle size and glucose tolerance with electrically stimulated resistance training in subjects with chronic spinal cord injury. Arch Phys Med Rehabil. 2005;86(7):1502-4.

[57] Lew RD. The effects of FNS on disuse osteoporosis. Proceedings of the 10th Annual Conference of Rehabilitation Engineering Society of North America; 1987; San Jose, CA. Washington (DC): RESNA Press; 1987. p. 616-17.

[58] Y Dionyssiotis, G Trovas, A Galanos, P Raptou, N Papaioannou, P Papagelopoulos, K Petropoulou, G P Lyritis (2007) Bone loss and mechanical properties of tibia in spinal cord injured men. *J Musculoskelet Neuronal Interact* 7: 1. 62-68 Jan/Mar

[59] Betz R, Boden B, Triolo R, Mesgarzadeh M, Gardner E, Fife R. Effects of functional electrical stimulation on the joints of adolescents with spinal cord injury. Paraplegia. 1996;34(3):127-36R. J. Weber, "Functional neuromuscular stimulation," in Rehabilitation Medicine: Principles and Practice. Philadelphia, PA: Lippincott, 1993

[60] Brindley G. The first 500 patients with sacral anterior root stimulator implants:General description. Paraplegia.1994;32:795–805

[61] Creasey GH, Grill JH, Hoi SU, et al. An Implantable neuroprosthesis for restoring bladder and bowel control to patients with spinal cord injuries: a multicenter trial. Arch Phys Med Rehabil. 2001;82:1512–1519. doi: 10.1053/apmr.2001.25911.

[62] Heruti RJ, Katz H, Menashe Y, et al. Treatment of male infertility due to spinal cord injury using rectal probe electroejaculation: the Israeli experience. Spinal Cord. 2001;39(3):168–175. doi: 10.1038/sj.sc.3101120.

[63] Finetech Medica, UK. http://finetech-medical.co.uk/

[64] M Possover, J Baekelandt, A Kaufmann, V Chiantera. Spinal Cord (2008) Laparoscopic endopelvic sacral implantation of a Brindley controller for recovery of bladder function in a paralyzed patient. 46; 70-73

[65] J Vastenholt, G Snoek, H Buschman, H van der Aa, E Alleman, M Ijzerman.A 7 year follow-up of sacral anterior root stimulation for bladder control in patients with a spinal cord injury; quality of life and users experiences. Spinal Cord (2003) 41; 397-402.

[66] Duffell LD et.al. (2008) Long-term intensive electrically stimulated cycling by spinal cord-injured people: effect on muscle properties and their relation to power output. Muscle Nerve, 38(4):1304-11.

[67] Janssen TWJ et.al. (1998) Clinical efficacy of electrical stimulation exercise training: effects on health, fitness and function. Topics in Spinal Cord Injury Rehabilitation, 3, 33-49

[68] Mohr T et.al. (1997) Long term adaption to electrically induced cycle training in severe spinal cord injured individuals. Spinal Cord, 35(1):1-16.

[69] Baldi JC, et.al. (1998) Muscle atrophy is prevented in patients with acute spinal cord injury using functional electrical stimulation. Spinal Cord, 36(7):463-9.

[70] Demchak TJ, et.al. (2005) Effects of functional electric stimulation cycle ergometry training on lower limb musculature in acute SCI individuals. J Sports Science Med, 4, 263-271.

[71] Sloan KE, et.al. (1994) Musculoskeletal effects on an electrical stimulation induced cycling programme in the spinal injured. Paraplegia, 32(6):407-15.

[72] Krause P, et.al. (2008) Changes in spastic muscle tone increase in patients with spinal cord injury using functional electrical stimulation and passive leg movements. Clinical Rehali, 22(7), 627-34.

[73] Van der Salm A, et.al. (2006) Comparison of electric stimulation methods for reduction of triceps suraespasticity in spinal cord injury. Arch Phys Med Rehabil, 87(2): 222-8.

[74] Griffin L, et.al. (2009). Functional electrical stimulation cycling improves body composition, metabolic and neural factors in persons with spinal cord injury. J Electromyogr Kinesiol. 19(4):614-22.

[75] Berry HR, et.al. (2008) Cardio-respiratory and power adaptations to stimulated cycle training in paraplegia.Medicine & Science in Sports & Exercise, 40(0), 1573-1580.

[76] Hettinga DM, Andrews BJ (2008). Oxygen consumption during functional electrical stimulation-assisted exercise in persons with spinal cord injury: implications for fitness and health. Sports Med, 38(10), 825-38.

[77] Gerrits HL, et.al. (2001) Peripheral vascular changes after electrically stimulated cycle training in people with spinal cord injury. Arch Phys Med Rehabil, 82(6):832-9.

[78] Janssen TWJ et.al. (1998) Clinical efficacy of electrical stimulation exercise training: effects on health, fitness and function. Topics in Spinal Cord Injury Rehabilitation, 3, 33-49.

Section 3

Complications and Special Musculoskeletal Issues in Paraplegia

Chapter 6

Malnutrition in Paraplegia

Yannis Dionyssiotis

Additional information is available at the end of the chapter

http://dx.doi.org/10.5772/58382

1. Introduction

Despite the advances in medical and nutritional science surveys show that 40-50% of patients admitted to hospitals are at risk of nutritional deficiency; one in three hospitalized patients are malnourished upon admission and up to 12% are severely malnourished [1, 2]. Malnutrition is a state in which a deficiency, excess or imbalance of energy, protein and other nutrients causes adverse effects on body form, function and clinical outcome [3, 4]. Studies report a variable prevalence of obesity from 40 to 66% in persons with SCI completing the spectrum of newly introduced concept in nutritional deficiency [5, 6, 7].

After the lesion paralysis and loss of function that usually occur and well documented hypercatabolic responses may lead to deleterious effects such as loss of lean body mass, obesity, increased susceptibility to infections, and reduced wound healing [5, 8, 9]. Unwanted weight gain should be prevented because induces the risk for diseases such as diabetes, coronary heart disease and dyslipidaimias in this population [8]. Mortality and pathogenesis of critically ill patients are affected by nutritional status. Body fat has been identified as a significant predictor of mortality. Moreover, some disorders such as carbohydrate intolerance, insulin resistance, lipid abnormalities, and heart disease occur prematurely and at a higher prevalence in disabled populations may be related to immobilization and skeletal muscle denervation [10]. According to the above the term malnutrition should include not only undernourishment but also obesity [11]. Therefore, the objective should be either the maintenance of optimal nutritional status of the patient, either to supplement the deficiencies in nutrients. Nutrition support therapy should be tailored to each patient. An optimal nutritional assessment and management of the disabled subject can minimize the complications associated with acute traumatic injury and long-term rehabilitation [12].

This chapter reviews methods of nutritional assessment and describes the physiopathological mechanisms of malnutrition, reviews specific nutritional studies, and the supplemental support which can be used in paraplegic subjects.

2. Nutritional assessment

For an initial assessment of nutritional status serial measurements to assess trends over time and then monitor the response to a dietary intervention may be useful. The proposed assessments should be interpreted collectively including the examination of possible factors that contribute to the nutritional status, such as age, sex, over-or under-hydration, interactions between drugs-food, metabolic stress, infection, and the existence of other diseases[13].

2.1. Diet history

During hospitalization adequate intake of nutrients is intercepted by many factors, and may be caused by anorexia, early satiety, immobility, depression. Moreover, gastrointestinal function is compromised: gastric dilatation and paralytic ileus occurs often, although the intestinal activity usually returns within the first week after injury.

2.2. Nutritional requirements

The provision of energy and nutritional requirements is a very important factor for patient management. Malnutrition, in this case undernourishment or over nutrition-obesity, can lead to muscle loss, atrophy of the lining of the intestine, immunochemical reduction, poor wound healing and fluid overload, hyperglycemia, high levels of urea nitrogen in blood, high triglycerides, elevated liver enzymes, respiratory exhaustion due to increased production of CO_2, and difficulty weaning from the oxygen, respectively. The assessment of nutritional requirements includes not only calculations but also the opinion of an expert clinician in order to assess the clinical and morphometric data before applying the equations that provide the energy and protein requirements [14].

There have been several methods for predicting energy expenditure (EE); the components and the methods for its determination and estimation, summarizing their main advantages and limitations have been recently reviewed [15]. However, because of various confusing factors such as infections and sepsis, hyper nutrition supportive nutritional diets, clinical procedures, postoperative medications, and changes in body weight such as sarcopenia, obesity, amputations and significant weight loss, the prediction equations can be complex and invalid [16].

A group of equations among these are Mifflin–St Jeor equation [17], the Harris-Benedict equation [18], the American College of Chest Physicians (ACCP) recommendation based on kcal/kg body weight [19], the Faisy equation [20], the Ireton-Jones equations [21, 22] and the Penn State equations [23, 24]. Because the Mifflin equation was designed for healthy people is not analyzed here.

The Harris-Benedict is calculated by sex with the following formula:

Men: Resting Metabolic Rate (RMR) (kcal/d)=67+Body Weight x 13.75+Height x 5 – Age x 6.8 [18, 24].

Women: RMR (kcal/d)=655+Body Weight x 9.6+Height x 1.85 – Age x 4.7 [25].

Ideal body weight is calculated by the Hamwi rule of thumb while metabolically active weight (MAW) is calculated as 25% of excess weight (actual weight – ideal weight) added to the ideal body weight [26]. The Ireton-Jones equations include one specifically for obese patients and one for general critical care populations:

Obesity: RMR (kcal/d)=Wt x 9+Gender x 606 – Age x 12+1844 [27].

Nonobese: RMR (kcal/d)=Wt x 5 – Age x 10+Gender x 281+Trauma x 292+1925 (for gender: male=1, female=0) [28].

To determine accurately the early energy expenditure after spinal cord injury, studies compared measurements of real resting energy expenditure (REE) with the Harris-Benedict equation (basic energy expenditure, BEE) [18]. During the first two weeks after the injury, the exact measurements of REE are similar to the estimated calorie needs, when used with BEE stressor/injury factor of 1.6. To avoid overestimation of calorie needs, the deletion of factor activity of 1.2 (rest in bed) is proposed. Kearns et al. reported that in 10 patients, the mean REE after acute injury was only 67% of BEE predicted by Harris-Benedict formula. They hypothesized that non-specific changes in neurogenic stimuli and reduced oxygen consumption by relaxing muscles contributed to their findings. Also, an interesting feature observed is that the REE was raised by 5% with the return of muscle tone [29]. Jeejeboy and Cerra proposed an alternative approach that uses body weight (kg) alone as a determining factor, and omits the variables of age, sex and height as used in HB equation. This type of assessment has proven to be accurate and efficient over time [30, 31]. Ireton-Jones and Owen et al. have developed specific formulas for the obese patient, which is common in SCI subjects. The predefined types may overestimate their needs due to increased fat mass in this population [21, 22, 32].

2.3. Assessment of subjects in the clinical setting

Patients admitted in the hospital should be examined for actual or potential occurrence of malnutrition because of an unintentional weight loss or gain. In the clinic this examination includes measurements of body weight depicting a loss of more than 10% of normal body weight within 6 months or loss of more than 5% of usual body weight within 1 month or 20% more or less than ideal body weight (IBW), calculation of body mass index (BMI) <18, depletion of visceral protein (serum albumin <3.5 g/dl, serum transferrin <200 mg/dl, serum cholesterol <160 mg/dl, serum pre – albumin <15 mg/ml, creatinine height index (CHI) <75% (measured by 24-hour creatinine excretion, which is typically associated with muscle mass of the patient as an indicator of malnutrition, especially in young men), and the presence of diet modifications (patient receives total parenteral nutrition (TPN) or enteral nutrition (EN), inadequate food intake due instructions for stopping any food by mouth (NPO), liquid diet, disorders of absorption, reduced swallowing capacity, increased metabolic needs, gastrointestinal disturbances (nausea, vomiting, diarrhea, constipation). Unintentional weight gain is an increase in body weight that occurs when a person takes in more calories than the body needs or uses [33, 34].

For able bodied persons the World Health Organization (WHO) advocates use of BMI as a population-level indicator of obesity which is not a direct measure of body fat, but a more accurate indicator of overweight and obesity than relying on weight alone. BMI is calculated using the equation weight (Kg)/height (m^2), which is a very practical and useful measure that allows the easy determination of categories of weight status. In able-bodied subjects overweight is defined as a BMI of 25–29.9 kg/m^2 and obesity as a BMI of ≥30.0 kg/m^2 and extreme obesity≥40 kg/m^2 (Table 1) [35, 36].

Classification	**BMI (kg/m²)**	**Obesity Category**
Underweight	<18.5	-
Normal	18.5-24.9	-
Overweight	25.0-29.9	-
Obesity	30, 0-34, 9	I
Moderate obesity	35.0-39.9	II
Extreme obesity	> 40.0	III

Table 1. Classifications based on the weight for BMI and obesity category (published with permission from Dionyssiotis Y. [36])

In a chronic SCI population with paraplegia values of body mass index (BMI, kg/m^2) were not significant vs. controls, which is a finding in line with the literature [10, 37]. Nevertheless, Gupta et al demonstrated the usefulness of BMI as an indicator of obesity [38]. Whether the criteria of BMI may assess obesity in people with spinal cord injury the latest studies show the opposite [39]. The applicability of conventional BMI cut off values is into question [40, 41]. Another critical issue is that the relationship between BMI and disease is typically U-or J-shaped with those in the middle categories of BMI having the lowest risk compared to the lowest extreme and upper levels of BMI. It is under question if the cut-points for underweight, normal, overweight, and obese used in able-bodied populations can be applied to disabled subjects [42]. Not many studies investigated BMI in patients with MS. Nevertheless, BMI was found statistically less compared to age comparable controls [43].

Anthropometric standards such as the ideal body weight (IBW), the triceps skin fold thickness and the middle arm circumference which are common tools for assessment of nutrition may not be valid for disabled subjects due to water changes, atrophy of muscles because of immobility, increased body fat, and the inevitable weight loss beyond the normal. Patients' early weight loss is mainly due to loss of muscle rather than fat which bias the results of validity. In chronic paraplegics, the ideal weight has been estimated to be 4.5 to 6.5 kg below their respective controls finding which is in line with our recently published results [37]. Indeed, height and weight measurements are the key elements in nutritional assessment. The IBW is determined by the height. No matter which method of calculation is used, the IBW should be adjusted for body type (frame sizes: small-IBW 10% reduction, middle size-no changes required, large size-IBW increased by 10%) and spinal cord injury (paraplegia-decrease IBW by 10-15%, tetraplegia-by 15-20%, respectively). The weight in admission is probably the most reliable measure of weight in determining the actual body weight (ABW) of the patient because is unreliable postoperatively or during an acute illness due to administration of fluids or due to edematous condition. As a chronic index, one can assume that the weight gain or loss is associated with an increase or decrease in lean body mass. To determine the weight which should be used on the nutritional calculations, first % IBW should be calculated through the equation: % IBW=actual body weight (actual body weight, ABW / ideal body weight (IBW) x 100. If the actual body weight (ABW) is less than IBW, use ABW, to define the nutritional requirements, if is greater than IBW, but less than 120%, it is necessary to determine nutritional needs using the adjusted relationship of body weight in the calculation needs: IBW+(ABW-IBW x 0.25). The nutritional status of patients can be categorized according to their ABW as a percentage of IBW as follows: over 200% of IBW (pathologic obesity), over 150% of IBW (obese), more than 120% IBW (overweight), 100% of IBW+/-10% (normal), 80-90% of IBW (mildly malnourished), 70-80% of IBW (moderately malnourished), less than 70% of IBW (severe nutritional deficiency–malnutrition), respectively [1].

3. Biochemical measurements

As with the visceral and somatic visceral proteins, non-dietary factors (i.e. blood loss, chronic infections, and fluid overload) should be considered as potential reasons for the reduction of serum concentrations [1]. Proteins are essential for tissue growth, maintenance and rebuilding their synthesis of hormones, enzymes, antibodies and cells transport molecules. In cases of protein excess protein is either metabolized for energy or stored as fat. The recommendations for protein intake in patients with spinal cord injury vary with respect to acute or chronic phase of the lesion and the presence of decubitus ulcers or not. Specific proteins (albumin, transferrin, and pre-albumin) are biochemical indicators used for assessing nutritional status [44].

The level of serum albumin is not a definitive measure of visceral protein status, but reflects the complex relationship between synthesis, degradation, and distribution. Given the long half-life of 21 days, serum albumin cannot be effectively used for monitoring the acute response to nutritional therapy. Therefore, albumin levels should be included in the initial profile for food control and monitoring purposes during hospitalization for measuring trends of visceral protein or as an indicator of chronic nutritional status. Beside this limitation there are many non-dietary factors that reduce the levels of albumin, regardless of nutritional status (inadequate composition: acute stress, hypoxia, impaired digestion, as in malabsorption, modified status as edematous fluid status and fluid overload, chronic loss of protein) (Table 2) [36].

Albumin (g/dl)	3.5-5	3-3.5	<3.5	<3.0	<2.5
nutritional status	normal	point that dietary intervention should be revised or adjusted	associated with poor outcome of surgery, rising costs of hospitalization and prolonged stay in ICU	severe malnutrition	increased morbidity and mortality

Table 2. Basic levels of albumin and nutritional status distribution (published with permission from Dionyssiotis Y. [36])

Due to the lower half-life (8-9 days) and the smaller size as a constituent body, transferrin is a better indicator of nutritional status of visceral protein from albumin. Normal levels of transferrin are between 200-400 mg/dl, and 150 mg/dl are considered nutritionally decision point or a point where nutritional support should be revised or adjusted. The transferrin levels are reduced in impaired synthesis as chronic infections, increased secretion, fluid overload, increased iron stores and increased in reduced iron stores as iron deficiency anemia and chronic blood loss, increased protein synthesis on estrogen therapy and oral contraception and dehydration. The serum concentration of transferrin is approximately 0.8 times the total iron binding capacity (TIBC). If direct measurement of transferrin is not possible due to the high cost and limited availability of equipment required, the level of transferrin can be easily calculated from TIBC, using the following formula: TIBC x 0.8-43=transferrin [45].

The third protein biochemical indicator is pre-albumin, which has very short half-life (2 days), making it an excellent nutritional index and due to this reason is increasingly used as an indicator of response to nutritional therapy. Reference values for pre-albumin are 16-35 mg/dl. A value of dietary intervention is 11 mg/dl because a value below this level means malnutrition. The failure of patients to increase pre-albumin above 11 mg/dl with dietary therapy is an indication that nutritional needs are not met. Concentrations should increase about 1 mg/dl per day or twice a week when the treatment is the appropriate. Non-dietary factors that reduce pre-albumin include stress, inflammation [46, 47, 48].

Physical measurements include protein nitrogen balance studies and measurement of creatinine / height index (CHI). Nitrogen balance studies measure the net change in total body protein. An assessment of nitrogen balance can be achieved by measurement of urinary urea (UUN) and compare it with the intake of nitrogen at the same time. The nitrogen balance is calculated as follows: N_2=balance intake N_2-N_2 elimination or=[protein (gr)]-(24 hour UUN+3) [6.25 gr nitrogen]. An "agent" of 3 is added to the equation for nitrogen losses in feces, skin, and the drainage of body fluids. When calculating the nitrogen balance a value of 0 meaning nitrogen balance (healthy adults), nitrogen balance> 0 (protein anabolism exceeds catabolism, usually consistent with pregnancy, growth, and recovery from disease or may indicate nutrient saturation, the goal in nutrition replenishment is a positive nitrogen balance of 4-6 grams per day and nitrogen balance <0 (the protein catabolism exceeds protein anabolism, occurs in situations of famine, increased catabolism due to trauma or surgery, and inadequate nutrition therapy), respectively. CHI measures the 24-hour creatinine excretion in urine and compares with an optimum value based on the ideal weight for height [49].

4. Malnutrition screening tools

Screening is important for the early detection of patients who are undernourished or at risk of developing malnutrition. Since January 2010, the Dutch Health Care Inspectorate (HCI) has defined under nutrition as a main care problem in rehabilitation centres, by establishing it as a Performance Indicator for Risk Steering Supervision. Dutch rehabilitation centres are now obligated to screen all rehabilitants for under nutrition on admission The Short Nutritional Assessment Questionnaire (SNAQ) is the recommended screening tool in this benchmark (Figure 1) [50]. However, various screening tools have been developed to detect a patient's nutritional status in many healthcare settings, but not in the rehabilitation setting. In the Netherlands, the SNAQ [51] and the Malnutrition Universal Screening Tool (MUST) are used for the hospital situation [52, 53]. The HCI advises the use of the SNAQ for under nutrition screening in rehabilitation centres [51]. Our results suggest the use of the SNAQ65+as a screening tool. This tool showed the best diagnostic accuracy of the quick and easy screening tools investigated (sensitivity 96%, specificity 77%) [52, 54].

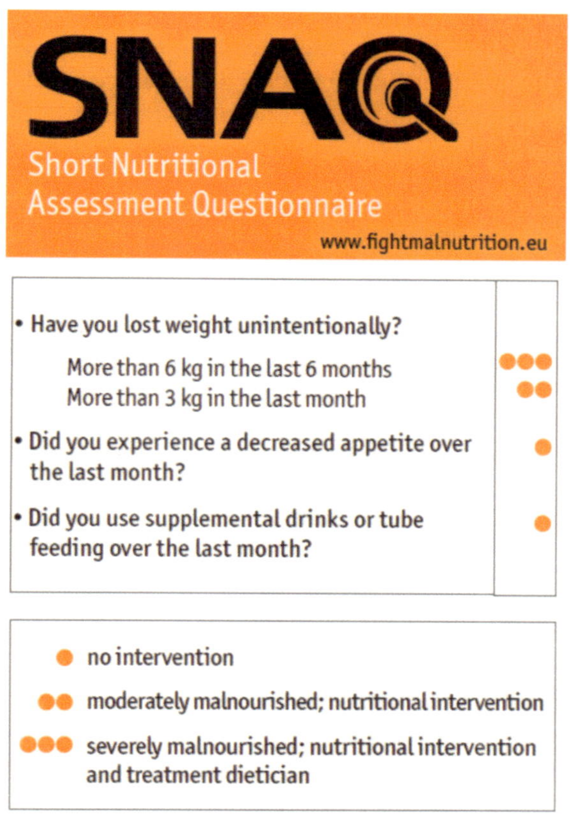

Figure 1. The Short Nutritional Assessment Questionnaire (SNAQ). Published with permission from: http://www.fight-malnutrition.eu/fight-malnutrition/screening-tools/

5. Monitoring

Healthcare professionals with relevant skills and training should review the indications, route, risks, benefits and goals of nutrition support at regular intervals. The time between reviews depends on the patient, care setting and duration of nutrition support. Intervals may increase as the patient is stabilised on nutrition support [55]. (NICE Clinical Guideline 32 Feb.2006 Nutrition Support in Adults: Oral Nutrition Support, Enteral Tube Feeding and Parenteral Nutrition, the whole guideline can be downloaded from: http://www.nice.org.uk/nicemedia/live/10978/29979/29979.pdf)

6. Physiopathological mechanisms of malnutrition

6.1. Malnutrition in the acute phase of paraplegia

Pathophysiological mechanisms of malnutrition in paraplegia are multifactorial. There is a dramatic increase in energy expenditure, endogenous protein catabolism and nitrogen excretion after lesion-injury. Extensive multiple organ trauma, soft tissue injuries and fractures, may further increase hyper catabolic reactions. Also, the body temperature and energy expenditure increases due to pulmonary infections or urinary tract infractions, and pancreatitis. The metabolic rate does not seem to be affected by the small reductions in thyroxin levels in plasma observed after the injury [56, 57].

Metabolic changes are also present with the elevated catabolic hormonal and cytokine responses including increased blood levels of counter regulatory hormones (e.g., cortisol, catecholamines, and glucagon), increased blood and tissue levels of proinflammatory cytokines (i.e., interleukin-1, interleukin-6, interleukin-8, and tumor necrosis factor α), and peripheral-tissue resistance to endogenous anabolic hormones (i.e., insulin and insulin-like growth factor 1) to be primarily responsible for the initial changes in metabolism [58-61].

Glucose intolerance, which cannot be readily apparent during the acute phase, but may be caused by complications and physiological processes of acute care such as the initial hyper metabolic-catabolic stress response, administration of steroids, the parenteral / enteral nutrition, and atrophy as a consequence of aponeurosis which results in gluconeogenesis [62]. Glucose and lipid metabolism disrupt in acute post-traumatic phase. Increased hepatic gluconeogenesis and regional response to insulin result in hyperglycemia. The metabolism of glucose in combination with acute nerve injury has been studied extensively, especially as related to ischemia. These studies suggest that hyperglycemia which follows immediately after head injury or spinal cord may worsen the outcome. High serum glucose levels increase the availability of substrate for anaerobic glycolysis, and thus the production of lactic acid, which may have the reverse effect on neurological recovery from injury. The prevention of hyperglycemia, particularly during the first 2 to 8 hours after injury, seems to be very critical for optimal recovery. After 2 to 8 hours after injury, elevated glucose levels may be beneficial, allowing the beginning of intestinal or parenteral feedings in a short time after the injury. It is also likely the serum triglyceride levels to be found elevated due to the accelerated lipogenesis, decreased lipoprotein lipase activity, and impaired clearance of triglycerides [63]. Glucose is the preferred energy molecule for the central nervous system, red blood cells, the cellular tissue, etc. A minimum quantity of 100-150 gr glucose per day is required for these functions and prevents the consumption of endogenous protein. The normal rate at which the body metabolizes carbohydrates or glucose is approximately 2-4 mg/ Kg/min. In times of severe stress, glucose metabolism may be increased to 3-5 mg/Kg/min. In most patients, administration of more than 400-500 gr glucose per day, exceeding the body's ability to metabolize and stored as energy. Sources of glucose include not only the liquid diet and peritoneal fluid filtration. Excess glucose is converted into fat (lipogenesis) and leads to an increased ratio of VCO_2/VO_2 (or RQ) [64].

The provision of lipids as a source of increased calories can facilitate protein maintenance, reduce the risk of excessive carbohydrates and reduce the total volume of liquid. Lipids are required to account for 30% of total calories supplied. In the acute phase after injury, large amounts of fat, especially as linoleic or omega-6 fatty acids have an immunosuppressive effect by triggering the release of arachidonic acid. This leads to synthesis of prostaglandins and then compresses the delayed hypersensitivity cell-regulated, proliferation of lymphocytes. In the presence of sepsis, high levels of serum triglycerides (250 gr/ml) indicate limited tolerance and decreased need for intravenous fluid delivery. A minimum of 4% of total energy requirements is necessary for the essential fatty acids to avoid deficiencies [65]. Unfortunately, although the hormonal cataract through increases in glycogenolysis and gluconeogenesis, is enhancing lipolysis, which provides endogenous glucose, amino acids, and free fatty acids that are required for cellular and organ function and wound healing and certain plasma levels of substrates are increased (i.e., glutamine) they could be insufficient to meet metabolic needs due to limited availability for use by peripheral tissues (because of factors such as insulin resistance and inhibition of lipoprotein lipase) [60, 61].

Acute post-traumatic nitrogen requirements are much higher than in normal state. Another serious metabolic issue is negative nitrogen balance, due to excessive secretion of nitrogen because of protein use by the body to meet energy needs in the first week, with a peak at 3 weeks and can last for a period of 7 weeks. This imbalance will respond only slightly increased protein intake and may be non-modifiable as a process during the acute phase. The more severe the injury the greater the amount of nitrogen excreted. The accelerated catabolism of muscle mass results in a supply of amino acids for the acute-phase of protein synthesis, gluconeogenesis, and the healing of wounds. Moreover, administration of glucocorticosteroids after injury may increase the catabolism of protein. The losses of nitrogen in the urine, mainly due to muscle atrophy because of paralysis, are increasing with the severity of the injury. On the other side, Cooper and Hoen stated that the secretion of more than 25 gr/day of nitrogen in the urine during the first two weeks after the injury is insufficient prognostic indicator for functional recovery of paralyzed muscles. The nitrogen losses after an injury are always present and last at least 7 weeks. In cases of acute injury, despite the provision of sufficient quantities of calories and protein usually occurs a negative nitrogen balance (NB), which peaks during the third week after injury. The same phenomenon has been observed in cases of severe poisoning with botulinum toxin (botulism) which resulted in paralysis of muscles. Negative nitrogen balance following injury, has been associated with further findings. During the first weeks after injury, many patients experience a transient positive nitrogen balance, possibly due to initial delays in the loss of nitrogen [66]. Four conscientious objectors were immobilized on pelvic corset and leg casts for 6 to 7 weeks in a metabolic chamber. All 4 subjects showed an increase in nitrogen excretion and negative nitrogen balance. However, it took 4 to 5 days to develop. In conclusion, acute immobilization of paralyzed patients contributes to increased excretion of nitrogen which starts about a week after the injury [67].

Deficiencies in zinc and vitamin C have been associated with poor wound healing. The provision of these micronutrients supplementation in patients with these deficits enhances the healing. Adequate quantities of salts and vitamins are usually provided in a balanced diet. The supplemental micro-nutrient dietary substances are necessary if we suspect shortcomings intake or increased requirements because of circumstances specific diseases. Zinc is often prescribed to improve stress ulcers, is known to be involved in structural integrity of collagen. However, zinc levels in serum is similar in patients taking supplements that contain sulfur (220 mg daily) and do not affect the healing process of ulcers sprawling over a period of 2-3 months. Opposite physiological effects, such as metabolism of copper, copper deficiency and anemia may be caused by long-term supplementation of large amounts of zinc [68]. The role of vitamin C in collagen synthesis is crucial. Although the supplementation with vitamin C did not accelerate the healing of decubitus ulcers in patients, dietary intake of vitamin C has not been associated with the development of decubitus ulcers. Moreover, given that the subclinical deficiencies are difficult to show up, the minimum recommended dietary intake is proposed to 60mg [69]. Excessive excretion of potassium and abnormal hyponatremia; hypercalcemia, due to immobilization, particularly in young men and hypercalciuria exceed the normal range in 4 weeks, with higher values at 16 weeks, which can persist for a long time. Hypercalcemia occurs with anorexia, abdominal cramps, nausea, vomiting, constipation, polydipsia, polyuria, dehydration and did not respond to diets which restrict the intake of calcium and need to be treated with medication, hydration, and mobilization [70].

Finally the effect of drugs such as analgesics and barbiturates is crucial. Drugs that are frequently administered to acute paraplegic patients may themselves increase skeletal-muscle breakdown (corticosteroids), decrease splanchnic blood flow (pressor agents), or increase urinary loss of electrolytes, minerals, and water-soluble vitamins (diuretics). Infection, operative trauma, and other stresses may increase energy expenditure and protein and micronutrient needs [71-74]. The average daily dietary needs are modified because of the altered physiology of each body system and psychological integrity of a patient susceptible to an injury, potentially at any age, which cannot exclude the possibility of a pre-existing disease causing nutritional problems [75].

Moreover, the frequent coexistence of injuries from other systems, such as brain injury, maxillofacial injuries, fractures, etc., disturbs the normal physiology further. Studies in malnourished patients stated that malnutrition before a spine stabilization surgery is leading to postoperative complications, hyperthermia, which increases the caloric needs of the patient, and denervation, leading to atrophy and paralysis, which supply amino acids for gluconeogenesis, which, in turn, supplies glucose to meet caloric needs [1].

Serum hemoglobin and hematocrit may reflect a general state of malnutrition. Anemia, defined by low hemoglobin levels (<14 mg/dl) and hematocrit (<36%) reduces the oxygen in the blood and impedes the wound healing. Anemia may be due to a preexisting condition or as the result of unbalanced production and distribution of blood cells as a result of reaction to stress, gastrointestinal bleeding or obvious bleeding due to other trauma [76]. Low levels of total serum protein (<6.4 mg/dl) and protein (<3.5 mg/dl), accelerate the development of edema, which causes a decrease in skin elasticity and prevent the transfer of oxygen and nutrients from the blood to the skin. Also, the swelling may increase local tissue pressure, causing loss of regional blood flow and tissue damage. The loss of protein and protein secretion in pressure ulcers increases the deficiencies in proteins. The paralytic ileus occurs as a result of disturbance of the autonomic and simultaneous or ischemia as a complication of hypokalemia, abdominal trauma or sepsis, generally persists for 72 hours-1 week and may restrict the movement of the diaphragm [77]. Parenteral nutrition is indicated if paralytic ileus persists for more than 3-5 days. Ulcers and bleeding, which occur as a result of paralytic vasodilatation with ischemia, steroids, nasogastric tube irritation, and other causes should be treated with oral or enteral feeding as soon as possible but may require parenteral nutrition [78].

6.2. Malnutrition in the chronic phase of paraplegia and during aging

During aging with paraplegia other complications are added in the physiopathological context of "malnourished paraplegics".

A neglected factor is muscle tonus: hypotonia (low muscle tone, floppiness) results in a lower resistance to muscle movement. The lower the resistance, the fewer calories burned during movement. Furthermore, hypertonia (high muscle tone, spasticity) is limiting muscle movement and reduces caloric needs. Lack of movement results in muscle atrophy and a lower lean body mass, which in turn reduces the number of calories burned even at rest [79].

In spinal cord injured subjects is mainly central or abdominal obesity leading to metabolic, cardiovascular issues etc. There is conflicting evidence about the contribution of visceral and subcutaneous adipose tissue to different metabolic disorders after SCI. Moreover subjects with longstanding disabilities (i.e. spinal cord injury) are at increased risk for cardiovascular disease and cardiopulmonary disease because of extensive fat intake and limiting activities. In generally, subjects with disabilities are prone to developing vitamin D deficiency. Earlier work by Bauman et al suggested that approximately 32% of veterans with spinal cord injury (SCI) were absolutely deficient in vitamin D (25 hydroxyvitamin D [25(OH)D]). Most subjects have a high incidence of vitamin D deficiency as defined by levels of 25(OH)D<20 ng/mL. The reasons might be due to a combination of low dietary vitamin D intake and avoiding sun exposure because of depression or sensitivity in drugs i.e. dantrolene [80]. The low intake of vitamin D, which is supplied by food either in vitamin D2 (ergocalciferol, activated ergosterol), found in yeast, or vitamin D3 (cholecalciferol), found in fish, can be bypassed through supplements [81].

Moreover, reduced mobility and immobilization for long period cause pressure ulcers of the skin and the wound but can be prevented by adequate intake of quantity of protein, vitamin E, zinc, and fluids to maintain skin integrity [82].

Pneumonia and paralysis of respiratory muscles through malnutrition may further weaken the respiratory muscles. On the other site excessive feeding may lead to increased oxidation of glucose and production of carbon dioxide to be eliminated and further stress on the respiratory system. The fluid overload or aggressive implementation of parenteral support can lead to pulmonary edema. The reduced hydration can lead to reduced drainage of secretions, atelectasis, and pneumonia. Abdominal distension due to unabsorbed food by mouth or enteral feeding or swallowing air during feeding can lead to compromise the functioning of the diaphragm and predisposes to hypoventilation or aspiration [83]. Neurogenic bowel requires the right amount of food, fiber and fluids in order to be successful retraining of the bowel, and prevent constipation, diarrhea, incontinence, and autonomic dysreflexia as a result of fecal impaction. Bowel function may be compromised by hyperosmolar feeding through a tube, lactose intolerance or pseudomembranous colitis, prolonged treatment with antibiotics, which can cause diarrhea and require parenteral nutritional support. For neurogenic bladder vitamin C and other supplements are necessary for the acidification of urine and prevention of infection of the urinary tract.

7. The nutritional support

The provision of a nutritional supplement is definitely not a frontline management technique for poor oral intake. Supplements when administered correctly to patients can easily optimize nutrition and should be an adjunctive to nutrition.

Per os feeding is recommended for patients who are weaned from tracheal tubes, which are awakened, may follow commands and have good swallowing and intestinal function. Patients with central nervous system (CNS) acute diseases are frequently in coma or have their swallowing reflexes impaired and need parenteral nutrition or enteral tube feeding [84, 85]. Enteral nutrition (EN) is recommended for patients who are tubed, not able to swallow or to receive adequate diet orally but have good bowel function.

Early nutrition support through the enteral route has been shown to blunt catabolism, reduce complications and reduce length of stay in a number of patient populations, including both surgical and non-surgical neuro patients [86, 87]. However, nutrition support must be initiated within the 48-to 72-hour period immediately following injury or surgical insult to achieve these benefits. Clinicians are often hesitant to feed critically ill neuro patients too soon. However, studies indicate patients with severe neurological deficits and clinically silent abdomens can tolerate low-rate jejunal feedings within 36 hours of injury with a gradual increase in feeding rate to meet initial caloric goals within two to four days [88, 89]. If jejunal feedings are initiated prior to induction of pentobarbital infusion, even patients in pentobarbital coma can be fed enterally [90].

Nasogastric or nasoenteric feeding tubes should not be used for periods longer than 4 weeks because of discomfort and the risk of nasal injury and sinusitis. Placement of a percutaneous endoscopic gastrostomy (PEG) tube should be considered for patients who continue to require enteral feeding beyond 4 weeks[90]. PeG is also indicated as firstline intervention in conditions

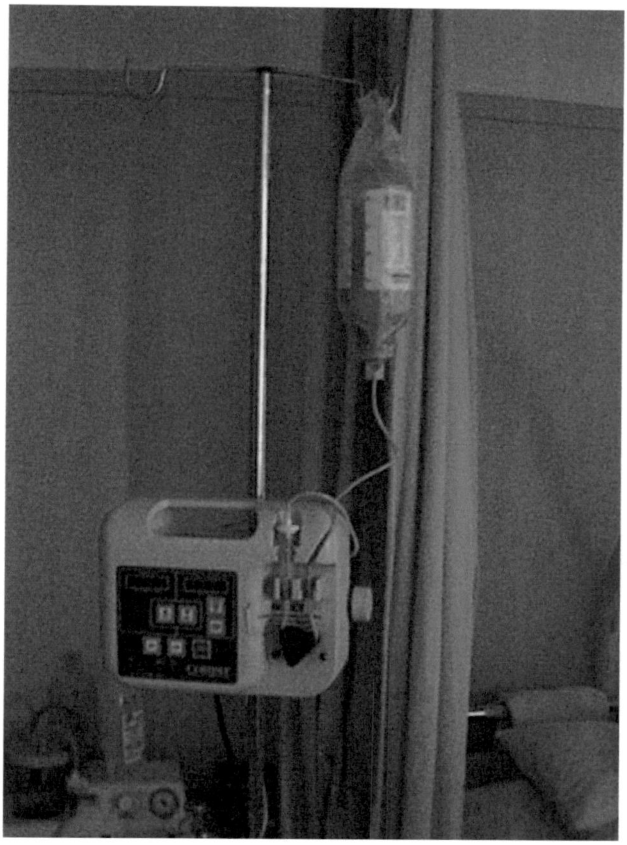

Figure 2. The enteral feeding pump type COMPAT (unpublished photo courtesy of Dionyssiotis Y). The system is a relatively simple, lightweight, easy to use for managing all types of enteral feeding. Have an audible and visual alarm that alerts you when each of the following conditions: empty container feeding, low battery, change the dose, or the existence of j free flow out of the system (waste). The memory of the pump retains infusion rate, volume delivered, dose limit even after turning it off. It is designed to provide precision dosing. Start enteral feeding schedule and progress.

where enteral feeding is expected to be required for longer than 2–4 weeks, for example in patients with acute stroke [91]. Although complications of PEG tube feeding are rare in stable patients, they become increasingly common in critically ill and debilitated patients. One of most feared complication of enteral feeding: aspiration hypoxia/ pneumonia. Clinically, gastric residual volume (GRV) measurement was frequently used as marker to predict aspiration & pneumonia. Elevated GRV: associated with comorbidities such as vasopressor use, sedation sepsis, vomiting. GRV: no significance between GRV> 200ml and GRV> 400ml, low sensitivity as a marker of aspiration [92].

With increasing frequency, nasogastric feeding tubes are replaced by PEG to provide semi-long-term enteral nutrition because of various advantages of a PEG in daily use [93-95]. In contrast to a nasogastric feeding tube, PEG does not interfere with the swallowing mechanism, which reduces the possibility of choking, especially when oral feeding is initiated during neurological recovery. The cosmetic advantage of a PEG, which can be worn invisibly underneath the patients' clothes, may play a psychological role during recovery. PEG placement is associated with a mortality rate of 1-3 per cent, major complication rates of 3-9 per cent and minor complication rates of 5-45 per cent. The risk of aspiration, frequently associated with nasogastric feeding tubes, has not been eliminated with PEG placement [96-100].

Another interesting issue is early compared with late introduction of the feed. With data limited to ICU patients there was no overall difference in mortality rates with either EN or PN with no apparent difference in mortality rates across groups receiving EN or PN (RR 1.08; 95% CI 0.70 to 1.65). As suggested compared with PN, EN was associated with a significant reduction in infectious complications (RR 0.61; 95% CI 0.44 to 0.84; p=0.003). The early compared with late introduction of enteral feed only suggested that early EN was associated with a trend toward a reduction in mortality (RR 0.52; 95% CI 0.25 to 1.08; p=0.08) when compared with delayed nutrient intake and infection risk was not different [101]. The compilation of 11 high quality studies comparing enteral and parenteral nutrition revealed a significant effect in favor of parenteral nutrition [odds ratio (OR) 0.51, 95% confidence interval (CI) 0.27–0.97]. A subgroup analysis of trials comparing parenteral nutrition with early or late enteral feeding showed that there was no survival benefit in parenteral nutrition when enteral nutrition was provided early. The benefit of parenteral nutrition was confined to trials comparing it with late enteral nutrition. Therefore, this metaanalysis confirms at least a finding already reported in earlier metaanalyses: there is no increased mortality risk with parenteral nutrition! [102].

A major concern with EN is the discrepancy between prescribed and delivered amount of nutrient, the major causes of which are diarrhea, vomiting or gastric stasis. Furthermore, enteral nutrient delivery is gradually increased in critically ill patients in order to avoid the possibility of gastrointestinal intolerance, so that a few days are required to achieve the caloric target. Administering the total nutritional requirement of mechanically ventilated medical patients starting on day 1 was associated with greater infectious complications and prolonged length of hospital stay compared to patients in whom a gradual approach was implemented [103]. Despite the caloric deficiency, EN is still superior to PN so that non-energetic effects of EN, such as immune modulation or protection of the intestinal mucosal barrier, seem to be of greater value in the critically ill than the mere energetic supply. The issue of the better enteral access (gastric vs. post-pyloric route) is not yet settled. However, available evidence does not support the routine insertion of post-pyloric tubes as long as the gastric route is effective [104, 105, 106].

Aside from the potential problems associated with receiving in adequate or excessive nutrition or medication therapy, additional injury to the patient may result from using the gut that is at risk for bacterial or candidal translocation. Therefore, enteral nutrition should be started only if the potential benefits outweigh the risks [107, 108].

However, nutritional support is not without adverse effects and risks. Early EN may be associated with high gastric residuals, bacterial colonization of the stomach, and increased risk of aspiration pneumonia. PN has been associated with gut mucosal atrophy, overfeeding, hyperglycemia, an increased risk of infectious complications and increased mortality rates in critically ill patients [104, 105].

8. Transition from parenteral to enteral feeding and vice versa

Malabsorption and maldigestion must be recognized early in the decision making process in the use of enteral nutrition. Weight loss, signs of macronutrient (i.e., decreased visceral protein status, hypoglycemia, and steatorrhea) and micronutrient (electrolytes, trace elements, and vitamins) abnormalities suggest that the intestine may not be optimally functioning [107].

The European Society for Clinical Nutrition and Metabolism guidelines recommends that: "All patients receiving less than their targeted enteral feeding after 2 days should be considered for supplementary parenteral nutrition" [108].

Despite considerable controversy in this field, physicians generally agree on two key aspects: firstly, the enteral route is preferable whenever possible, and secondly, if possible, enteral nutritional support should be started early (within 24–48 h after admission) [101, 108, 109].

The American Society for Parenteral and Enteral Nutrition (ASPEN) and Society of Critical Care Medicine (SCCM) guidelines recommend that parenteral nutrition be initiated after 1 week, unless the patient is severely malnourished. By contrast, the European Society of Enteral and Parenteral (ESPEN) guidelines recommend consideration of a combination of enteral and parenteral nutrition after only 2–3 days in the ICU if enteral nutrition alone is insufficient at that time [108, 110].

In the early phase of rehabilitation enteral feeding solutions with low osmolarity (<300 mOsm/l) to prevent hyperosmolar diarrhea (appeared in case of long time left unfeeded intestine, and low calorie <1Kcal/ml) are usually used (Table 3).

Products	Novartis Novasource start 500ml	Nutricia Pre-nutrison 500ml	Fresenius Intestamin 500ml	Abbott Osmolite HP
Energy Kcal/ml	0, 75	0, 5	0, 5	1
Protein g/100ml	5 27%	2 16%	8, 5 68%	5, 2 20, 8%
Gluamine g/100ml	1	N.A.	6	1, 4
Carbohydrates g/100ml	8 43%	6, 1 49%	17, 7 54%	16, 4 64, 9%
Fat g/100ml	2, 5 30%	1, 95 35%	0, 2 2%	1, 5 13, 3%
Fibers	0, 5	0	0	0
Osmolarity	250	140	N.A.	269

Table 3. Starters for enteral nutrition

The rate of early products' infusion is shown in the Table 4. Moreover, Table 5 depicts most used enteral products according to categories and their characteristics.

Day	Rate	Drops per minute (20 drops=1ml)	Total Volume
1	30ml/h	10	max 500ml
2	40ml/h	10	max 1000ml
3	60ml/h	20	max 1500ml
4	90ml/h	30	max 2000ml
5	100ml/h	30	max 2000ml

Table 4. Starting enteral nutrition rate

Categories	Products	Characteristics
Isotonic	Osmolite HN (Abbott) Pediasure (Abbott) Frebini (Fresenius) Fresubin Original (Fresenius) Isosource Standard (Novartis) Nutrison Standard (Nutricia) Nutrini Standard (Nutricia) Tetrini Standard (Nutricia)	1 kcal/ml
Enriched with fibers	Jevity FOS (Abbott)	1 kcal/ml
	Fresubin Energy Fibre (Fresenius)	1, 5 kcal/ml
	Fresubin Original Fibre (Fresenius)	1 kcal/ml
	Novasource Forte (Novartis)	1, 5 kcal/ml
	Novasource Gl Control (Novartis)	1, 1 kcal/ml
	Cubison (Nutricia)	1 kcal/ml
	Nutrison Multifibre (Nutricia)	
	Stresson Multi Fibre (Nutricia)	1 kcal/ml
Hypercaloric	Ensure Plus (Abbott) Fresubin Energy (Fresenius) Fresubin HP Energy (Fresenius)	1, 5 kcal/ml

Categories	Products	Characteristics
	Novasource Forte (Novartis)	
	Nutrison Energy (Nutricia)	
	Nutridrink (Nutricia)	
Hyperprotein	Perative (Abbott)	1, 31 kcal/ml
	Fresubin HP Energy (Fresenius)	1, 5 kcal/ml
	Intestamin (Fresenius)	0.5 kcal/ml)
	Infatrini (Nutricia	1 kcal/ml

Table 5. Most used enteral solution products per company

The goal of rehabilitation is to return through a gradual transition from the feeding tube back in swallowing if possible. The steps for neurocognitive and neuromuscular patients are based in a clinical algorithm proposed by Buchholz [111].

The initial (preparatory) phase focuses on physiologic readiness for oral nutrition and incorporates medical and nutrition stability (normal swallowing function and nutrition values in normal range), and includes implementation of intermittent tube feeding, and swallowing assessment. The second (weaning) phase is described as a graduated increase in oral feeding, with corresponding decreases in tube feeding. In a patient able to consume more than 75% of his nutrition requirements consistently by mouth for 3 days, all tube feedings are discontinued. Subjects during weaning phase are being continuously evaluated for specific clinical parameters including weight, hydration, and swallowing ability, focusing on respiratory complications [111, 112].

Author details

Yannis Dionyssiotis[1,2*]

1 Rehabilitation Center "Aghios Loukas o Iatros", Trikala Thessaly, Greece

2 University of Athens, 1st Department of Orthopaedics, General University Hospital Attikon, Athens, Greece

References

[1] Dawodu TS, Scott DD, Chase M. Nutritional management in the rehabilitation setting. http://emedicine.medscape.com/article/318180-overview

[2] Leistra E, Neelemaat F, Evers AM, van Zandvoort MH, Weijs PJ, van Bokhorst-de van der Schueren MA, Visser M, et al. Prevalence of undernutrition in Dutch hospital outpatients. Eur J Intern Med 2009;20(5):509-13.

[3] Harris D, Haboubi N. Malnutrition screening in the elderly population. J R Soc Med 2005;98(9):411-4.

[4] Stratton RJ, Green CJ, Elia M. Disease Related Malnutrition: an Evidence Based Approach to Treatment. Oxford: CABI, 2003

[5] Anson CA, Shepherd C. Incidence of secondary complications in spinal cord injury. Int J Rehabil Res 1996;19(1):55-66.

[6] Chen YM, Ho SC, Lam SS, Chan SS. Validity of body mass index and waist circumference in the classification of obesity as compared to percent body fat in Chinese middle-aged women. Int J Obes (Lond) 2006;30(6):918-25.

[7] Liang H, Chen D, Wang Y, Rimmer JH, Braunschweig CL. Different risk factor patterns for metabolic syndrome in men with spinal cord injury compared with able-bodied men despite similar prevalence rates. Arch Phys Med Rehabil 2007;88(9): 1198-204.

[8] Dufoo M Jr., Oseguera AC, Dufoo-Olvera M, Lopez OG, Palacios JL, Trejo AA, Toledo GC, et al. Metabolic changes and nutritional status in the spinal cord injured patient ASIA A. Evaluation and monitoring with routine laboratories, a feasible option. Acta Ortop Mex 2007;21(6):313-7.

[9] Rodriguez D. Nutritional Assessment and Management in spinal cord injury patients. In Charles Tator and Edward Benzel (Eds). Contemporary Management of Spinal Cord Injury: From Impact to Rehabilitation.), 2nd edition, Publisher: Thieme / AANS; 2000.

[10] Dionyssiotis Y. Body Composition in Disabilities of Central Nervous System. In: El Maghraoui, Editor. Dual Energy X-Ray Absorptiometry, Rijeka: InTech; 2012.p 75-94.

[11] Shetty P. Malnutrition and Under nutrition. Medicine.2003;31(4):18-22.

[12] Peiffer SC, Blust P, Leyson JF. Nutritional assessment of the spinal cord injured patient. J Am Diet Assoc 1981;78(5):501-5.

[13] McClave SA, Martindale RG, Vanek VW, et al. Guidelines for the provision and assessment of nutrition support therapy in the adult critically ill patient: Society of Critical Care Medicine (SCCM) and American Society for Parenteral and Enteral Nutrition (A.S.P.E.N.). JPEN J Parenter Enteral Nutr 2009;33(3):277-316.

[14] Pinheiro Volp AC, Esteves de Oliveira FC, Duarte Moreira Alves R, Esteves EA, Bressan J. Energy expenditure: components and evaluation methods. Nutr Hosp 2011;26(3):430-40.

[15] Williams RR, Fuenning CR. Circulatory indirect calorimetry in the critically ill. JPEN J Parenter Enteral Nutr 1991;15(5):509-12.

[16] Long CL, Schaffel N, Geiger JW, Schiller WR, Blakemore WS. Metabolic response to injury and illness: estimation of energy and protein needs from indirect calorimetry and nitrogen balance. JPEN J Parenter Enteral Nutr 1979;3(6):452-6.

[17] Mifflin MD, St Jeor ST, Hill LA, et al. A new predictive equation for resting energy expenditure in healthy individuals. Am J Clin Nutr 1990;51(2):241-7.

[18] Harris JA, Benedict FG. A Biometric Study of Human Basal Metabolism. Proc Natl Acad Sci USA 1918;4(12):370-3.

[19] Cerra FB, Benitez MR, Blackburn GL, Irwin RS, Jeejeebhoy K, Katz DP, et al. Applied nutrition in ICU patients. A consensus statement of the American College of Chest Physicians. Chest 1997;111(3):769-78.

[20] Faisy C, Guerot E, Diehl JL, Labrousse J, Fagon JY. Assessment of resting energy expenditure in mechanically ventilated patients. Am J Clin Nutr 2003;78(2):241-9.

[21] Ireton-Jones CS, Turner WW, Liepa GU, Baxter CR. Equations for estimation of energy expenditures in patients with burns with special reference to ventilator status. J Burn Care Rehab 1992;13(3):330-3.

[22] Ireton-Jones CS, Turner WW. Actual or ideal body weight: which should be used to predict energy expenditure? J Am Diet Assoc 1991;91(2):193-5.

[23] Frankenfield DC, Coleman A, Alam S, Cooney RN. Analysis of estimation methods for resting metabolic rate in critically ill adults. JPEN J Parenter Enteral Nutr 2009;33(1):27-36.

[24] Frankenfield DC. Validation of an equation for resting metabolic rate in older obese, critically ill patients. JPEN J Parenter Enteral Nutr 2011;35:264-9.

[25] Frankenfield DC, Ashcraft CM, Galvan DA. Longitudinal prediction of metabolic rate in critically ill patients. JPEN J Parenter Enteral Nutr 2012;36(6):700-12.

[26] Hamwi GL. Therapy: changing dietary concepts. In: Danowski TS, ed. Diabetes Mellitus: Diagnosis and Treatment. New York, NY: American Diabetes Association; 1964.

[27] Frankenfield DC, Hise M, Malone A, Russell M, Gradwell E, Compher C.Prediction of resting metabolic rate in critically ill adult patients: results of a systematic review of the evidence. J Am Diet Assoc 2007;107(9):1552-61.

[28] Campbell CG, Zander E, Thorland W. Predicted vs. measured energy expenditure in critically ill, underweight patients. Nutr Clin Pract 2005;20(2):276-80.

[29] Kearns PJ, Thompson JD, Werner PC, Pipp TL, Wilmot CB. Nutritional and metabolic response to acute spinal-cord injury. JPEN J Parenter Enteral Nutr 1992;16(1):11-5.

[30] Jeejeebhoy KN. Total parenteral nutrition at home. Can J Surg 1976;19(6):477-8.

[31] Cerra FB, Shronts EP, Raup S, Konstantinides N. Enteral nutrition in hypermetabolic surgical patients. Crit Care Med 1989;17(7):619-22.

[32] Owen OE, Kavle E, Owen RS, et al. A reappraisal of caloric requirements in healthy women. Am J Clin Nutr 1986;44(1):1-19.

[33] Jeejeebhoy KN, Baker JP, Wolman SL, Wesson DE, Langer B, Harrison JE, et al. Critical evaluation of the role of clinical assessment and body composition studies in patients with malnutrition and after total parenteral nutrition. Am J Clin Nutr 1982 ; 35(5 Suppl):1117-27.

[34] Klein JD, Hey LA, Yu CS, Klein BB, Coufal FJ, Young EP, et al. Perioperative nutrition and postoperative complications in patients undergoing spinal surgery. Spine (Phila Pa 1976). 1996;21(22):2676-82.

[35] Alpers DH, Klein S. Approach to the patient requiring nutritional supplementation. In Yamada T, ed. Textbook of Gastroenterology, 4th edn. Baltimore: Lippincott Williams & Wilkins, 2003.

[36] Dionyssiotis Y. Malnutrition in spinal cord injury: more than nutritional deficiency. J Clin Med Res 2012;4(4):227-36.

[37] Dionyssiotis Y, Petropoulou K, Rapidi CA, Papagelopoulos PJ, Papaioannou N, Galanos A, Papadaki P, and Lyritis GP. Body Composition in Paraplegic Men. Journal of Clinical Densitometry 2008;11(3):437-43.

[38] Gupta N, White KT, Sandford PR. Body mass index in spinal cord injury – a retrospective study. Spinal Cord. 2006;44(2):92-4.

[39] McDonald CM, Abresch-Meyer AL, Nelson MD, Widman LM. Body mass index and body composition measures by dual x-ray absorptiometry in patients aged 10 to 21 years with spinal cord injury. J Spinal Cord Med. 2007;30:S97-104.

[40] Jones LM, Legge M, Goulding A Healthy body mass index values often underestimate body fat in men with spinal cord injury. Arch Phys Med Rehab 2003;84(7): 1068-71

[41] Buchholz AC, Bugaresti JM. A review of body mass index and waist circumference as markers of obesity and coronary heart disease risk in persons with chronic spinal cord injury. Spinal Cord. 2005;43(9):513-8.

[42] Laughton GE, Buchholz AC, Martin Ginis KA Lowering body mass index cutoffs better identifies obese persons with spinal cord injury. Spinal Cord 2009;47(10):757-62.

[43] Formica CA, Cosman F, Nieves J, Herbert J, Lindsay R. Reduced bone mass and fat-free mass in women with multiple sclerosis: effects of ambulatory status and glucocorticoid Use. Calcif Tissue Int 1997;61(2):129-33.

[44] Charney P. Nutrition assessment in the 1990s: where are we now? Nutr Clin Pract. 1995;10(4):131-9.

[45] Ingenbleek Y, Van Den Schrieck HG, De Nayer P, De Visscher M. Albumin, transferrin and the thyroxinebinding prealbumin/retinol-binding protein (TBPARBP) complex in assessment of malnutrition. Clin Chim Acta 1975;63(1):61-7.

[46] Devoto G, Gallo F, Marchello C, Racchi O, Garbarini R, Bonassi S, et al. Prealbumin serum concentrations as a useful tool in the assessment of malnutrition in hospitalized patients. Clin Chem 2006;52(12):2281-5.

[47] Mears E. Linking serum prealbumin measurements to managing a malnutrition clinical pathway. J Clin Ligand Assay 1999;22:296-303.

[48] Robinson MK, Trujillo EB, Mogensen KM, Rounds J, McManus K, Jacobs DO. Improving nutritional screening of hospitalized patients: the role of prealbumin. JPEN J Parenter Enteral Nutr 2003;27(6):389-95;

[49] Frankenfield D. Energy expenditure and protein requirements after traumatic injury. Nutr Clin Pract 2006;21(5):430-7.

[50] Hertroijs D, Wijnen C, Leistra E, Visser M, van der Heijden E, Kruizenga H. Rehabilitation patients: undernourished and obese? J Rehabil Med 2012;44(8):696-701.

[51] [Set Performance Indicator rehabilitation centers.] Commissie Prestatie-indicatoren, Revalidatie Nederland en Nederlands Vereniging van Revalidatieartsen 2011 (in Dutch).

[52] Kruizenga HM, Seidell JC, de Vet HCW, Wierdsma NJ, van Bokhorst-de van der Schueren. Development and validation of a hospital screening tool for malnutrition: the short nutritional assessment questionnaire (SNAQ). Clin Nutr 2005; 24(1):75–82.

[53] Stratton RJ, Hackston A, Longmore D, Dixon R, Price S, Stroud M. Malnutrition in hospital outpatients and inpatients: prevalence concurrent validity and ease of use of the 'Malnutrition Universal Screening Tool' ('MUST') for adults. Br J Nutr 2004; 92(5): 799–808.

[54] Kruizenga HM, de Vet HC, Van Marissing CM, Stassen EE, Strijk JE, Van Bokhorst-de Van der Schueren MA, et al. The SNAQ(RC), an easy traffic light system as a first step in the recognition of undernutrition in residential care. J Nutr Health Aging 2010;14(2):83-9.

[55] National Collaborating Centre for Acute Care (UK). Nutrition Support for Adults: Oral Nutrition Support, Enteral Tube Feeding and Parenteral Nutrition. London: National Collaborating Centre for Acute Care (UK); 2006 Feb.

[56] Kolpek JH, Ott LG, Record KE, Rapp RP, Dempsey R, Tibbs P, Young B. Comparison of urinary urea nitrogen excretion and measured energy expenditure in spinal cord injury and nonsteroid-treated severe head trauma patients. JPEN J Parenter Enteral Nutr 1989 ;13(3):277-80.

[57] Claus-Walker J, Halstead LS. Metabolic and endocrine changes in spinal cord injury: IV. Compounded neurologic dysfunctions. Arch Phys Med Rehabil 1982;63(12):632-8.

[58] Wilmore DW. Catabolic illness: strategies for enhancing recovery. N Engl J Med 1991;325(10):695-702.

[59] Burnham EL, Moss M, Ziegler TR. Myopathies in critical illness: characterization and nutritional aspects. J Nutr 2005;135(7):1818S-23S.

[60] Bongers T, Griffiths RD, McArdle A. Exogenous glutamine: the clinical evidence. Crit Care Med 2007;35(9 Suppl):S545-52.

[61] Cree MG, Wolfe RR. Postburn trauma insulin resistance and fat metabolism. Am J Physiol Endocrinol Metab 2008;294(1):E1-9.

[62] Thibault-Halman G, Casha S, Singer S, Christie S. Acute management of nutritional demands after spinal cord injury. J Neurotrauma 2011;28(8):1497-507.

[63] Robertson CS, Grossman RG. Protection against spinal cord ischemia with insulin-induced hypoglycaemia. J Neurosurg 1987;67(5):739-44.

[64] Burr RG, Clift-Peace L, Nuseibeh I. Haemoglobin and albumin as predictors of length of stay of spinal injured patients in a rehabilitation centre. Paraplegia 1993;31(7):473-8.

[65] Gottschlich MM, Matarese LE, Shronts EP. Nutrition Support Dietetics Core Curriculum. 2 ed. Silver Springs, MD: A.S.P.E.N., 1993.

[66] Cooper IS, Hoen TI. Metabolic disorders in paraplegics. Neurology 1952;2(4):332-40.

[67] Whedon GD, Dietrick JE, Shorr E. Modification of the effects of immobilization upon metabolic and physiologic functions of normal men by the use of an oscillating bed. Am J Med 1949;6(6):684-711.

[68] Eleazer GP, Bird L, Egbert J, Ryan C, Wei M, Guest K. Appropriate protocol for zinc therapy in long term care facilities. J Nutr Elder 1995;14(4):31-8.

[69] ter Riet G, Kessels AG, Knipschild PG. Randomized clinical trial of ascorbic acid in the treatment of pressure ulcers. J Clin Epidemiol 1995;48(12):1453-60.

[70] Peruzzi WT, Shapiro BA, Meyer PR Jr, Krumlovsky F, Seo BW. Hyponatremia in acute spinal cord injury. Crit Care Med 1994;22(2):252-8.

[71] De Jonghe B, Appere-De-Vechi C, Fournier M, Tran B, Merrer J, Melchior JC, et al. A prospective survey of nutritional support practices in intensive care unit patients: what is prescribed? What is delivered? Crit Care Med 2001;29(1):8-12.

[72] Nardo P, Dupertuis YM, Jetzer J, Kossovsky MP, Darmon P, Pichard C. Clinical relevance of parenteral nutrition prescription and administration in 200 hospitalized patients: a quality control study. Clin Nutr 2008;27(6):858-64.

[73] Shaw JH, Wildbore M, Wolfe RR. Whole body protein kinetics in severely septic patients: the response to glucose infusion and total parenteral nutrition. Ann Surg 1987;205(3):288-94.

[74] Streat SJ, Beddoe AH, Hill GL. Aggressive nutritional support does not prevent protein loss despite fat gain in septic intensive care patients. J Trauma 1987 ;27(3): 262-6.

[75] Monroe MB, Tataranni PA, Pratley R, Manore MM, Skinner JS, Ravussin E. Lower daily energy expenditures as measured by a respiratory chamber in subjects with spinal cord injury compared with control subjects. American Journal of Clinical Nutrition 1998; 68(6):1223-7.

[76] Perkash A, Brown M. Anaemia in patients with traumatic spinal cord injury. Paraplegia 1982;20(4):235-6.

[77] Blissitt PA. Nutrition in acute spinal cord injury. Crit Care Nurs Clin North Am 1990;2(3):375-84.

[78] Braunschweig C, Levy P. Sheean P, Wang X. Enteral compared to parenteral nutrition: a meta analysis American Journal of Clinical Nutrition 2001;74(4):534-42.

[79] Yin L, McLennan M, Bellou TF. Overweight in children with intellectual disabilities: No Simple Matter. ICAN: Infant, Child, & Adolescent Nutrition April 2013 5: 92-6.

[80] Bauman WA, Zhong YG, Schwartz E. Vitamin D deficiency in veterans with chronic spinal cord injury Metabolism 1995; 44(12):1612–6.

[81] Dionyssiotis Y. Bone loss and fractures in multiple sclerosis: focus on epidemiologic and physiopathological features. Int J Gen Med 2011;4:505-9.

[82] Maklebust J, Magnan MA. Risk factors associated with having a pressure ulcer: a secondary data analysis. Adv Wound Care 1994;7(6):25, 27-8, 31-4 passim.

[83] Fishburn MJ, Marino RJ, Ditunno JF Jr. Atelectasis and pneumonia in acute spinal cord injury. Arch Phys Med Rehabil 1990;71(3):197-200.

[84] Endersbe LA. Nutrition Support in Neurologic Impairment. In: Shronts, Eva P, editors. Nutrition support dietetics. Maryland, Aspen: Silver Spring, p.107-18, 1989.

[85] Jacksic T, Blakburn GL. Nutrition and CNS disease, the unconscious patient. In: Jeejeebhoy KN, editor. Current therapy in nutrition. Toronto, Philadelphia: B C Decker Inc., p.269-78, 1988.

[86] Minard G, Kudsk K A. Is early feeding beneficial? How early is early? New horizons (Baltimore, Md.), 2(2), p. 156-63, 1994.

[87] Nyswonger GD, Helmchen RH. Early enteral nutrition and length of stay in stroke patients. J Neurosci Nurs 1992; 24(4):220-3.

[88] Kirby DF, Clifton GL, Turner H, Marion DW, Barrett J, Gruemer HD. Early enteral nutrition after brain injury by percutaneous endoscopic gastrojejunostomy. JPEN J Parenter Enteral Nutr 1991;15(3):298-302.

[89] Grahm TW, Zadrozny DB, Harrington T: The benefits of early jejunal hyperalimentation in the head-injured patient. Neurosurgery 1989; 25(5):729-35.

[90] Magnuson B, Hatton J, Zweng TN, Young B. Pentobarbital coma in neurosurgical patients: nutrition considerations. Nutr Clin Pract 1994;9(4):146-50.

[91] O'Keefe SJ. A guide to enteral access procedures and enteral nutrition. Nat Rev Gastroenterol Hepatol 2009;6(4):207-15.

[92] Zaloga GP. The myth of the gastric residual volume. Crit Care Med 2005;33(2):449-50.

[93] Park RH, Allison MC, Lang J, Spence E, Morris AJ, Danesh BJ, et al.Randomised comparison of percutaneous endoscopic gastrostomy and nasogastric tube feeding in patients with persisting neurological dysphagia. BMJ 1992;30:(304):1406-9.

[94] Wicks C, Gimson A, Vlavianos P, Lombard M, Panos M, Macmathuna P, et al. Assessment of the percutaneous endoscopic gastrostomy feeding tube as part of an integrated approach to enteral feeding. Gut 1992;33(5):613-6.

[95] Allison MC, Morris AJ, Park RH, Mills PR. Percutaneous endoscopic gastrostomy tube feeding may improve outcome of late rehabilitation following stroke. J R Soc Med 1992;85(3):147-9.

[96] Larson DE, Burton DD, Schroeder KW, DiMagno EP. Percutaneous endoscopic gastrostomy. Gastroenterology, 1987; 93(1), 48-52.

[97] Miller RE, Castlemain B, Lacqua FJ, Kotler DP. Percutaneous endoscopic gastrostomy. Results in 316 patients and review of literature. Surg Endosc 1989;3(4):186-90.

[98] Burtch GD, Shatney CH. Feeding gastrostomy. Assistant or assassin? Am Surg 1985;51(4):204-7.

[99] Fay DE, Poplausky M, Gruber M, Lance P. Long-term enteral feeding: a retrospective comparison of delivery via percutaneous endoscopic gastrostomy and nasoenteric tubes. Am J Gastroenterol 1991;86(11):1604-9.

[100] Marik PE, Zaloga GP. Early enteral nutrition in acutely ill patients: a systematic review. Crit Care Med 2001;29(12):2264-70. Erratum in: Crit Care Med 2002;30(3):725.

[101] Heyland DK, Dhaliwal R, Drover JW, Gramlich L, Dodek P; Canadian Critical Care Clinical Practice Guidelines Committee. Canadian clinical practice guidelines for nutrition support in mechanically ventilated, critically ill adult patients. JPEN J Parenter Enteral Nutr 2003;27(5):355-73.

[102] Simpson F, Doig GS. Parenteral vs. enteral nutrition in the critically ill patient: a meta-analysis of trials using the intention to treat principle. Intensive Care Med 2005;31(1):12-23.

[103] Kudsk KA, Croce MA, Fabian TC, Minard G, Tolley EA, Poret HA, et al. Enteral versus parenteral feeding. Effects on septic morbidity after blunt and penetrating abdominal trauma. Ann Surg 1992;215(5):503-11; discussion 511-3.

[104] Heyland DK, Konopad E, Alberda C, Keefe L, et al. How well do critically ill patients tolerate early, intragastric enteral feeding? Results of a prospective, multicenter trial. Nutr Clin Pract 1999;14(1):23-8.

[105] Rello J, Quintana E, Ausina V, Castella J, Luquin M, Net A, et al. Incidence, etiology, and outcome of nosocomial pneumonia in mechanically ventilated patients. Chest 1991;100(2):439-44.

[106] Heyland DK, Macdonald S, Keefe L, Drover JW. Total parenteral nutrition in the critically ill patient: a meta analysis. JAMA 1998; 280(23):2013-9.

[107] Baumgartner TG, Cerda JJ, Somogyi L, Baumgartner SL. Enteral Nutrition in Clinical Practice Croatian Med J 1999;40(4):515-27.

[108] Singer P, Berger MM, Van den Berghe G, Biolo G, Calder P, Forbes A, Griffiths R, Kreyman G, Leverve X, Pichard C, ESPEN. ESPEN Guidelines on Parenteral Nutrition: intensive care. Clin Nutr 2009;28(4):387-400.

[109] Martindale RG, McClave SA, Vanek VW, McCarthy M, Roberts P, Taylor B, et al. American College of Critical Care Medicine; A.S.P.E.N. Board of Directors. Guidelines for the provision and assessment of nutrition support therapy in the adult critically ill patient: Society of Critical Care Medicine and American Society for Parenteral and Enteral Nutrition: Executive Summary. Crit Care Med 2009;37(5): 1757-61.

[110] Vincent JL, Preiser JC. When should we add parenteral to enteral nutrition? Lancet 2013;381(9864):354-5.

[111] Buchholz AC. Weaning patients with dysphagia from tube feeding to oral nutrition: a proposed algorithm. Can J Diet Pract Res 1998;59(4):208–14.

[112] Crary MA, Groher ME. Reinstituting oral feeding in tube-fed adult patients with dysphagia. Nutr Clin Pract 2006;21(6):576-86.

Chapter 7

Body Composition in Paraplegia

Yannis Dionyssiotis

Additional information is available at the end of the chapter

http://dx.doi.org/10.5772/58539

1. Introduction

Paraplegia leads to immobilisation associated with profound changes in body composition. The potential risks involved with these changes i.e. loss of lean tissue mass (LM) and bone mineral density (BMD) vs. gain in fat mass (FM) in body composition have implications for the health of the disabled individuals [1]. Body fat has been identified as a significant predictor of mortality in humans making body composition measurement to quantify nutritional and health status an important issue for human health [2-4]. Moreover, some disorders such as carbohydrate intolerance, insulin resistance, lipid abnormalities, and heart disease occur prematurely and at a higher prevalence in disabled populations may be related to adverse changes in body composition that result from immobilization and skeletal muscle denervation [5]. To standardize or index physiological variables, such as resting metabolic rate and power fat free mass (FFM) is usually used [4]. Skeletal muscle represents 50% of the non fat component in the total body [6, 7] and exact quantification of the amount of skeletal muscle is important to assess nutritional status, disease risk, danger of illnesses, physical function, atrophic effects of aging, and muscle-wasting diseases [8, 9].

A paraplegic subject could be wheelchair bound, may have an alternated walking gait pattern but may also be unable to walk at all [10, 11]. In addition to these differences and according to osteoporosis the role of factors which do not change, such as race or gender of patients has not been yet clarified, although there are few studies in women debating that bone mass in women with paraplegia is more affected than men [12, 13]. Similar findings of reduced muscle mass and increased intramuscular fat have been also published in individuals with incomplete spinal cord injury (SCI) [14].

Therefore, the purpose of this chapter was to present the bone-mineral density, bone-mineral content, and bone-mineral-free lean and fat tissue mass alterations of ambulatory and non-ambulatory subjects with paraplegia.

2. Body composition measurements

2.1. Anthropometric and various techniques of body composition measurements

Similar body mass indices were found between paraplegics and controls; although there were significant decreases in the lean muscle mass of the paraplegics (16% less). The analysis of body composition with dual-energy X-ray absorptiometry (DXA) has also revealed large increases in fat in people who do not appear to be obese, yet they carry large amounts of fat tissue and in the group of paraplegic subjects fat mass was 47% higher [15]. Furthermore, where authors performed a research in the usage of the body mass index (BMI) in anthropometric measurements, the conclusion was that BMI, widely used as an obesity measurement tool, is not capable of distinguishing the weight components among people so that the fat percentage is degraded in the population of paraplegic in comparison to the control group [16].

In a study which investigated a chronic paraplegic population the values of BMI did not present statistical significance in relation to the controls, which is a finding in line with the literature [17, 18, 19]. Moreover, the values of BMI in both paraplegics and controls were below values consider to signify obesity (BMI>27.8) [19, 20, 21]. This finding could be acceptable for the population of the controls, but raises questions regarding the paraplegics. It is known from literature that paraplegics are obese [22]. Nevertheless, there are studies which demonstrate the usefulness of BMI as an indicator of obesity, in body composition in people with spinal cord injury [23]. These studies, however, included in their sample both tetraplegics and middle-aged people unlike the Greek one which included relatively young individuals [19]. Whether the criteria of BMI may assess obesity in people with spinal cord injury the latest studies show the opposite [24].

Similarly to the healthy population values of BMI are positively correlated with obesity. This emerged from a study, conducted by whole body DXA Norland X-36, only when the findings of total fat in paraplegics were correlated with BMI. Employing whole body DXA Norland XR-36 it was found that the total fat mass was statistically significantly higher for any given BMI value in paraplegics compared with controls [19], finding that strongly supports the studies held by the whole body DXA Hologic QDR-2000 method [5, 25].

The studies illustrated statistically significantly higher total fat mass and fat percentages for any given unit of body mass index in paraplegics in comparison to controls. Increased fat per body mass index unit was found in a study of monozygotic twins, one with SCI compared with a non-SCI co-twin by the above authors also [25]. Adjustments in classifications of normal, overweight, obese, and morbid obesity by BMI are needed for persons with SCI [26].

In addition, by analysis between paraplegics with high and low neurological level injuries not statistically significant differences in BMI were highlighted. However, when data from the analysis undertaken in areas measured by the method of whole body DEXA were compared in the same patients there were differences between paraplegics with high and low neurological level of injury. This finding is new and reinforces those views on the inability of BMI usage in the analysis of body composition of paraplegics [19].

BMI of the male paraplegic group was slightly greater than that of the male tetraplegic group (25.2 vs. 24.7 kg/ m^2; $p<0.01$). Proportion of overweight or obese was comparable between men with SCI and that observed in men in the US general population. Distribution of BMI by level of injury was similar with 37.5% and 40.5% of the male tetraplegic and male paraplegic groups, respectively, falling into the recommended BMI range. Approximately 50% in each male group were overweight by BMI, and 12.5% and 10.8%, respectively, were classified as obese. Overall, when compared with the general population-observed distribution by BMI, a greater proportion of men with SCI fell into the desirable BMI range and fewer fell into the obese category [26].

No differences were found in BMI between paraplegics in the acute phase of injury and controls, which is a finding in accordance with other studies reported in chronic paraplegic patients and controls, in which despite the same BMI the body composition and the distribution of fat and fat free mass were alterated in patients with spinal cord damage, with the fat free mass being statistically significantly lower in paraplegic patients in total body composition and in the lower, but not the upper limbs. As far as the fat mass is concerned, it was statistically significantly higher (kilograms and %) in the total body composition in the upper and lower limbs [27].

These findings show that using the BMI does not contribute substantially in determining the body composition of paraplegics and lowers the percentage of fat in this population, finding that agrees with other studies and shows that the anthropometric measurement with BMI in paraplegics, underestimates fat in body composition when measurements are compared with healthy subjects [1].

Changes in body composition in spinal cord injured subjects can be assessed with various techniques including isotope-labelled water [1] total body potassium counting (Lussier et al 1983; Spungen et al 1992) anthropometric measures [16] hydrodensitometry [28] dual photon absorptiometry (DPA) [29] and dual energy X-ray absorptiometry (DXA) [1]. However, some of these methods are not particularly suitable for use in the SCI population.

The hydrodensitometric model was regarded as the "gold standard" for body composition assessment. This model partitions the body into two compartments of constant densities [fat mass: 0.9007 g/cm^3 and FFM: 1.100 g/cm^3] and assumes that the relative amounts of the FFM components [water, protein, protein, bone mineral (BM), and non-BM] are fixed [4]. Hydrodensitometry is clearly inappropriate for individuals who deviate from these fixed and/or assumed values (e.g., children, elderly, blacks, obese), and its application is, therefore, somewhat limited [30, 31].

Bioelectrical impedance analysis has been used to measure cerebral palsy subjects. However, the inclusion of weight in the BIA predictive equation may reduce its accuracy in determining change in lean body mass. The inability of BIA to accurately predict percentage body fat in the sample may be related to several factors. In the BIA method where the impedance of a geometrical system (i.e., the human body) is dependent on the length of the conductor (height) and its configuration, it is almost impossible to measure accurately height in subjects with CP because of their muscle contractures. An over-or underestimation of height by 2.5 cm can result in a 1.0-L error in the estimation of TBW, producing a small error in the estimation of percentage body fat (< 5%). The second major problem is body asymmetry which renders the assumption of a symmetrical configuration of the human body invalid in this case [20, 32].

Isotope dilution measures the water compartment of the whole body rather than a single area assumed to mimic the composition of the whole body. Thus, the use of a stable isotope to measure body composition is ideal for people with CP because it is non-invasive, does not require the subject to remain still for the measurement, and is independent of height and body symmetry. However, the prohibitive cost of the isotopes and the need for a mass spectrometry facility and highly trained technicians make this method impractical for routine clinical use [32].

To determine whether bioelectrical impedance analysis (BIA) and anthropometry can be used to determine body composition for clinical and research purposes in children with cerebral palsy 8 individuals (two female, mean age=10 years, mean gross motor function classification=4.6 [severe motor impairment]) recruited from an outpatient tertiary care setting underwent measurement of fat mass, fat-free mass, and percentage body fat using BIA, anthropometry (two and four skinfold equations), and dual-energy x-ray absorptiometry. Correlation were excellent for determination of fat-free mass for all methods (i.e., all were above 0.9) and moderate for determination of fat mass and percent body fat (range=0.4 to 0.8). Moreover, skinfolds were better predictors of percent body fat, while bioelectrical impedance was a better predictor for fat mass [33]. On the contrary another study investigated the pattern of body composition in 136 subjects with spastic quadriplegic cerebral palsy, 2 to 12 years of age, by anthropometric measures, or by anthropometric and total body water (TBW) measures (n=28), compared with 39 control subjects. Body composition and nutritional status indicators were significantly reduced. Calculation of body fat from two skinfolds correlated best with measures of fat mass from TBW [34].

Magnetic resonance imaging (MRI) provides remarkably accurate estimates of skeletal muscle in vivo [7]. MRI and also quantitative computed tomography (QCT) have been validated in studies of humancadavers in the assessment of regional skeletal muscle [35]. Although, these devices have disadvantages of high radiation exposure and are expensive.

2.2. Dual-energy X-ray absorptiometry (DXA)

Recently, dual-energy X-ray absorptiometry (DXA) has gained acceptance as a reference method for body composition analysis [36, 37]. Originally designed to determine bone density, DXA technology has subsequently been adopted for the assessment of whole body composition and offers estimation rapidly, non-invasively and with minimal radiation exposure [4, 19]. Moreover, is well tolerated in subjects who would be unable to tolerate other body composition techniques, such as underwater weighing (hydro-densitometry). DXA software determines the bone mineral and soft tissue composition in different regions of the body being a three-compartment model that quantifies: (i) bone mineral density and content (BMD, BMC), (ii) fat mass (FM); and (iii) lean mass (LM), half of which is closely correlated with muscle mass and also yields regional as well as total body values [38] for example in the arms, legs, and trunk (figure 1).

http://dx.doi.org/10.5772/58539

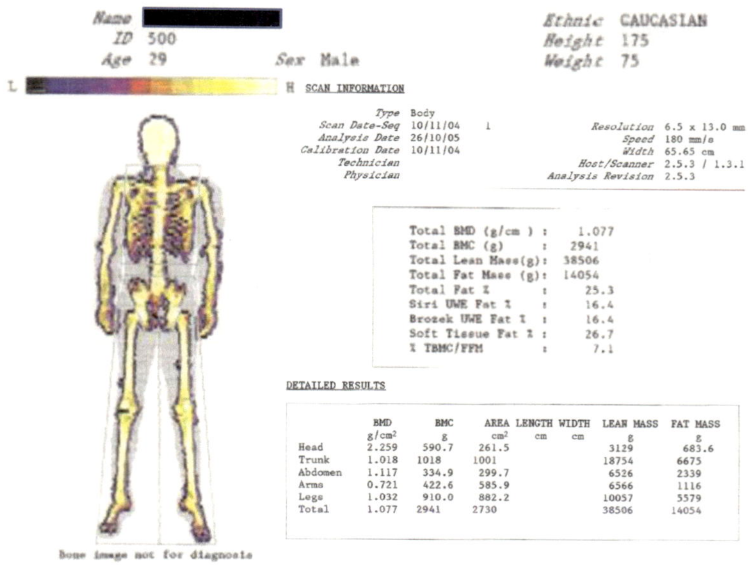

Figure 1. Whole body and regional distribution of fat mass, lean mass, bone mineral content (BMC) and bone mineral density (BMD) from paraplegic subject thoracic 6 using whole body DXA (Norland X-36, Fort Atkinson, Wisconsin, USA) and values of measured parameters. Modified and translated with permission from Dionyssiotis Y, Doctoral Dissertation, Laboratory for Research of the Musculoskeletal System, University of Athens, 2008 [39].

DXA analyzes differently the dense pixels in body composition. Soft tissue pixels are analyzed for two materials: fat and fat-free tissue mass. Variations in the fat mass/fat free tissue mass composition of the soft tissue produce differences in the respective attenuation coefficients at both energy levels. The ratio at the two main energy peaks is automatically calculated of the X-ray attenuation providing separation of the soft tissue compartment into fat mass and fat-free tissue mass (lean mass) [40, 41]. A bone-containing pixel is analyzed for "bone mass" (bone mineral content, BMC) and soft tissue as the two materials. Thus, the fat mass/fat free tissue mass of the soft tissue component of the bone pixels cannot be measured, but only estimated [42].

The important issue on this the investigation of distribution of bone mineral, fat and mass throughout the body. These changes induce the risk for diseases such as diabetes, coronary heart disease, dyslipidaimias and osteoporosis [22, 43, 44, 45]. There is a need to quantify the alterations in body composition to prevent these diseases and their complications. Studies also reported that bone density measurements at one site cannot usefully predict the bone density elsewhere [46] because different skeletal regions, even with similar quantities of trabecular or cortical bone, may respond variably in different physiopathological conditions [47].

In disabled conditions the accuracy of skeletal muscle measured by DXA may be compromised when muscle atrophy is present. A lower ratio of muscle to adipose-tissue-free mass indicates a lower proportion of muscle in the fat-free soft tissue mass. Cross-sectional area of skeletal muscle in the thighs after SCI is extensively reduced [48]. If this is the case muscle mass would be overestimated by prediction models that assume that muscle represents all or a certain proportion of the fat-free soft tissue mass, i.e. in spinal cord injured subjects [7]. DXA technique has been used in assessment of SCI and appears to be tolerated well by this population [49, 50, 51].

Name [redacted]
ID 2210
Age 36 Sex Male
Ethnic cauc
Height 180
Weight 125

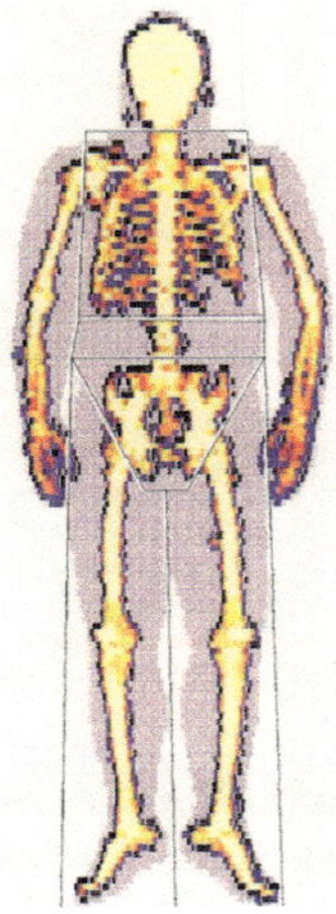

Total BMD (g/cm) :	1.256
Total BMC (g) :	3527
Total Lean Mass(g):	79838
Total Fat Mass (g):	40884
Total Fat % :	32.9
Siri UWE Fat % :	29.6
Brozek UWE Fat % :	28.6
Soft Tissue Fat % :	33.9
% TBMC/FFM :	4.2

DETAILED RESULTS

	BMD g/cm²	BMC g	AREA cm²	LENGTH cm	WIDTH cm	LEAN MASS g	FAT MASS g
Head	2.218	586.9	264.6			4142	1035
Trunk	1.254	1181	942.0			40251	24108
Abdomen	1.542	564.3	365.8			17188	12251
Arms	0.781	456.0	583.7			8784	4205
Legs	1.280	1302	1017			26661	11536
Total	1.256	3527	2807			79838	40884

Figure 2. Whole body and regional distribution of fat mass, lean mass, bone mineral content (BMC) and bone mineral density (BMD) from controls male subject using whole body DEXA Norland X-36 and values of measured parameters. Modified and translated with permission from Dionyssiotis, Doctoral Dissertation, Laboratory for Research of the Musculoskeletal System, University of Athens, 2008 [39].

3. Physiopathological context

Spinal cord injury (SCI) always results in substantial and rapid bone loss predominately in areas below the neurological level of injury. The predominant finding of SCI on bone is a large loss of bone during the first year of injury [5] and an ongoing demineralisation 3 years after trauma in tibia [52] with a progressive bone loss over 12 to 16 months prior to stabilizing [53] was demonstrated.

Cancellous bone is more affected than cortical bone after SCI. In a prospective study, six acute tetraplegics were followed up for 12 months, and the trabecular and cortical BMD's of the tibia were found to be decreased by 15 and 7% [54], while in paraplegics trabecular metaphyseal-epiphyseal areas of the distal femur and the proximal tibia are the most affected sites [55]. A cross-sectional study [56] in SCI subjects demonstrated a significant demineralization at the distal femur (-52%) and the proximal tibia (-70%), respectively.

There is no demineralization of the upper limbs in paraplegics. On the contrary, a minor increase of BMD (6%) in the humerus was reported in a cross-sectional study of 31 male chronic paraplegics 1 year post injury. With reliance on the upper limbs to provide movement for activities of daily living in the SCI population, this area could be subjected to greater site-specific loading, and thus increasing osteogenesis, than in the corresponding able-bodied population. At the lumbar spine, the trabecular bone demineralization remains relatively low compared to the cortical bone demineralization of long bones [56]. Normal [52, 57] or even higher than normal [58] values of BMD in the lumbar spine have been reported a phenomenon is named "dissociated hip and spine demineralization" [54]. One reason for preservation of bone mass in the vertebral column is because of its continued weight-bearing function in paraplegics. In a cross-sectional study of 135 SCI men, BMD in the lumbar spine was found to be stable with an insignificant decline in the tetraplegic population at 1±5 years post injury in the 20–39-year age group, whereas in the 40-59-year age group and the 60+-year age group, bone mass in the lumbar spine remained unchanged or even increased with age [49]. However, several factors may affect the results of BMD measurement: lumbar spine arthrosis, bone callus, vertebral fracture, aortic calcification, osteosynthesis material, etc. Degenerative changes in the spine may be the most possible reason to give falsely higher values of BMD [56]. An interesting question is why we don't see osteoporotic vertebral fractures in SCI patients to the extent it occurs in post-menopausal osteoporotic women or senile osteoporotic men?

Figure 3 depicts the analysis of bone mineral density (BMD) in high and low level paraplegics and controls. A statistically significant reduction in total BMD ($p<0.001$) and lower limbs BMD in body composition compared to able-bodied males was observed. On the contrary, upper limbs BMD was higher in low paraplegics and controls, an unexpected finding explained in the paper of Dionyssiotis et al. [19].

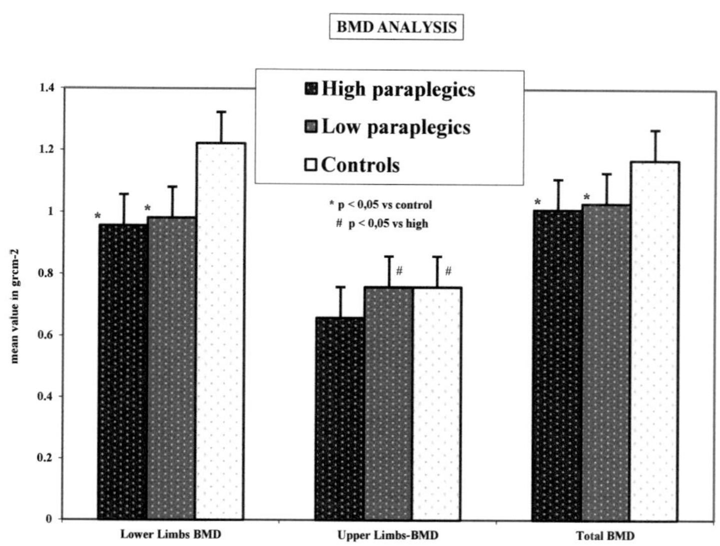

Figure 3. Analysis of bone mineral density (BMD) in high and low level paraplegics and controls. Diagram modified and translated from Dionyssiotis Y [39].

The neurological level of the lesion i.e. the extent of impairment of motor and sensory function is important, because tetraplegics are more likely to lose more bone mass throughout the skeleton than paraplegics [60]. In paraplegics legs' BMC was reduced vs. controls, independently of the neurological level of injury and negatively correlated with the duration of paralysis in total paraplegic group, but after investigation according to the neurological level of injury this correlation was due to the strong correlation of high paraplegics' legs BMC with the duration of paralysis, meaning that the neurological level of injury determines the extent of bone loss [61]. The similar severity of demineralization in the sublesional area was shown between paraplegics and tetraplegics, and the extent of the bone loss may be variable [56, 60, 62].

In addition, in those SCI individuals with complete lesions (an absence of sensory or motor function below the neurological level, including the lowest sacral segment) bone loss is more severe than subjects with incomplete lesions (partial preservation of motor and/or sensory function below the neurological level, including the lowest sacral segment) [62, 63]. In a cross-sectional study of 11 patients with complete SCI and 30 patients with incomplete SCI noticed a significant osteopenia in patients with complete SCI than in patients with incomplete SCI [62].

The duration of paralysis has an inverse relationship with leg percentage-matched BMD and trunk percentage-matched BMD [64]. In addition in complete paraplegics, with high (thoracic 4-7) and low (thoracic 8-12) neurological level of injury, upper limbs FM and lower limbs BMD were correlated with the duration of paralysis in total paraplegic group but after investigation according the neurological level of injury this correlation was due to the strong correlation of high paraplegics' lower limbs BMD with the duration of paralysis. The explanation of this strong correlation could possibly lie on higher incidence of standing in the group of low paraplegics and direct effect of loading lower limbs while standing and walking with orthotic equipment. Moreover, the association of the duration of paralysis with parameters below and above the neurological level of injury (upper limbs FM) raises the question of the existence of a hormonal mechanism as an influential regulator in paraplegics' body composition [19, 61, 65].

Is there a time after injury where bone loss ceases? Some authors reported that approximately 2 years after SCI, a new steady state level between bone resorption and formation would be re-established [52, 57], whereas others [66] found that there was no sign of a new steady state in bone formation in the lower extremities 2 years after the SCI. If a new steady state of bone remodelling is re-established after SCI still remains controversial.

Inconsistent results have been reported regarding the effect of muscle spasms on BMD in SCI patients. Those with spasticity were found with higher BMD when compared with flaccid individuals [62], and a significant correlation between the degree of spasticity measured with modified Ashworth scale and BMD was reported. Thus, it was concluded that spasticity may be protective against bone loss in SCI patients [67]; however, without any preserving effect in the tibia [65, 67]. A possible explanation for that could lie in the fact paraplegics to be above thoracic (T)12 level with various degrees of spasticity according to the Ashworth scale. In addition, muscle spasms affecting the lower leg would mainly be extension spasms resulting in plantar flexion thus creating little resistance to the contracting muscles. Furthermore, the measuring sites of the tibia did not include any muscle insertions of either the knee or the ankle extensor muscles [65]. Other investigators have not established a correlation between BMD and muscle spasticity [68].

Studies also emphasize the contribution of aging to bone loss in complete SCI patients. Moderate correlation between age and femoral BMD was observed in a cross-sectional study of 30 patients with SCI of 1-year duration or less [69]. On the other side bone loss in eight pairs of identical male twins with SCI of duration ranging from 3 to 26 years appeared to be independent of age [70].

Muscular loading of the bones has been thought to play a role in the maintenance of bone density. The ability to stand or ambulate itself does not improve BMD and does not prevent osteoporosis after SCI, although exercise increases site-specific osteogenesis in able-bodied individuals [71]. There was only one study demonstrating that standing might reduce the loss of trabecular bone after SCI. In this prospective study of 19 acute SCI patients, the patients involved in early loading intervention exercise lost almost no bone mineral, whereas the immobilization patients lost 6.9 to 9.4% of trabecular bone [66].

Muscles rather than body weight are causing the greatest loads on bone [72]. It is difficult to translate in vivo bone strains from animal work to a gross loading environment for humans. However, the pioneering work in animal models [73] suggests that if the active–resistive standing exercise can indeed transmit loads at an appropriate frequency and strain-rate, compressive loads approaching 240 % body weight may have the potential to be osteogenic [73, 74].

FES cycling [75] and quadriceps muscle training [76] have been able to increase force-generating capability and to improve muscular endurance with training after SCI [75]. Conversely, cycling with FES has been reported to induce only small improvements in BMD [77, 78] as well as have no effect [78] on lower extremity BMD measurements in individuals with SCI. Additionally, neither passive standing, ambulation with long-leg braces, nor ambulation with FES have yet to exhibit any improvement in lower extremity BMD in chronically injured subjects [79]. The subject populations of previous BMD studies were comprised almost exclusively of individuals with chronic rather than acute SCI. these interventional BMD studies may have utilized sub-threshold mechanical stimuli. The use of relatively low bone loading regimens is not unexpected due to the extensive atrophy of chronically paralyzed muscle [80, 81] and concerns of fracture, which have been reported to occur with physical interventions [82, 83].

The role of leptin: The hormone leptin is secreted by fat cells and help regulate body weight and energy consumption [84]. The amount of leptin in the circulation is positively correlated with the percentage of fat in people [85]. In paraplegics, when compared with healthy subjects, higher levels of leptin have been found, possibly due to greater fat tissue storage [86, 87]. Leptin activates the sympathetic nervous system (SNS) through a central administration. The disruption of the sympathetic nervous system may modify the secretion and activity of the leptin, because the sympathetic preganglionic neurons become atrophic in high paraplegics [88, 89]. The irritation thus, below the neurological level of injury, from the leptin is disturbed. In addition, extensive obesity is known to reduce lipolytic sensitivity [89, 90, 91]. Given that in the high level of neurological paraplegia there is a problem of disorder of the autonomic nervous system and in combination with the existence of scientific evidence that the hormone leptin activates the sympathetic nervous system through central control, was formulated, that the closure <of paths> of the central nervous system disrupts the effect of leptin and possibly increases the risk of obesity in paraplegic patients with high-level injury [92, 93].

However, after separation of SCI subjects into those with an injury above or below Thoracic (T) 6, leptin levels were significantly higher in the former group. T6 appears to be the lowest level of injury in most patients with SCI to develop autonomic dysreflexia. With SCIs above the level of T6, there is reduced SNS outflow and supraspinal control to the splanchnic outflow and the lower-extremity blood vessels. Multiple regression analysis showed that serum leptin levels in men with SCI correlated not only with BMI but also with the neurologic deficit. This finding supports the notion that decentralization of sympathetic nervous activity relieves its inhibitory tone on leptin secretion, because subjects with tetraplegia have a more severe deficit of sympathetic nervous activity [94].

Actually, little is known regarding the nature and time frame of the influence of complete SCI on human skeletal muscle because published data are coming from cross-sectional studies, where different groups with few subjects have been examined at different times, usually in the chronic phase of paralysis. Disuse was thought to be the mechanism responsible for the skeletal muscle atrophy in paraplegics, but muscle fibres following SCI begin to change their functional properties early post injury. Muscle fiber cross-sectional area (CSA) has been suggested to decline from 1 to 17 months after injury and thereafter to reach its nadir. Conversion to type II fibers has been suggested to occur between 4 months and 2 years after injury, resulting in even slow-twitch muscle becoming predominantly fast twitch thereafter (Castro et al 1999). Metabolic enzymes levels in skeletal muscle might be expected to be reduced after SCI because of inactivation. In support of this contention, succinic dehydrogenase (SDH) activity, a marker of aerobic-oxidative capacity, has been reported to be 47–68% below control values in fibers of tibialis anterior muscle years after injury in support of this contention [95].

The muscle atrophy in SCI is of central type and depends on the disuse and loss of upper connections of the lower motor neuron, sometimes associated to the loss of anterior horn cells and transinaptic degeneration. The last alteration may be responsible for the denervation changes seen in early stages post SCI. In the later stages (10-17 months post SCI) diffuse muscle atrophy with reduction of the muscle fascicle dimension is associated to fat infiltration and endomysial fibrosis. In all stages post SCI, almost all patients showed myopathic changes, as internal nuclei, fibre degeneration and cytoplasmic vacuolation due to lipid accumulation [95].

It is evident that other co-factors as spasticity and microvascular damage, contribute to the induction of the marked morphological and enzyme histochemical changes seen in the paralyzed skeletal muscle [95]. Small fibers, predominantly fast-twitch muscle, and low mitochondrial content have been reported years after injury in cross-sectional studies. These data have been interpreted to suggest that human skeletal muscle shows plasticity [48].

On the contrary, force loss during repetitive contractions evoked by surface electrical stimulation (ES) of skeletal muscle in humans does not appear to be altered within a few months of injury [80] but it is greater a year or more after SCI (Hillegass and Dudley, unpublished observations). The greater fatigue, when evident, was partially attributed to lower metabolic enzyme levels [95].

Muscular loading of the bones has been thought to play a role in the maintenance of bone density [65, 66]. However, the ability to stand or ambulate itself does not improve BMD or prevent osteoporosis after SCI.

4. Conclusions

Other important issues according alterations of body composition are the completeness of lesions (an absence of sensory or motor function below the neurological level, including the lowest sacral segment), because body composition seems to be worse than subjects with incomplete lesions (partial preservation of motor and/or sensory function below the neurological level, including the lowest sacral segment) and aging which contributes to major alterations of body composition [62, 63].

In disabled subjects the most important issue according to body composition is how to promote optimal body weight to reduce risk of diseases such as coronary heart disease, non-insulin dependent diabetes mellitus, lipid abnormalities and fractures because of bone loss. Dietary changes, individualized physical activity programs and medication should be taken in mind in therapy when we deal with this subgroup of subjects. However, self-management of dietary changes to improve weight control and disease should be the case, which means they need to follow diets with lower energy intake and at the same time to eat regularly foods rich in nutrients [26].

We need to take in mind that healthy BMI values often underestimate body fat and may mask the adiposity and spasticity did not defend skeletal muscle mass and bone, supporting the concept that in neurologic disabilities the myopathic muscle could not recognize correctly the stimulation because of the neurogenic injury. Moreover, disabled subjects mostly transfer much of the weight-bearing demands of daily activities to their upper extremities reducing the weight-bearing of the affected paralyzed muscles triggering a cycle of added muscle atrophy which interacts with the continuous catabolic action caused by the neurogenic factor. Finally, an irreversible (once established) decline in bone mineral density, bone mineral content as well as geometric characteristics of bone is expected and the duration of lesion-injury is positively correlated with the degree of bone loss.

Further research about body composition is needed in all physical disabilities and more longitudinal studies to quantitate and monitor body composition changes and to modify our therapeutic interventions. However, prevention rather than treatment may have the greatest potential to alleviate these major complications. Therapies should focus on how to perform weight bearing, standing or therapeutically walking activities early in the rehabilitation program to gain benefits according to muscles and bones.

Author details

Yannis Dionyssiotis[1,2*]

1 Rehabilitation Center "Aghios Loukas o Iatros", Trikala Thessaly, Greece

2 University of Athens, 1st Department of Orthopaedics, General University Hospital Attikon, Athens, Greece

References

[1] Jones LM, Goulding A, Gerrard DF. DEXA: a practical and accurate tool to demonstrate total and regional boneloss, lean tissue loss and fat mass gain in paraplegia. Spinal Cord. 1998;36:637-40

[2] Seidell JC, Verschuren WM, van Leer EM, Kromhout D. Overweight, underweight, and mortality. A prospective study of 48.287 men and women. Arch Intern Med. 1996;156:958-63.

[3] Bender R, Trautner C, Spraul M, Berger M. Assessment of excess mortality in obesity. Am J Epidemiol. 1998;147:42-8.

[4] Van Der Ploeg GE, Withers RT, Laforgia J. Percent body fat via DEXA: comparison with a four-compartment model. J Appl Physiol. 2003;94:499-506.

[5] Spungen AM, Adkins RH, Stewart CA, Wang J, Pierson RN Jr, Waters RL, Bauman WA. Factors influencing body composition in persons with spinal cord injury: a cross-sectional study. J Appl Physiol. 2003;95: 2398–2407.

[6] Clarys JP, Martin AD, Drinkwater DT. Gross tissue weights in the human body by cadaver dissection. Hum Biol. 1984;56:459-73.

[7] Modlesky CM, Bickel CS, Slade JM, Meyer RA, Cureton KJ, Dudley GA. Assessment of skeletal muscle mass in men with spinal cord injury using dual-energy X-ray absorptiometry and magnetic resonance imaging. J Appl Physiol. 2004;96:561-5.

[8] Forbes GB. Human body composition: growth, aging, nutrition, and activity. New York: Springer-Verlag; 1987.

[9] Mojtahedi MC, Valentine RJ, Arngrímsson SA, Wilund KR, Evans EM. The association between regional body composition and metabolic outcomes in athletes with spinal cord injury. Spinal Cord. 2008;46:192-7.

[10] Dionyssiotis Y. (2011). Bone Loss in Spinal Cord Injury and Multiple Sclerosis. In: JH Stone, M Blouin, editors. International Encyclopedia of Rehabilitation, av. online: http://cirrie.buffalo.edu/encyclopedia/en/article/340/

[11] Dionyssiotis Y. Spinal cord injury-related bone impairment and fractures: an updateon epidemiology and physiopathological mechanisms. J Musculoskelet Neuronal Interact. 2011;11:257-65.

[12] Smeltzer SC, Zimmerman V, Capriotti T. Osteoporosis risk and low bone mineral density in women with physical disabilities. Arch Phys Med Rehabil. 2005;86:582-6.

[13] Coupaud S, McLean AN, Allan DB. Role of peripheral quantitative computed tomography in identifying disuse osteoporosis in paraplegia. Skeletal Radiol. 2009; 38:989-95.

[14] Gorgey AS, Dudley GA. Skeletal muscle atrophy and increased intramuscular fat after incomplete spinal cord injury. Spinal Cord. 2007;45:304–9.

[15] Jones LM, Legge M, Goulding A. Healthy body mass index values often underestimate body fat in men with spinal cord injury. Arch Phys Med Rehabil. 2003;84:1068-71.

[16] Bulbulian R, Johnson RE, Gruber JJ, Darabos B. Body composition in paraplegic male athletes. Med Sci Sports Exerc. 1987;19:195-201.

[17] Maggioni M, Bertoli S, Margonato V, Merati G, Veicsteinas A, Testolin G. Body composition assessment in spinal cord injury subjects. Acta Diabetol. 2003;40:S183-6.

[18] Mamoun L, Puech AM, Manetta J, Badiou S, Paris F, Ohanna F, Rossi M, Sultan C. Circulating leptin concentrations can be used as a surrogate marker of fat mass in acute spinal cord injury patients. Metabolism. 2004;53:989-94.

[19] Dionyssiotis Υ, Petropoulou K, Rapidi CA, Papagelopoulos PJ, Papaioannou N, Galanos A, Papadaki P, and Lyritis GP. Body Composition in Paraplegic Men. Journal of Clinical Densitometry. 2008;11: 437-43.

[20] National Institutes of Health Consensus Development Conference Statement. Health implications of obesity. Natl Inst Health Consens Dev Conf Consens Statement. 1985;5:1-7.

[21] Schulte PA, Wagner GR, Ostry A, Blanciforti LA, Cutlip RG, Krajnak KM, Luster M, Munson AE, O'Callaghan JP, Parks CG, Simeonova PP, Miller DB. Work, obesity,and occupational safety and health. Am J Public Health. 2007;97:428-36.

[22] Kocina P. Body composition of spinal cord injured adults. Sports Medicine. 1997;23:48-60.

[23] Gupta N, White KT, Sandford PR. Body mass index in spinal cord injury -- a retrospective study. Spinal Cord. 2006;44:92-4.

[24] McDonald CM, Abresch-Meyer AL, Nelson MD, Widman LM. Body mass index and body composition measures by dual x-ray absorptiometry in patients aged 10 to 21 years with spinal cord injury. J Spinal Cord Med. 2007;30:S97-104.

[25] Spungen AM, Wang J, Pierson RN, Jr., Bauman WA. Soft tissue body composition differences in monozygotic twins discordant for spinal cord injury. J Appl Physiol. 2000;88:1310-5.

[26] Groah SL, Nash MS, Ljungberg IH, Libin A, Hamm LF, Ward E, Burns PA, Enfield G. Nutrient intake and body habitus after spinal cord injury: an analysis by sex and level of injury. J Spinal Cord Med. 2009;32:25-33.

[27] Maimoun L, Fattal C, Micallef JP, Peruchon E, Rabischong P. Bone loss in spinal cord-injured patients: from physiopathology to therapy. Spinal Cord. 2006;44:203-10.

[28] Lussier L, Knight J, Bell G, Lohman T, Morris AF. Body composition comparison in two elite female wheelchair athletes. Paraplegia. 1983;21:16-22.

[29] Spungen AM, Bauman WA, Wang J, Pierson RN. Reduced quality of fat free mass in paraplegia. Clin Research. 1992;40:280A.

[30] Womersley J, Durnin JV, Boddy K, Mahaffy M. Influence of muscular development, obesity, and age on the fat-free mass of adults. J Appl Physiol. 1976;41:223-9.

[31] Fuller NJ, Sawyer MB, Laskey MA, Paxton P, Elia M: Prediction of body composition in elderly men over 75 years of age. Ann Hum Biol. 1996;23:127-47.

[32] Hildreth HG, Johnson RK, Goran MI, Contompasis SH. Body composition in adults with cerebral palsy by dual-energy X-ray absorptiometry, bioelectrical impedance analysis, and skinfold anthropometry compared with the 18O isotope-dilution technique. Am J Clin Nutr. 1997;66:1436-42.

[33] Liu LF, Roberts R, Moyer-Mileur L, Samson-Fang L. Determination of body composition in children with cerebral palsy: bioelectrical impedance analysis and anthropometry vs dual-energy x-ray absorptiometry. J Am Diet Assoc. 2005;105:794-7.

[34] Kuperminc MN, Stevenson RD. Growth and nutrition disorders in children with cerebral palsy. Dev Disabil Res Rev. 2008;14:137-46.

[35] Mitsiopoulos N, Baumgartner RN, Heymsfield SB, Lyons W, Gallagher D, and Ross R. Cadaver validation of skeletal muscle measurement by magnetic resonance imaging and computerized tomography. J Appl Physiol. 1998;85:115–22.

[36] Mahon AK, Flynn MG, Iglay HB, Stewart LK, Johnson CA, McFarlin BK, Campbell WW. Measurement of body composition changes with weight loss in postmenopausal women: comparison of methods. J Nutr Health Aging. 2007;11:203-13.

[37] LaForgia J, Dollman J, Dale MJ, Withers RT, Hill AM. Validation of DXA body composition estimates in obese men and women. Obesity (Silver Spring). 2009;17:821-6.

[38] Rittweger J, Beller G, Ehrig J, Jung C, Koch U, Ramolla J, Schmidt F, Newitt D, Majumdar S, Schiessl H, Felsenberg D. Bone-muscle strength indices for the human lower leg. Bone. 2000;27:319-26.

[39] Dionyssiotis Y. Changes in bone density and strength of the tibia and alterations of lean and fat mass in chronic paraplegic men. Doctoral Dissertation Laboratory for Research of the Musculoskeletal System, University of Athens, Athens 2008.

[40] Peppler WW, Mazess RB. 1981. Total body bone mineral and lean body mass by dual-photon absorptiometry. Calcif Tissue Int 33:353-359

[41] Pietrobelli A, Formica C, Wang AM, Heymsfield SB. 1996. Dual-energy X-ray absorptiometry body composition model: review of physical concepts. Am J Physiol 271 (Endocrinol Metab 34): E941-E951

[42] Ferretti J.L., Cointry G.R., Capozza R.F., Zanchetta J.R. Dual energy X-ray absorptiometry. Skeletal Muscle: Pathology, Diagnosis and Management of Disease. V.R.Preedy, T.J.Peters (eds),Greenwich Medical Media, Ltd., London, 2001; p.451-458.

[43] Bauman WA, Spungen AM, Raza M, Rothstein J, Zhang RL, Zhong YG, Tsuruta M, Shahidi R, Pierson RN Jr, Wang J, et al. Coronary artery disease: metabolic risk factors and latent disease in individuals with paraplegia. Mt Sinai J Med. 1992;59:163-8.

[44] Bauman WA, Spungen AM. Disorders of carbohydrate and lipid metabolism inveterans with paraplegia or quadriplegia: A model of premature aging. Metabolism. 1994;43:749-56.

[45] Garland DE, Stewart CA, Adkins RH, Hu SS, Rosen C, Liotta FJ, Weinstein DA Osteoporosis after spinal cord injury. J Orthop Res. 1992;10:371-8.

[46] Heymsfield SB, Wang J, Heshka S, Kehayias JJ, Pierson RN. Dual-photon absorptiometry: comparison of bone mineral and soft tissue mass measurements in vivo with established methods. Am J Clin Nutr.1989;49:1283-9.

[47] Laskey MA. Dual-energy X-ray absorptiometry and body composition. Nutrition. 1996;12:45-51.

[48] Castro MJ, Apple DF Jr, Staron RS, Campos GE, Dudley GA. Influence of complete spinal cord injury on skeletal muscle within 6 mo of injury. J Appl Physiol.1999; 86:350-8.

[49] Szollar SM, Martin EM, Parthemore JG, Sartoris DJ, Deftos LJ. Densitometric patternsof spinal cord injury associated bone loss. Spinal Cord. 1997;35:374-82.

[50] Uebelhart D, Demiaux-Domenech B, Roth M, Chantraine A. Bone metabolism in spinal cord injured individuals and in others who have prolonged immobilisation. A review.Paraplegia. 1995;33:669-73.

[51] Chow YW, Inman C, Pollintine P, Sharp CA, Haddaway MJ, el Masry W, Davie MW.Ultrasound bone densitometry and dual energy X-ray absorptiometry in patients with spinal cord injury: a cross-sectional study. Spinal Cord. 1996;34:736-41.

[52] Biering-Sorensen F, Bohr H, Schaadt O. Bone mineral content of the lumbar spine and lower extremities years after spinal cord lesion. Paraplegia. 1988 ;26:293-301.

[53] Lazo MG, Shirazi P, Sam M, Giobbie-Hurder A, Blacconiere MJ, Muppidi M. Osteoporosis and risk of fracture in men with spinal cord injury. Spinal Cord. 2001;39:208-14.

[54] Frey-Rindova P, de Bruin ED, Stussi E, Dambacher MA, Dietz V. Bone mineral density in upper and lower extremities during 12 months after spinal cord injury measured by peripheral quantitative computed tomography. Spinal Cord. 2000;38:26–32.

[55] Jiang SD, Dai LY, Jiang LS. Osteoporosis after spinal cord injury. Osteoporos Int. 2006;17:180-92.

[56] Dauty M, Perrouin Verbe B, Maugars Y, Dubois C, Mathe JF. Supralesional and sublesional bone mineral density in spinal cord-injured patients. Bone. 2000;27:305-9.

[57] Chantraine A, Nusgens B, Lapiere CM. Bone remodelling during the development of osteoporosis in paraplegia. Calcif Tissue Int. 1986;38:323-7.

[58] Ogilvie C, Bowker P, Rowley DI. The physiological benefits of paraplegic orthotically aided walking. Paraplegia. 1993;31:111-5.

[59] Leslie WD, Nance PW. Dissociated hip and spine demineralization: a specific finding in spinal cord injury. Arch Phys Med Rehabil. 1993; 74:960-4.

[60] Tsuzuku S, Ikegami Y, Yabe K. Bone mineral density differences between paraplegic and quadriplegic patients: a cross-sectional study. Spinal Cord. 1999; 37:358-61.

[61] Dionyssiotis Y, Lyritis GP, Papaioannou N, Papagelopoulos P, Thomaides T. Influence of neurological level of injury in bones, muscles, and fat in paraplegia. J Rehabil Res Dev. 2009;46:1037-44.

[62] Demirel G, Yilmaz H, Paker N, Onel S. Osteoporosis after spinal cord injury. Spinal Cord. 1998;36:8

[63] Sabo D, Blaich S, Wenz W, Hohmann M, Loew M, Gerner HJ. Osteoporosis in patients with paralysis after spinal cord injury: a cross sectional study in 46 male patients with dual-energy X-ray absorptiometry. Arch Orthop Trauma Surg. 2001;121:75–8.

[64] Clasey JL, Janowiak AL, Gater DR Relationship between regional bone density measurements and the time since injury in adults with spinal cord injuries. Arch Phys Med Rehabil. 2004;85:59–64

[65] Dionyssiotis Y, Lyritis GP, Mavrogenis AF, Papagelopoulos PJ. Factors influencingbone loss in paraplegia. Hippokratia. 2011;15:54-9.

[66] de Bruin ED, Vanwanseele B, Dambacher MA, Dietz V, Stussi E. Long-term changes in the tibia and radius bone mineral density following spinal cord injury. Spinal Cord. 2005;43:96-101.

[67] Eser P, Frotzler A, Zehnder Y, Schiessl H, Denoth J. Assessment of anthropometric, systemic, and lifestyle factors influencing bone status in the legs of spinal cord injured individuals. Osteoporos Int. 2005;16:26-34.

[68] Löfvenmark I, Werhagen L, Norrbrink C. Spasticity and bone density after a spinal cord injury. J Rehabil Med. 2009;41:1080-4.

[69] Kiratli BJ, Smith AE, Nauenberg T, Kallfelz CF, Perkash I. Bone mineral and geometric changes through the femur with immobilization due to spinal cord injury. J Rehabil Res Dev. 2000;37:225-33.

[70] Wood DE, Dunkerley AL, Tromans AM. Results from bone mineral density scans in twenty-two complete lesion paraplegics. Spinal Cord. 2001;39:145–8.

[71] Kunkel CF, Scremin AM, Eisenberg B, Garcia JF, Roberts S, Martinez S. Effect of ''standing'' on spasticity, contracture, and osteoporosis in paralyzed males. Arch Phys Med Rehabil. 1993;74:73–8.

[72] Frost HM. Bone "mass" and the "mechanostat": a proposal. Anat Rec. 1987;219:1-9.

[73] Frost HM. Skeletal structural adaptations to mechanical usage (SATMU): 2. Redefining Wolff's law: the remodeling problem. Anat Rec. 1990;226:414-22.

[74] Frost HM. Perspectives: on a "paradigm shift" developing in skeletal science. Calcif Tissue Int. 1995;56:1-4.

[75] Ragnarsson KT, Pollack S, O'Daniel W Jr, Edgar R, Petrofsky J, Nash MS. Clinical evaluation of computerized functional electrical stimulation after spinal cord injury: a multicenter pilot study. Arch Phys Med Rehabil. 1988;69:672-7.

[76] Belanger M, Stein RB, Wheeler GD, Gordon T, Leduc B. Electrical stimulation: can it increase muscle strength and reverse osteopenia in spinal cord injured individuals? Arch Phys Med Rehabil. 2000;81:1090-8.

[77] Bloomfield SA, Mysiw WJ, Jackson RD. Bone mass and endocrine adaptations to training in spinal cord injured individuals. Bone. 1996;19:61-8.

[78] BeDell KK, Scremin AM, Perell KL, Kunkel CF. Effects of functional electrical stimulation-induced lower extremity cycling on bone density of spinal cord-injured patients. Am J Phys Med Rehabil. 1996;75:29-34.

[79] Needham-Shropshire BM, Broton JG, Klose KJ, Lebwohl N, Guest RS, Jacobs PL. Evaluation of a training program for persons with SCI paraplegia using the Parastep 1 ambulation system: part 3. Lack of effect on bone mineral density. Arch Phys Med Rehabil. 1997;78:799-803.

[80] Shields RK. Muscular, skeletal, and neural adaptations following spinal cord injury. J Orthop Sports Phys Ther. 2002;32:65-74.

[81] Shields RK, Dudley-Javoroski S. Musculoskeletal adaptations in chronic spinal cord injury: effects of long-term soleus electrical stimulation training. Neurorehabil Neural Repair. 2007;21:169-79.

[82] Valayer-Chaleat E, Calmels P, Giraux P, Fayolle-Minon I. Femoral fracture and iatrogenic hyperthyroidism in spinal cord injury. Spinal Cord. 1998;36:593-5.

[83] Frey Law LA, Shields RK. Femoral loads during passive, active, and active-resistive stance after spinal cord injury: a mathematical model. Clin Biomech. (Bristol, Avon). 2004;19:313-21.

[84] Fruhbeck G, Jebb SA, Prentice AM. Leptin: physiology and pathophysiology. Clin Physiol. 1998;18:399-419.

[85] Maffei M, Halaas J, Ravussin E, Pratley RE, Lee GH, Zhang Y, Fei H, Kim S, Lallone R, Ranganathan S, et al. Leptin levels in human and rodent: measurement of plasma leptin and ob RNA in obese and weight-reduced subjects. Nat Med. 1995;1:1155-61.

[86] Bauman WA, Spungen AM, Zhong YG, Mobbs CV. Plasma leptin is directly related to body adiposity in subjects with spinal cord injury. Horm Metab Res. 1996;28:732-6.

[87] Correia ML, Morgan DA, Mitchell JL, Sivitz WI, Mark AL, Haynes WG. Role of corticotrophin-releasing factor in effects of leptin on sympathetic nerve activity and arterial pressure. Hypertension. 2001;38:384-8.

[88] Elias CF, Lee C, Kelly J, Aschkenasi C, Ahima RS, Couceyro PR, Kuhar MJ, Saper CB, Elmquist JK. Leptin activates hypothalamic CART neurons projecting to the spinal cord. Neuron. 1998;21:1375-85.

[89] Haque MS, Minokoshi Y, Hamai M, Iwai M, Horiuchi M, Shimazu T. Role of the sympathetic nervous system and insulin in enhancing glucose uptake in peripheral tissues after intrahypothalamic injection of leptin in rats. Diabetes. 1999;48:1706-12.

[90] Horowitz JF, Coppack SW, Paramore D, Cryer PE, Zhao G, Klein S. Effect of short-term fasting on lipid kinetics in lean and obese women. Am J Physiol. 1999;276:E278-84.

[91] Horowitz JF, Klein S. Whole body and abdominal lipolytic sensitivity to epinephrine is suppressed in upper body obese women. Am J Physiol Endocrinol Metab. 2000;278:E1144-52.

[92] Krassioukov AV, Bunge RP, Pucket WR, Bygrave MA. The changes in human spinal sympathetic preganglionic neurons after spinal cord injury. Spinal Cord. 1999;37:6-13.

[93] Jeon JY, Steadward RD, Wheeler GD, Bell G, McCargar L, Harber V. Intact sympathetic nervous system is required for leptin effects on resting metabolic rate in people with spinal cord injury. J Clin Endocrinol Metab. 2003;88:402-7.

[94] Wang YH, Huang TS, Liang HW, Su TC, Chen SY, Wang TD. Fasting serum levels of adiponectin, ghrelin, and leptin in men with spinal cord injury. Arch Phys Med Rehabil. 2005;86:1964-8.

[95] Scelsi R. Skeletal Muscle Pathology after Spinal Cord Injury: Our 20 Year Experience and Results on Skeletal Muscle Changes in Paraplegics, Related to Functional Rehabilitation Basic Appl Myol. 2001;11:75-85.

Chapter 8

Paraplegia Related Osteoporosis

Yannis Dionyssiotis

Additional information is available at the end of the chapter

http://dx.doi.org/10.5772/57969

1. Introduction

Osteoporosis is characterized by low bone mass and destruction of the micro architecture of bone tissue, resulting in increased bone fragility and susceptibility to fractures. [1]

The World Health Organisation (WHO) created an operational definition of postmenopausal osteoporosis based on a bone mineral density (BMD)-based T-score measurement. The most widely validated technique to measure BMD is dual energy X-ray absorptiometry (DXA), and diagnostic criteria based on the T-score for BMD are a recommended entry criterion for the development of pharmaceutical interventions in osteoporosis. (2) The ranking system of the WHO is commonly used in the literature and in all discussions with respect to bone diseases. According to WHO criteria, the general categories for making a diagnosis are the following: 1) normal: BMD of not less than one standard deviation (SD) than the average young adult (T-score>-1), 2) osteopenia: BMD between one and 2.5 SD below the average for young adults (-1<T-score<-2.5), 3) osteoporosis: BMD 2.5 SD or more below the average for young adults (T-score>-2.5) and 4) severe or established osteoporosis: BMD 2.5 SD or more below the average for young adults and the presence of one or more fractures. [2, 3]

Because of the unique and individually-based approach needed in the management of each disabled subject with a spinal cord lesion and their complications according to bone loss the new term "paraplegia-related bone impairment, (Para-related BI)" is used throughout this chapter. The term bone impairment is more appropriate than bone disorder because includes terminology from Rehabilitation Science a specialty which interferes with all complications of spinal cord injury (SCI) and follows these patients during aging with paralysis. It is not used here for the 1st time. Very experienced scientists and researchers chose this term to describe "osteoporosis" in SCI. [4]

2. Paraplegia related bone impairment

2.1. Epidemiology

According to the literature, spinal cord injury-related bone impairment (SCI-related BI) occurs in 75% of patients with complete SCI. [5] Twenty five out of 41 patients with SCI (61%) met WHO criteria for osteoporosis; eight (19.5%) were osteopenic and only eight (19.5%) showed normal values.[6] In SCI children (boys and girls), values for BMD at the hip were approximately 60% of normal, or had a Z-score that indicated a 1.6-1.8 SD reduction in BMD compared with age-and sex-matched peers. [7] The decrease in BMD was probably the dominant cause for the high prevalence of SCI-related BI in the long femur or proximal tibia and explains why these areas are often fracture site. [6, 8, 9] For example, a reduction in bone mineral density in the femoral neck of about 0.1 g/cm^2 increases fracture risk by 2.2 times. This decrease in bone mass is associated with alterations in bone material, reduced bone elasticity and is connected to the origin of pathological fractures with minimal injury, in which these patients are vulnerable and exposed. [8, 9]

2.2. Bone mineral density

In individuals with SCI bone loss begins immediately after injury. [10, 11] SCI-related BI below the level of injury is much greater compared with other conditions (i.e. age, immobilization, bed rest, lack of gravity environment). A reduction of bone mineral content during the first years after the injury of 4% per month in regions rich in cancellous bone, and 2% per month on sites containing mainly cortical bone is reported. [12] According to another study 25 out of 41 patients with SCI (61%) met WHO's criteria for osteoporosis, eight (19.5%) were osteopenic and only eight (19.5%) showed normal values. [6] In SCI children (boys and girls) values for BMD at the hip were approximately 60% of normal, or had a Z-score that indicated a 1.6-1.8 SD reduction in BMD compared with age-and sex-matched peers. [7]

Bone loss measured with peripheral quantitative computed tomography (p QCT) in SCI subjects in the femur's and tibia's epiphyses was 50% and 60% vs. 35% and 25% in the diaphyses, respectively, meaning that bone loss in the epiphyses almost doubled the loss in the diaphyses. [13] This study also showed that bone loss between trabecular and cortical bone compartment differs in mechanism, i.e. in the epiphyses bone is lost due to the decrease in trabecular, while in diaphysis, the cortical bone density is maintained and bone is lost due to endocortical resorption. In line with the previous study, another p QCT study, performed in complete paraplegics with high (thoracic 4-7) and low (thoracic 8-12) neurological level of injury at the tibia, found a loss of trabecular (57.5% vs. 51%, in high vs. low paraplegics, respectively) and cortical bone (3.6% and 6.5%, respectively), suggesting that trabecular bone is more affected during the years of paralysis in comparison with cortical bone. [14] In the same study both paraplegic groups had a similar loss of total BMD (46.90% vs. 45.15%, in high vs. low paraplegics, respectively) suggesting that a homogenously deficit pattern occurs in the epiphyseal area, especially in the group of low paraplegics because the central and the peripheral of the cross sectional area of bone were similarly affected. On the contrary, in high paraplegics' group trabecular bone loss was higher suggesting an increasing endocortical remodeling keeping the total BMD similar. Concerning cortical geometric properties the results had shown an increased endosteal circumference between both paraplegic groups vs. controls leading to reduction of cortical thickness, 19.78% vs. 16.98% in paraplegic groups respectively, whereas periosteal circumference was comparable to controls (Fig. 1).

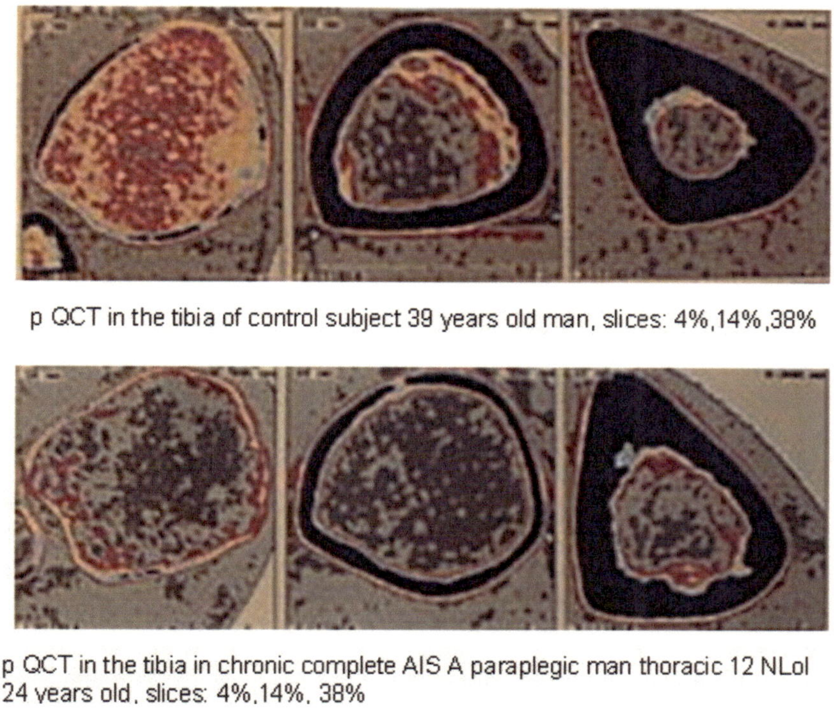

Figure 1. Peripheral quantitative computed tomography (p QCT) tibia slices in control (a) and paraplegic subject (b), (scanner XCT 3000 Stratec, Medizintechnik, Pforzheim, Germany). Areas in red represent trabecular bone, while areas in grey represent fat; pQCT allows the measurements of true volumetric densities at a minimum exposure to X-rays, assess cortical and trabecular bone density separately as well as to evaluate the geometrical properties of long bones non-invasively, adapted from: Dionyssiotis Y. (15) (with permission).

Regarding tetraplegic patients statistically significant differences were found in BMD of the spine, trochanteric region and upper limbs between paraplegic and tetraplegic patients but not in the femoral neck, pelvis, and lower extremities. [16] Indeed, the effects on spinal BMD differed from previously published work in which the investigation was mainly focused in paraplegics. [17-19]

The importance of mechanical loading and site specificity to maintain or increase BMD is already shown. [20] According to bone loss there are some interesting features in spinal cord injured subjects; demineralization is area dependent, occurs exclusively in the areas below the level of injury, affecting mainly paralyzed extremities and increasing from proximal to distal regions i.e. in paraplegics weight bearing skeleton regions, as the distal end of femur and proximal tibia, which are rich in cancellous bone, while region of the diaphysis of the femur and tibia, rich in cortical bone is reserved. [13, 14, 21] Moreover, bone loss between trabecular and cortical bone compartment differs in mechanism, i.e. in the epiphyses is due to decrease in trabecular but in diaphysis cortical bone is maintained and bone is lost through endocortical resorption by reducing cortical wall thickness. [13, 14]

2.2.1. The additional risk factor of feminine gender

Women with disabilities have a higher risk of losing bone mass compared to men because of the inevitable reduction in estrogen levels that occurs at menopause. Findings that women with serious disabilities have low bone density are not surprising and are probably related to the lack of activity (reduced mobility, reduced loading on bone) and worsening of the disability. [22] Regarding women with complete SCI, the initial bone loss in the lumbar spine is negligible. Post injury over a period of years BMD in SCI women is maintained or increases compared with non-injured age-matched women, in whom BMD decreases during aging.

2.2.2. Biochemical changes in bone after spinal cord injury

After SCI, osteoblast activity slightly increases, while a significant increase in osteoclast activity within a maximum of 10 weeks after injury and at level up to 10 times greater than normal is present. The imbalance between bone resorption and bone formation below the level of the lesion or injured area may be due to decreased blood flow and venous stasis, arteriovenous anastomoses and tissue oxidation. [23] SCI-related BI can be enhanced by a lack of muscular tension on bone or other neuronal factors associated with the lesion. The parathyroid glands are inactive with low levels of parathyroid hormone (PTH) observed up to one year after injury. The hypercalcemia that occurs immediately after injury is responsible for low levels of PTH. Gradually, in a range of one to nine years after injury, the function of the parathyroid is restored. The result is an increase in bone resorption associated with dysfunction of the parathyroid glands in the chronic phase of injury. This mechanism of SCI-related BI during the chronic phase tends to be balanced by an increase in bone mineral density (BMD) in areas of the body with increased loading (upper limbs, spinal column) and adds bone density (transferring bone mineral) compared to a loss in the chronic non-loadable areas of the skeleton (pelvis, lower limbs and upper limbs in tetraplegics). Hormonal changes (parathyroid hormone, glucocorticoids and calcitonin) and metabolic disorders (increased alkaline phosphatase, hypercalcemia/hypercalciuria and hydroxyproline excretion) may be secondary to the loss of bone density. [10, 24] Hypercalciuria is seen in the first 10 days after neurological injury and reaches its maximum value after one to six months and is two to four times greater that the hypercalciuria observed after prolonged bed rest. The significant increase of calcium in the urine is the result of an imbalance between bone formation and bone resorption. [25] The rate of formation or resorption of bone matrix can be determined by quantifying the enzyme activity of bone cells or by measuring the components of the matrix that are released into the circulation during the process of absorption. It should be noted that these indices of bone activity are somewhat non-specific. The intact procollagen I N-terminal propeptide (PINP) molecule is the amino end of type I procollagen before excision and the formation of fibrils and is a measure of the total synthesis of collagen in the body, all of which is related to bone matrix. Osteocalcin is a non-collagen protein which is a primary constituent of osteoblasts, and may also be released during apoptosis of osteoclasts and indicates either formation when resorption and formation are coupled or turnover in decoupling. [26, 27] Urinary excretion of cross-linked pyridoline type I collagen is recognised as a sensitive marker of bone resorption, and pyridoline quality tests including measurement of the aminoterminal (NTx) and carboxyterminal (CTx) intermolecular cross-linking domain of bone type-1 collagen provide a good indicator of bone resorption. [28, 29] Others studied markers of bone metabolism for six months after acute spinal cord injury and observed an increase in ionised serum calcium above the upper limit of normal and suppression of serum PTH. [30] The indices of bone resorption (total pyridoline, deoxypiridoline [total and free] and NTx) recorded a significant increase (even 10 times above the upper limit of normal) after acute immobilisation, with the highest values found 10 to 16 weeks after injury. The markers of bone formation (total alkaline phosphatase and osteocalcin) showed an insignificant increase, which remained within the normal limits. [10] Moreover, Nance et al. observed that values of NTx in the urine were lower during the first months in patients receiving pamidronate compared with the control group, but this finding did not reach significance. [31] Regarding the lack or insufficiency of vitamin D, it has been reported that 64% of paraplegics are deficient (<15ng/ml). [32]

Mechanical unloading (paralysis) in acute SCI subjects causes greater sclerostin levels than those observed in the able bodied. This increase is associated with reduced bone formation during the acute phase of SCI. The ability to walk (mechanical loading) modulates the response of bone to paralysis by causing a smaller increase in sclerostin levels, thereby partially protecting against bone loss. In the chronic phase, bone wasting results in lower sclerostin levels than those observed in the able bodied. This effect is due to the reduction of sclerostin-producing osteocytes in the osteoporotic bone. In the chronic phase, similar to the acute phase, the ability to walk partially protects against bone loss. Sclerostin causes up-regulation of RANKL (key factor that promotes the differentiation of osteoclasts) and down regulation of osteoprotegerin (a key inhibitor of osteoclast differentiation) expression in osteocytes, which leads to increased osteoclast activity and bone resorption. [33]

2.2.3. Duration of paralysis and bone steady state

The duration of paralysis affects the degree of bone loss in regions below the level of injury. A study of 21 men with SCI with an average duration of 10.6 years, using DEXA, expressed at various levels of injury an inverse relationship between BMD in the legs and the duration of the lesion, while others found a weaker relationship regarding the microarchitecture of the distal end of tibia. [34, 35]

In a study which included paraplegics with duration of paralysis of 14 ± 11.5 years a positive correlation between the duration of paralysis and the degree of bone loss was found. [13] The length of immobilization in the acute posttraumatic period increased bone loss in the legs, particularly in the proximal tibia; over 50% of bone mass was lost (in the affected areas) in the period of ten years after the injury. [21] When subjects categorized depending on the length of the lesion (0-1, 1-5, 6-9, 10-19, 20-29, 30-39, 40-49, and 50-59 years after the injury), in all age groups bone mineral density of the proximal femur declined and was detected a year after the injury. [24]

Using DXA and QUS (quantitative ultrasound) measurements in 100 men with SCI, aged 18 to 60 years, it was found that bone density decreases over time in all measured points, while bone loss followed a linear pattern in the femoral neck and distal epiphysis, stabilized within three years after the injury. On the contrary, Z-scores of the distal region of the diaphysis of the tibia continued to decrease even beyond ten years after the injury. [36] Duration of paralysis related bone loss in the legs of monozygotic twins with chronic paraplegia in comparison with their able-bodied co-twins has been also reported. [37]

The results of a comparison of chronic complete paraplegic men vs. controls in another study found a reduction of BMD in paraplegics' legs independent of the neurological level of lesion. BMD of the legs was negatively correlated with the duration of paralysis in the total paraplegic group, but after investigation according to the neurological level this correlation was due to the strong correlation of high paraplegics' legs BMD with the duration of paralysis, suggesting a possible influence of the neurological level of injury on the extent of bone loss. [38] A significant inverse relationship between percentage-matched in BMD leg, arm and trunk values and time since injury was found when varying levels of SCI were analyzed. [34]

Studies are supporting the concept of a new bone steady state at 16-24 months after injury, especially for bone metabolic process, but BMD decreases over the years at different areas and is inversely related to the time of the injury, which means continuous bone loss beyond the first two years after the injury (Fig. 2). [11, 13, 14, 24, 38-41]

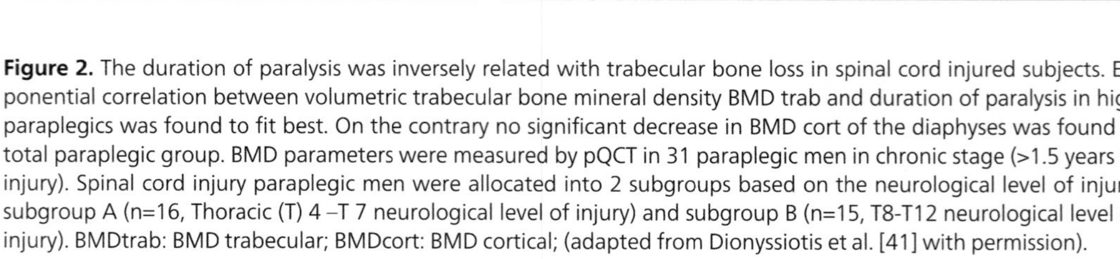

Figure 2. The duration of paralysis was inversely related with trabecular bone loss in spinal cord injured subjects. Exponential correlation between volumetric trabecular bone mineral density BMD trab and duration of paralysis in high paraplegics was found to fit best. On the contrary no significant decrease in BMD cort of the diaphyses was found in total paraplegic group. BMD parameters were measured by pQCT in 31 paraplegic men in chronic stage (>1.5 years of injury). Spinal cord injury paraplegic men were allocated into 2 subgroups based on the neurological level of injury; subgroup A (n=16, Thoracic (T) 4 –T 7 neurological level of injury) and subgroup B (n=15, T8-T12 neurological level of injury). BMDtrab: BMD trabecular; BMDcort: BMD cortical; (adapted from Dionyssiotis et al. [41] with permission).

The role played by factors such as race or gender of patients is not yet clear documented, but studies indicated more loss in women than men. [42] Loss of bone is closing fracture threshold from 1 to 5 years after injury and risk factors for fractures after spinal cord injury are gender (women are more at risk than men), age and duration of injury (increasing age and duration of injury increases the risk of fracture with a statistically significant increase in 10 years after injury), the type of injury (complete SCI subjects have more fractures than incomplete), low body mass index (BMI) and low bone density in the tibia. [6, 24, 43]

2.2.4. The role of central nervous system

2.2.4.1. Sympathetic denervation in SCI

Spinal cord injury is a dynamic process that is related to alterations in both the central and peripheral sympathetic nervous system (SNS). Sympathetic denervation in SCI may cause arteriovenous shunts and a slowdown of intraosseous blood flow, thus increasing bone resorption. [44] With high-level spinal cord lesions the SNS is disproportionately involved when compared with the parasympathetic nervous system. In a complete high-level SCI, functioning in the isolated spinal cord below the lesion becomes independent of supraspinal control and has been termed "decentralization" of the sympathetic nervous system. [45]

Loss of supraspinal control leads to dysregulation of those homeostatic mechanisms normally influenced by the SNS through loss of facilitation or lack of inhibition. [46] Today there is clinical evidence that the sympathetic regulation of bone does exist in humans and plays a clinically important role in diseases characterized by excessive sympathetic activity. [47] The scientific finding about sympathetic innervations of bone tissue and its role in the regulation of bone remodelling is of major interest in situations where uncoupling between osteoclasts and osteoblasts occurs. [48-50]

2.2.4.2. Spasticity

So far, spasticity has been considered by many researchers as a prophylactic factor for bone. It is well known that voluntary muscle contraction is effective in the prevention of osteoporosis. [51, 52] Although muscle loading plays a vital role in maintaining bone density, conflicting results regarding the effect of muscle spasms in the form of spasticity have been reported in SCI patients. [53-56] Controversial results have also been reported regarding the effect of spasticity on BMD in paraplegics. A cross-sectional study of 41 paraplegics reported less reduction of BMD in the spastic compared to the flaccid paraplegic SCI patients. [53-55] Other investigators suggested that muscle spasms can slow bone loss based on the theory of a single basic muscle/bone unit. [56] Muscle spasms and muscle tension in the presence of spasticity put force on bone. This is likely to play a regulatory role in maintaining bone density. These studies concluded that spasticity may be a protective factor against bone loss in SCI. Other researchers, however, could not find a correlation between bone density and spasticity. [55] Moreover, in 18 motor complete SCI men matched for time since injury, gender and age (nine had severe spasticity and nine had spasticity that was either mild or not present) no difference was found in BMD depending on the level of spasticity. [57] A pQCT study investigating the tibia in complete paraplegics above the thoracic 12 (T12) level with various degrees of spasticity according to the Ashworth scale found no effect on volumetric BMD measurements.[41] Others have reported that spasticity may be protective against bone loss in SCI patients, however, without any preserving effect on the tibia. [55] A possible explanation for this could lie in the fact that studies include various SCI subjects with various degrees of spasticity. In addition, in studies examining the lower leg, muscle spasms affecting the lower leg would mainly be extension spasms resulting in plantar flexion, thus creating little resistance to the contracting muscles. Furthermore, the measuring sites of the tibia did not include any muscle insertions of either the knee or the ankle extensor muscles. Patients without spasticity usually have more fractures. At the same time, excessive spasticity may cause fractures through uncontrolled limb movements, i.e. in a wheelchair. Therefore, the effect of spasticity on bone is probably two-sided: a low grade of spasticity is beneficial while a high grade is harmful. [41]

3. Interventions for prevention of bone impairment

3.1. Weight bearing activities – Body weight supported treadmill – Cycling

The effect of standing in bone after SCI has been investigated by many researchers. A beneficial effect on bone mass using passive mechanical loading has been shown on preservation of bone mass in the region of the femoral shaft, but not at the proximal hip of standing and non-standing patients and relatively better-preserved densities in patients standing with braces than in those using a standing frame or standing wheelchair. [58] A slower rate of bone loss in paraplegic subjects who did standing was expressed in a prospective study of 19 patients in acute SCI phase participated in early standing training program which showed benefits concerning the reduction of cancellous bone loss compared to immobilized subjects, while no correlation for passive standing-training to bone status was found in another p QCT study. [59, 60] Protection afforded by standing in the femoral diaphysis stands in contrast with the loss of bone in the proximal femur. This suggests that the transmission of forces through trabecular and cortical bone varies; so the less effective strain for the initiation of bone remodeling reaches faster cortical bone. [61] Others also supported the concept of different strain thresholds during bone remodeling control. [62-64] There is level 2 evidence (from 1 non-randomized prospective controlled trial) that Functional Electrical Stimulation (FES)-cycling did not improve or maintain bone at the tibial midshaft in the acute phase. [65] Moreover, there is level 4 evidence (from 1 pre-post study) that 6 months of FES cycle ergometry increased regional lower extremity BMD over areas stimulated. [66] Body weight supported treadmill training (BWSTT) did not alter the expected pattern of change in bone biochemical markers over time and bone density at fracture-prone sites. [67]

3.2. Whole body vibration

At a meeting of the American Society for Bone and Mineral Research the results of a small randomised, placebo-controlled study among 20 children with cerebral palsy who used a similar, commercially available vibrating platform for 10 min per day, 5 days per week for 6 months, reported a significant increase in tibial, but not lumbar-spine bone density in the treated group despite the simplicity, short duration of the "vibration, the young age of the children and the poor compliance. [68, 69]

After 6 months of whole body vibration (WBV) therapy in twenty children (14 boys-6 girls) with cerebral palsy (age 6.2 to 12.3 years) randomized to either continue their school physio-

http://dx.doi.org/10.5772/57969

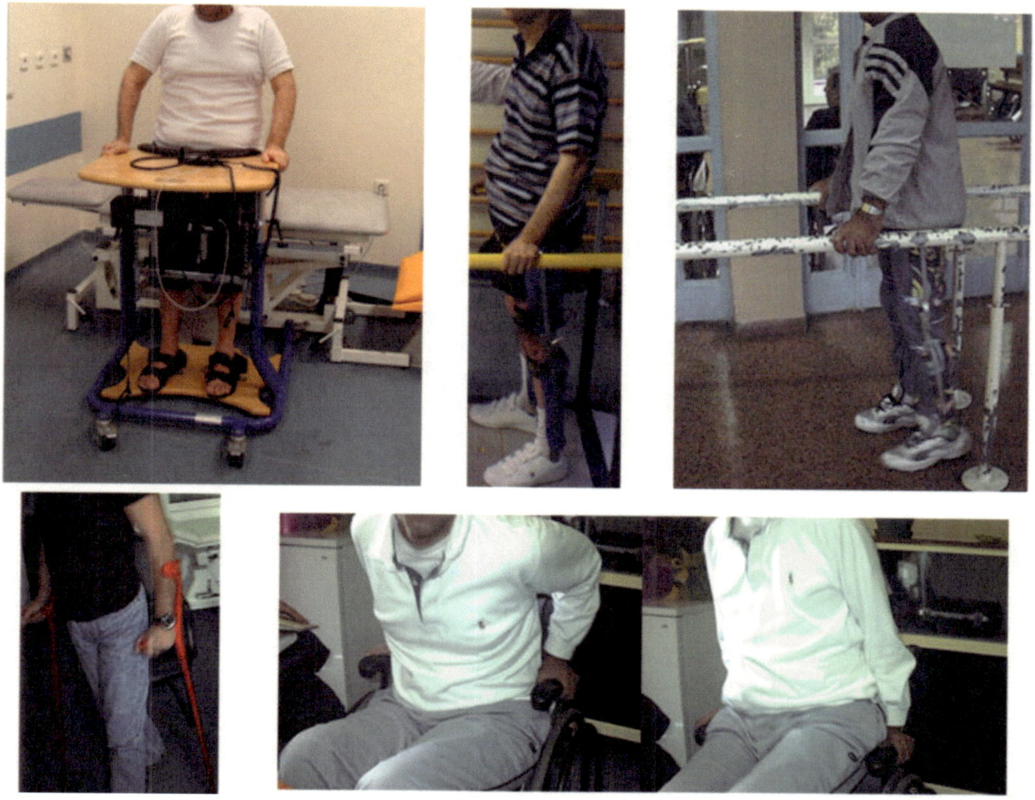

Figure 3. Weight bearing in disabled subjects; using standing frames, functional walking with orthoses between bars and crutches, even push-ups in the wheelchair (in case of multiple sclerosis with a clinical equivalent like tetraplegia) bone can be loaded and bone loss rate would be slower (unpublished photos of Dionyssiotis Y).

therapy program unchanged or to receive 9 minutes of side-alternating WBV (Vibraflex Home Edition II®, Orthometrix Inc) no effect on areal BMD at the lumbar spine was observed, while areal BMD seemed to decrease somewhat in the cortical region of the femoral diaphysis. Authors explained that mechanical stimulation increases intracortical bone remodeling and thereby cortical porosity; moreover changes occurred in ways that are not reflected by areal BMD, but might be detectable by more sophisticated techniques such as such as peripheral quantitative computed tomography. [70] Low-intensity vibration (LIV) has shown to be associated with improvement in bone mineral density in post-menopausal women and children with cerebral palsy. Seven non-ambulatory subjects with SCI and ten able-bodied controls underwent transmission of a plantar-based LIV signal (0.27+/-0.11 g; 34 Hz) from the feet through the axial skeleton as a function of tilt-table angle (15, 30, and 45 degrees). SCI subjects and controls demonstrated equivalent transmission of LIV, with greater signal transmission observed at steeper angles of tilt which supports the possibility of the utility of LIV as a means to deliver mechanical signals in a form of therapeutic intervention to prevent/reverse skeletal fragility in the SCI population. [71]

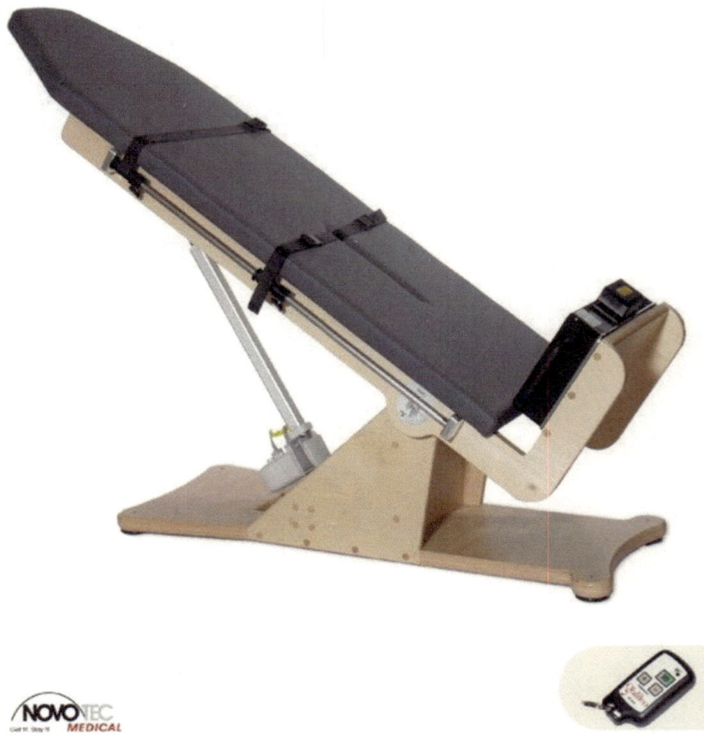

Figure 4. The Galileo Delta A TiltTable offers a wide variety of applications from relaxation to muscle training for a diverse range of patients who are unable to stand without support. The motor driven adjustable tilt angle of the Galileo Delta TiltTable (90°) allows vibration training with reduced body weight from 0 to 100%. This is ideal for deconditioned and disabled patients for gradually increasing training weights up to full body weight. System for application in adults (max. body height: 1.90 m) and children (max. body height: 1.50 m).The Galileo Delta A TiltTable is exclusively available from the manufacturer Novotec Medical GmbH. (published with permission).

3.3. Pulsed Electromagnetic Fields (PEMF)

Huang et al recently reviewed the effects of low-frequency pulsed electromagnetic fields (PEMFs) on chronic bony pain, bone mineral density (BMD), bone strength and biochemical markers of bone metabolism in the patients of osteoporosis. [72] Two studies are analyzed in SCI subjects: In a study that consisted of 6 male patients with complete spinal cord injury of a minimum of 2 years duration the time of therapy of PEMFs continued for 6 months and at 3 months BMD increased in the stimulated knees by 5.1% and declined in the control knees by 6.6% (P <0.05 and P <0.02, respectively). By 6 months the BMD returned to near baseline values and at 12 months both knees had lost bone at a similar rate. It was demonstrated that PEMFs can delay bone loss and there may exist both a local and a systemic response. [73] Another study consisted of 24 patients with SCI who were then divided into two groups, BMD of the total proximal femur and trochanter of patients in the treatment group were increased significantly compared with the control group. [74] Both of the trials indicated that the increase in BMD effects of PEMFs may relate to the features of the subjects. People with spinal cord injury are younger than osteoporosis patients, the osteoblasts and osteoclasts of patients with spinal cord injury may be more sensitive to the PEMFs stimulation than that of the old people.

Clinical examination and management of bone loss in paraplegia	
• history of the patient (co morbidities, neurologic complications, use of drugs which impair bone metabolism, alcohol, smoking and information about the level of injury, duration of paralysis, immobilization period, onset of rehabilitation, use of assistive devices and orthoses).	• pharmacological treatment with bisphosphonates p.os and i.v. that have been studied in patients with spinal cord injuries and had positive effects on bone parameters. • Use of calcium supplements (monitoring renal function) and vitamin D.
• anthropometric parameters (age, weight, body mass index, BMI)• clinical examination (level of injury according to American Spinal Injury Association Impairment Scale, AIS) and assessment of spasticity)	• Education on falls prevention • Counseling regarding osteoporosis and related factors and identification of fractures in regions of impaired sensation.
• imaging (bone densitometry by DXA at the hip and spine, and if possible, p QCT at the the tibia or femur)	• physical therapy including: a) range of motion exercises, b) loading of the skeleton to reduce bone loss, d) therapeutic standing-walking with orthoses, e) passive-active cycling
• measurement of bone turnover indices in the serum (parathyroid hormone, alkaline phosphatase, calcium, vitamin D, PINP molecule, osteocalcin) and urinary excretion of 24 hour (calcium, hydroxyproline, aminoterminal (NTx) and carboxylterminal (CTx) intermolecular cross-linking domain of bone type-1 collagen), which provide a good indicator of bone resorption.	• dietary interventions to improve dietary intake of calcium and nutrition indices.

Table 1. An algorithm for the screening and management of osteoporosis in subjects with spinal cord injury (should be read top to bottom starting with the left column); adapted from: Dionyssiotis Y. (84) (with permission).

3.4. Drugs

Calcitonin in varying doses and methods of administration has given variable results in paraplegia (preferred dosage regimen, treatment duration, and administration route for adequate efficacy in SCI patients' remains unclear). [75, 76] Likewise, the outcome using bisphosphonates has been variable. Etidronate produced long-term benefit in lower limb bone mineral density (BMD) in selected walking SCI patients; whereas tiludronate appeared effective in reducing bone resorption and preserving bone mass in a histomorphometric study in 20 paraplegic patients. [77, 78] Intravenous pamidronate has been shown to attenuate bone loss in SCI and normalize serum calcium in immobilization hypercalcemia. [79] Alendronate

(1000 times more potent than etidronate), in an open observational study, reversed BMD loss in men with established SCI increased both axial and trabecular bone density and has proven efficacy and safety in men treated for osteoporosis, prevents hypercalciuria and bone loss after bed rest and lower leg fracture. [80, 81] Six months after using zolendronic acid in the treatment group BMD showed differences in the response to treatment between the mixed trabecular/ cortical regions (narrow neck and intertrochanteric) and the purely cortical shaft. With respect to cross-sectional geometry, bone cross-sectional area and sectional modulus (indices of resistance to axial and bending loads, where higher values would indicate a positive effect of treatment) increased at the hip and buckling ratio (an index of the instability of thin-walled cross sections, where lower values would suggest that the treatment is improving stability) decreased consistent with improved bone outcomes; at 12 months, narrow-neck femur values declined and intertrochanteric and femoral shaft BMD was maintained vs. placebo group which showed a decrease in bone outcomes and an increase in buckling ratio at the hip at 6 and 12 months, while with respect to bone prevention 4 mg i.v. were effective and well-tolerated to prevent BMD loss at the total hip and trochanter for up to 12 months following SCI. [82, 83]

Author details

Yannis Dionyssiotis[1,2]

1 Rehabilitation Center "Aghios Loukas o Iatros", Trikala Thessaly, Greece

2 University of Athens, 1st Department of Orthopaedics, General University Hospital Attikon, Athens, Greece

References

[1] NIH Consensus Development Panel on Osteoporosis JAMA 285 (2001): 785-95

[2] World Health Organisation. Assessment of fracture risk and its implication to screening for postmenopausal osteoporosis: Technical report series 843. Geneva: WHO, 1994.

[3] Sambrook, P., Schrieber, L., Taylor, T., & Ellis, A. (2001). The musculoskeletal system. Edinburgh: Churchill Livingstone.

[4] Garland DE, Adkins RH, Stewart CA. 2013. Bone Impairment and Spinal Cord Injury. In: JH Stone, M Blouin, editors. International Encyclopedia of Rehabilitation. Available online: http://cirrie.buffalo.edu/encyclopedia/en/article/108/

[5] Claus-Walker J, Halstead LS. Metabolic and endocrine changes in spinal cord injury: IV. Compounded neurologic dysfunctions. Arch Phys Med Rehabil 1982;63:632-8.

[6] Lazo MG, Shirazi P, Sam M, Giobbie-Hurder A, Blacconiere MJ, Muppidi M. Osteoporosis and risk of fracture in men with spinal cord injury. Spinal Cord 2001;39:208-14.

[7] Lauer R, Johnston TE, Smith BT, Mulcahey MJ, Betz RR, Maurer AH. Bone mineral density of the hip and knee in children with spinal cord injury. J Spinal Cord Med. 2007;30 Suppl 1:S10-4.

[8] Ragnarsson KT, Sell GH. Lower extremity fractures after spinal cord injury: a retrospective study. Arch Phys Med Rehab 1981;62: 418–23.

[9] Nottage WM. A review of long-bone fractures in patients with spinal cord injuries. Clin Orthop 1981;155:65–70.

[10] Uebelhart D, Demiaux-Domenech B, Roth M, Chantraine A. Bone metabolism in spinal cord injured individuals and in others who have prolonged immobilisation. A review. Paraplegia 1995;33:669–73.

[11] Bauman WA, Garland DE, Schwartz E. Calcium metabolism and osteoporosis in individuals with spinal cord injury. Top Spinal Cord Inj Rehabil 1997;2:84-96.

[12] Wilmet E, Ismail AA, Heilporn A, Welraeds D, Bergmann P. Longitudinal study of bone mineral content and of soft tissue composition after spinal cord injury. Paraplegia 1995;33: 674–7.

[13] Eser P, Frotzler A, Zehnder Y, Wick L, Knecht H, Denoth J, Schiessl H. Relationship between the duration of paralysis and bone structure: a pQCT study of spinal cord injured individuals. Bone 2004;34:869-80.

[14] Dionyssiotis Y, Trovas G, Galanos A, Raptou P, Papaioannou N, Papagelopoulos P, Petropoulou K, Lyritis GP. Bone loss and mechanical properties of tibia in spinal cord injured men. J Musculoskelet Neuronal Interact 2007;7:62-8.

[15] Dionyssiotis Y. Spinal cord injury-related bone impairment and fractures: an update on epidemiology and physiopathological mechanisms. J Musculoskelet Neuronal Interact. 2011 Sep;11(3):257-65.

[16] Tsuzuku S, Ikegami Y, Yabe K. Bone mineral density differences between paraplegic and quadriplegic patients: a cross-sectional study. Spinal Cord 1999;37:358-61.

[17] Biering-Sorensen F, Bohr HH, Schaadt OP. Longitudinal study of bone mineral content in the lumbar spine, the forearm and the lower extremities after spinal cord injury. Europ J Clin Invest 1991;20:330-5.

[18] Biering-Sorensen F, Bohr HH, Schaadt OP. Bone mineral content of the lumbar spine and lower extremities years after spinal cord lesions. Paraplegia 1988;26:293-301.

[19] Leslie WD, Nance PW. Dissociated hip and spine demineralization: a specific finding in spinal cord injury. Arch Phys Med Rehabil 1993;74:960-4.

[20] Lanyon LE, Rubin CT, Baust G. Modulation of bone loss during calcium insufficiency by controlled dynamic loading. Calcif Tissue Int 1986;38:209-16.

[21] Dauty M, Perrouin Verbe B, Maugars Y, Dubois C, Mathe JF. Supralesional and sublesional bone mineral density in spinal cord-injured patients. Bone 2000;27:305-9.

[22] Smeltzer SC, Zimmerman V, Capriotti T. Osteoporosis risk and low bone mineral density in women with physical disabilities. Arch Phys Med Rehabil. 2005;86:582-6.

[23] Rauch F, Rittweger J. What is new in neuro-musculoskeletal interactions? J Musculoskelet Neuronal Interact 2005;5:91-4.

[24] Szollar SM, Martin EM, Sartoris DJ, Parthemore JG, Deftos LJ. Bone mineral density and indexes of bone metabolism in spinal cord injury. Am J Phys Med Rehabil 1998;77:28-35.

[25] Bauman WA, Spungen AM, Morrison N, Zhang RL, Schwartz E. Effect of a vitamin D analog on leg bone mineral density in patients with chronic spinal cord injury. J Rehabil Res Dev. 2005;42:625-34.

[26] Delmas PD. Markers of bone formation and resorption. In: Favus MJ, editor. Primer on the metabolic bone diseases and disorders of mineral metabolism. 2d ed. New York: Raven Press; 1993. p. 108-12.

[27] Raisz LG, Kream BE, Lorenzo JA. Metabolic bone disease. In: Wilson JD, Foster DW, Kronenberg HM, Larsen PR, editors. Williams textbook of endocrinology. 9th ed. Philadelphia (PA): W.B. Saunders Company; 1998. p. 1220-21.

[28] Gertz BJ, Shao P, Hanson DA, Quan H, Harris ST, Genant HK, Chesnut CH 3rd, Eyre DR. Monitoring bone resorption in early postmenopausal women by an immunoassay for cross-linked collagen peptides in urine. J Bone Miner Res 1994;9:135-42.

[29] Rosen HN, Dresner-Pollak R, Moses AC, Rosenblatt M, Zeind AJ, Clemens JD, Greenspan SL. Specificity of urinary excretion of cross-linked N-telopeptides of type I collagen as a marker of bone turnover. Calcif Tissue Int 1994;54:26-9.

[30] Roberts D, Lee W, Cuneo RC, Wittmann J, Ward G, Flatman R, McWhinney B, Hickman PE. Longitudinal study of bone turnover after acute spinal cord injury. J Clin Endocrinol Metab 1998;83:415-22.

[31] Nance PW, Schryvers O, Leslie W, Ludwig S, Krahn J, Uebelhart D. Intravenous pamidronate attenuates bone density loss after acute spinal cord injury. Arch Phys Med Rehabil. 1999;80:243-51.

[32] Bauman WA, Zhong YG, Schwartz E Vitamin D deficiency in veterans with chronic spinal cord injury. Metabolism 1995;44:1612–6.

[33] Morse LR, Sudhakar S, Danilack V, Tun C, Lazzari A, Gagnon DR, Garshick E, Battaglino RA. Association between sclerostin and bone density in chronic spinal cord injury. J Bone Miner Res. 2012;27:352-9.

[34] Clasey JL, Janowiak AL, Gater DR. Relationship between regional bone density measurements and the time since injury in adults with spinal cord injuries. Arch Phys Med Rehabil 2004;85:59-64.

[35] Modlesky CM, Bickel CS, Slade JM, Meyer RA, Cureton KJ, Dudley GA. Assessment of skeletal muscle mass in men with spinal cord injury using dual-energy X-ray absorptiometry and magnetic resonance imaging. J Appl Physiol 2004;96:561-5.

[36] Zehnder Y, Lüthi M, Michel D, Knecht H, Perrelet R, Neto I, Kraenzlin M, Zäch G, Lippuner K. Long-term changes in bone metabolism, bone mineral density, quantitative ultrasound parameters, and fracture incidence after spinal cord injury: a cross-sectional observational study in 100 paraplegic men. Osteoporos Int. 2004;15:180-9.

[37] Bauman WA, Spungen AM, Wang J, Pierson RN Jr, Schwartz E. Continuous loss of bone during chronic immobilization: a monozygotic twin study. Osteoporos Int 1999;10:123–7.

[38] Dionyssiotis Y, Petropoulou K, Rapidi CA, Papagelopoulos P, Papaioannou N, Galanos A, Papadaki P, Lyritis GP. Body composition in paraplegic men. J Clin Densitom 2008;11:437-43.

[39] Coupaud S, McLean AN, Allan DB. Role of peripheral quantitative computed tomography in identifying disuse osteoporosis in paraplegia. Skeletal Radiol 2009; 38(10): 989-95.

[40] Clasey JL, Janowiak AL, Gater DR. Relationship between regional bone density measurements and the time since injury in adults with spinal cord injuries. Arch Phys Med Rehabil 2004;85:59-64.

[41] Dionyssiotis Y, Lyritis GP, Mavrogenis AF, Papagelopoulos PJ. Factors influencing bone loss in paraplegia Hippokratia 2011;15:54-9.

[42] Garland DE, Adkins RH, Stewart CA, Ashford R, Vigil D. Regional osteoporosis in women who have a complete spinal cord injury. J Bone Joint Surg Am 2001;83 A: 1195-200.

[43] Garland DE, Foulkes G, Adkins RH, Hu SS, Rosen C, Liotta FJ, Weinstein DA. Regional osteoporosis following incomplete spinal cord injury. J Orthop Res 1992;10:371-8.

[44] Chantraine A, van Ouwenaller C, Hachen HJ, Schinas P. Intra-medullary pressure and intra-osseous phlebography in paraplegia. Paraplegia 1979;17:391-9.

[45] Karlsson AK, Friberg P, Lonnroth P, Sullivan L, Elam M Regional sympathetic function in high spinal cord injury during mental stress and autonomic dysreflexia. Brain 1998;121:1711–9.

[46] Teasell RW, Arnold JM, Krassioukov A, Delaney GA. Cardiovascular consequences of loss of supraspinal control of the sympathetic nervous system after spinal cord injury. Arch Phys Med Rehabil. 2000;81:506-16.

[47] Schwarzman RJ. New treatments for reflex sympathetic dystrophy. N Engl J Med 2000;343:654–6.

[48] Takeda S, Elefteriou F, Levasseur R, Liu X, Zhao L, Parker KL, Armstrong D, Ducy P, Karsenty G. Leptin regulates bone formation via the sympathetic nervous system. Cell 2002;111:305-17

[49] Kondo H, Nifuji A, Takeda S, Ezura Y, Rittling SR, Denhardt DT, Nakashima K, Karsenty G, Noda M. Unloading induces osteoblastic cell suppression and osteoclastic cell activation to lead to bone loss via sympathetic nervous system. J Biol Chem. 2005;280:30192-200.

[50] Levasseur R, Sabatier JP, Potrel-Burgot C, Lecoq B, Creveuil C, Marcelli C. Sympathetic nervous system as transmitter of mechanical loading in bone. Joint Bone Spine 2003;70:515-9

[51] Engelke K, Kemmler W, Lauber D, Beeskow C, Pintag R, Kalender WA. Exercise maintains bone density at spine and hip EFOPS: a 3-year longitudinal study in early postmenopausal women. Osteoporos Int 2006;17:133-42.

[52] Kraemer WJ. Endocrine responses and adaptations to strength training. In: Strength & Power in Sport, P.V. Komi (Editor). Oxford: Blackwell Scientific Publications, 1992; pp. 291-304.

[53] Demirel G, Yilmaz H, Paker N, Onel S. Osteoporosis after spinal cord injury. Spinal Cord 1998;36:822-5.

[54] Frey-Rindova P, de Bruin ED, Stussi E, Dambacher MA, Dietz V. Bone mineral density in upper and lower extremities during 12 months after spinal cord injury measured by peripheral quantitative computed tomography. Spinal Cord 2000;38:26-32.

[55] Eser P, Frotzler A, Zehnder Y, Schiessl H, Denoth J. Assessment of anthropometric, systemic, and lifestyle factors influencing bone status in the legs of spinal cord injured individuals. Osteoporos Int 2005;16:26-34.

[56] Rittweger J, Gerrits K, Altenburg T, Reeves N, Maganaris CN, de Haan A. Bone adaptation to altered loading after spinal cord injury: a study of bone and muscle strength. J Musculoskelet Neuronal Interact 2006;6:269-76.

[57] Löfvenmark I, Werhagen L, Norrbrink C. Spasticity and bone density after a spinal cord injury. J Rehabil Med. 2009; 41: 1080-4.

[58] Goemaere S, Van Laere M, De Neve P, Kaufman JM. Bone mineral status in paraplegic patients who do or do not perform standing. Osteoporos Int 1994 May;4:138-43.

[59] de Bruin ED, Frey-Rindova P, Herzog RE, Dietz V, Dambacher MA, Stüssi E.Changes of tibia bone properties after spinal cord injury: effects of early intervention. Arch Phys Med Rehabil 1999 Feb;80:214-20.

[60] Frey-Rindova P, de Bruin ED, Stüssi E, Dambacher MA, Dietz V. Bone mineral density in upper and lower extremities during 12 months after spinal cord injury measured by peripheral quantitative computed tomography. Spinal Cord 2000;38:26-32.

[61] Frost HM. Bone's mechanostat: a 2003 update. Anat Rec A Discov Mol Cell Evol Biol 2003 ;275:1081-101.

[62] LeBlanc AD, Spector ER, Evans HJ, Sibonga JD. Skeletal responses to space flight and the bed rest analog: a review. J Musculoskelet Neuronal Interact 2007;7:33-47.

[63] LeBlanc AD, Spector ER, Evans HJ, Sibonga JD. Skeletal responses to space flight and the bed rest analog: a review. J Musculoskelet Neuronal Interact 2007;7:33-47.

[64] Smith SM, Zwart SR, Heer MA, Baecker N, Evans HJ, Feiveson AH, Shackelford LC, Leblanc AD. Effects of artificial gravity during bed rest on bone metabolism in humans. J Appl Physiol (1985) 2009;107:47-53.

[65] Eser P, de Bruin ED, Telley I, Lechner HE, Knecht H, Stüssi E. Effect of electrical stimulation-induced cycling on bone mineral density in spinal cord-injured patients. Eur J Clin Invest 2003;33:412-9.

[66] Chen SC, Lai CH, Chan WP, Huang MH, Tsai HW, Chen JJ. Increases in bone mineral density after functional electrical stimulation cycling exercises in spinal cord injured patients. Disabil Rehabil 2005 30;27:1337-41.

[67] Giangregorio LM, Thabane L, Debeer J, Farrauto L, McCartney N, Adachi JD, Papaioannou A. Body weight-supported treadmill training for patients with hip fracture: a feasibility study. Arch Phys Med Rehabil 2009;90:2125-30.

[68] Ward K, Alsop C, Caulton J, Rubin C, Adams J, Mughal Z. Low magnitude mechanical loading is osteogenic in children with disabling conditions. J Bone Miner Res 2004;19:360-9.

[69] Eisman JA. Good, good, good... good vibrations: the best option for better bones? Lancet 2001 8;358:1924-5.

[70] Ruck J, Chabot G, Rauch F. Vibration treatment in cerebral palsy: A randomized controlled pilot study. J Musculoskelet Neuronal Interact 2010;10:77-83.

[71] Asselin P, Spungen AM, Muir JW, Rubin CT, Bauman WA. Transmission of low-intensity vibration through the axial skeleton of persons with spinal cord injury as a potential intervention for preservation of bone quantity and quality. J Spinal Cord Med 2011;34:52-9.

[72] Huang LQ, He HC, He CQ, Chen J, Yang L. Clinical update of pulsed electromagnetic fields on osteoporosis. Chin Med J (Engl). 2008;121:2095-9.

[73] Garland DE, Adkins RH, Matsuno NN, Stewart CA. The effect of pulsed electromagnetic fields on osteoporosis at the knee in individuals with spinal cord injury. J SpinalCord Med 1999;22:239-45.

[74] Cong F, Ji SR, Xu JB, Su GD, Du Y, Chang H, et al. Effect ofpulsed electromagnetic fields on bone mineral density of spinal cord injuried patients. Chin J Rehabil Theory Practice (Chin) 2005; 11: 250-1.

[75] Chantraine A, Heynen G, Franchimont P. Bone metabolism, parathyroid hormone, and calcitonin in paraplegia. Calcif Tissue Int 1979;27:199-204.

[76] Minaire P, Depassio J, Berard E, Meunier PJ, Edouard C, Pilonchery G, Goedert G.Effects of clodronate on immobilization bone loss. Bone 1987;8 Suppl 1:S63-8.

[77] Roux C, Oriente P, Laan R, Hughes RA, Ittner J, Goemaere S, Di Munno O, Pouillès JM, Horlait S, Cortet B. Randomized trial of effect of cyclical etidronate in the prevention of corticosteroid-induced bone loss. Ciblos Study Group. J Clin Endocrinol Metab 1998;83:1128-33.

[78] Chappard D, Minaire P, Privat C, Berard E, Mendoza-Sarmiento J, Tournebise H, Basle MF, Audran M, Rebel A, Picot C, et al. Effects of tiludronate on bone loss inparaplegic patients. J Bone Miner Res 1995;10:112-8.

[79] Bauman WA, Wecht JM, Kirshblum S, Spungen AM, Morrison N, Cirnigliaro C, Schwartz E. Effect of pamidronate administration on bone in patients with acute spinal cord injury. J Rehabil Res Dev 2005;42:305-13.

[80] Moran de Brito CM, Battistella LR, Saito ET, Sakamoto H. Effect of alendronate on bone mineral density in spinal cord injury patients: a pilot study. Spinal Cord 2005;43:341-8.

[81] Zehnder Y, Risi S, Michel D, Knecht H, Perrelet R, Kraenzlin M, Zäch GA, Lippuner K. Prevention of bone loss in paraplegics over 2 years with alendronate. J Bone Miner Res 2004;19:1067-74.

[82] Bubbear JS, Gall A, Middleton FR, Ferguson-Pell M, Swaminathan R, Keen RW. Early treatment with zoledronic acid prevents bone loss at the hip following acute spinal cord injury. Osteoporos Int 2011;22:271-9.

[83] Shapiro J, Smith B, Beck T, Ballard P, Dapthary M, BrintzenhofeSzoc K, Caminis J. Treatment with zoledronic acid ameliorates negative geometric changes in the proximal femur following acute spinal cord injury. Calcif Tissue Int 2007;80:316-22.

[84] Dionyssiotis Y. Bone loss in paraplegia: A diagnostic and therapeutic protocol. Osteoporos Int 2009;20:S23-S176.

Chapter 9

Estimating Renal Function in Paraplegia

Jennifer Pai Lee

Additional information is available at the end of the chapter

http://dx.doi.org/10.5772/57231

1. Introduction

The National Kidney Disease Education Program recommends using either the Cockcroft–Gault creatinine clearance (CL_{CG}) or Modification of Diet in Renal Disease (MDRD) equation when determining dosages of drugs that are primarily eliminated by the kidneys [1]. Both methods attempt to better predict creatinine clearance (CL_{CR}) or glomerular filtration rate (GFR) by taking into account different variables such as age, weight, gender, race, and serum creatinine (SCr), however neither equation captures the key factor of paraplegia. Over time, individuals with paraplegia develop low SCr concentrations relative to their actual CL_{CR} due to significantly reduced muscle mass as a result of chronic immobility and muscle atrophy. Both Cockcroft–Gault (CG) and MDRD formulas have SCr in their denominator inversely proportional to CL_{CR} or GFR, therefore low SCr in paraplegia would result in gross overestimation of their renal function. Based on falsely high CL_{CR} or GFR, clinicians could potentially prescribe renally eliminated medications at dosages higher than recommended, resulting in undesirably high drug concentrations leading to drug toxicity and/or adverse drug reactions (ADRs). For example, supratherapeutic vancomycin and aminoglycosides (AG) serum concentrations, especially if combined with other nephrotoxic and/or ototoxic medications, could drastically increase the risk of nephrotoxicity and/or ototoxicity. This could be devastating to many individuals with paraplegia who have existing renal insufficiency.

In addition to high prevalence of traditional risk factors for CKD such as advanced age, diabetes, hypertension, and cardiovascular disease, individuals with paraplegia have elevated incidence of recurrent and chronic urinary tract infections, neurogenic bladder dysfunction, and nephrolithiasis that put them at risk for developing CKD [2-6]. Fischer et al. conducted cross-sectional analyses of data on 9333 Veterans with spinal cord injury and disorder (SCI/D) and found that the prevalence of CKD in SCI/D was approximately 35%, considerably higher based on the modified MDRD for SCI/D than 10% based on the original MDRD formula [7]. Underrecognition of CKD in paraplegia makes it more crucial to use accurate tools to estimate renal function in this population.

Currently, there is no accepted standard method for determining renal dosing regimens for patients with paraplegia, and data on estimating renal function in such population is scarce. However clearance of drugs primarily eliminated by the kidneys such as vancomycin and AG nearly mirror that of the creatinine, hence could be used to assess renal function in paraplegia.

The aims of this chapter are: (1) to review the current literature on assessing renal function in paraplegia, (2) to evaluate different methods of estimating CL_{CR} or GFR compared with patient-specific vancomycin and AG clearance (CL_{DRUG}) in individuals with paraplegia, (3) to assess whether there is a difference in the estimation of renal function between the two anatomical degrees of SCI/D when compared with CL_{DRUG}, and (4) to present the "Spinal Cord Injury Equation" that more accurately estimates renal function in paraplegia.

2. Review of the current literature on assessing renal function in paraplegia

Tables 1 and 2 show, respectively, comparison of equations to predict CL_{CG} or GFR from SCr and review of the current literature on assessing renal function in paraplegia. Each equation and study will be discussed in detail below.

Equation 1: Cockcroft-Gault equation (CL_{CG}) [8]

GFR = CL_{CR} (mL/min) = [(140 – age) x IBW in kg] / (72 x SCr); (multiply 0.85 for females)

Equation 2: Modified Cockcroft-Gault equation (CL_M) [16]

GFR = CL_{CR} (mL/min) = [(140 – age) x IBW in kg] / (72 x SCr); (multiply 0.85 for females)

SCr rounded to 1 mg/dL for patients with SCr < 1 mg/dL while using the actual SCr for patients with SCr ≥ 1 mg/dL

Equation 3: MDRD equation [11-13*]

GFR (mL/min/1.73 m²) = 175 x standardized $SCr^{-1.154}$ x $age^{-0.203}$ x 1.212 (if black) x 0.742 (if female)

Equation 4: CKD-EPI equation [14*]

GFR (mL/min/1.73 m²) = 141 x min $(SCr/\kappa, 1)^{\alpha}$ x max $(SCr/\kappa, 1)^{-1.209}$ x 0.993^{Age} x 1.018 [if female] x 1.159 [if black]

where κ is 0.7 for females and 0.9 for males, α is -0.329 for females and -0.411 for males, min indicates the minimum of SCr/κ or 1, & max indicates the maximum of SCr/κ or 1.

Equation 5: 24-Hour endogenous creatinine clearance (CL_{24H}) [8]

GFR = CL_{24H} (mL/min) = [urine creatinine x urine volume (mL)] / [SCr x time (hours) x 60]

*To enable the expression of comparisons among different methods in the same unit (mL/min), GFR values normalized to a BSA of 1.73 m² need to be converted to uncorrected values.

Table 1. Comparison of Equations to Predict Creatinine Clearance (CL_{CR}) or Glomerular Filtration Rate (GFR) from Serum Creatinine Concentration

Characteristics	Macdi-armid et al. (2000) [9]	Mirah-madi et al. (1983) [10]	Chikka-lingaiah et al. (2010) [15]	Lee and Dang (2011) [16]	Lavezo et al. (1995) [18]	Lee and Yang (2013) [19]
SCI/D: Paraplegics (P) Tetraplegics (T) Non-SCI/D (control)	36 25 11 --	58 22 36 22	116 64 52 --	141 52 89 --	14 -- -- 14	87 54 33 --
Age (yr.) (mean ± SD)	38 (24-68)	P: 48 ± 17 T: 47 ± 14	63 ± 1	66 ± 11	53 ± 12	65 ± 16
Male (n [%])	--	SCI/D: 58 [100] Control: 11 [50]		140 [99]		87 [100]
Race (n [%]) White and other Black	--	--			75 [65] 41 [35]	71 [82] 16 [18]
BMI (kg/m²) (mean ± SD)	--	--		25 ± 6		27 ± 5
CL_{CG} (mL/min) (mean [SD])		P: 82 ± 46 T: 70 ± 23		91 ± 37	63 ± 26	93 ± 47
MDRD GFR (mL/min/ 1.73 m²) (mean ± SD)	--	--			76 ± 33	
SCr (mg/dL) (mean ± SD)	--	P: 1 ± 0.4 T: 0.8 ± 0.3		0.74 ± 0.29	SCI/D: 0.8 ± 0.4 Control: 1.1 ± 0.3	0.88 ± 0.40
Methodology	CL_{CG} vs. CL_{24H} vs. mea-sured CL_{CR} by ^{99m}Tc-DTPA	CL_{CG} vs. CL_{24H}	CL_{CG} vs. CL_{24H} vs. MDRD	CL_{CG} vs. CL_{M} vs. CL_{24H} vs. MDRD vs. CKD-EPI	SCI/D vs. Non-SCI/D CL_{VANCO}	CL_{SCI} vs. CL_{CG} vs. CL_{M} vs. CL_{24H} vs. MDRD vs. CKD-EPI
Findings/ Recommen-dations	CL_{24H} more accurate than CL_{CG}	Correction factor: 0.8 for paraplegic 0.6 for tetraple-gic	Correction factor: 0.7 for MDRD 0.8 for CL_{CG}	All methods over-estimate CL_{DRUG} (P< 0.001). Devel-opment of CL_{SCI}	↑half-life in SCI/D	Verifi-cation of CL_{SCI}: CL_{SCI} un-biased and more precise.

Table 2. Review of the Current Literature on Assessing Renal Function in Paraplegia

a. **The Cockcroft-Gault (CG) equation (CL_{CG})**

CL_{CG}(mL/min) = [(140 – age) x IBW in kg] / (72 x SCr);

(multiply 0.85 for females)

The CG equation was derived from a study of 236 males aged 18-92 years based on their 24-hour creatinine excretion. Since the publication in 1976, it has been exclusively used to estimate CL_{CR} based on SCr to calculate dosing regimens for renally cleared medications including vancomycin and AG. However it may not extrapolate to individuals with paraplegia because the CG study excluded 31 patients with 24-h creatinine excretion < 10 mg/kg, and it didn't reveal whether the study population included paraplegia and to what extent [8].

The review of current literature reports significant overestimation of renal function by CL_{CG}, thus does not recommend using the original equation in paraplegia [9-10].

Macdiarmid et al. studied 25 paraplegic and 11 tetraplegic patients and sought to compare their CL_{CG} and 24-hour endogenous creatinine clearance (CL_{24H}) to the measured CL_{CR} by ^{99m}Tc-DTPA clearance technique [9]. The investigators found that the CG method did not correlate well with that of the CL_{24H} (r=0.426) or ^{99m}Tc-DTPA clearance (r=0.366) [9]. The mean difference between CL_{CG} and CL_{24H} was 41.9%, and the difference between CL_{CG} and ^{99m}Tc-DTPA clearance 50.7% where CG formula overestimated CL_{CR} [9]. On the other hand, the difference between CL_{24H} and ^{99m}Tc-DTPA clearance was 17.7% with good correlation (r=0.71) [9]. The authors concluded that the CG formula significantly overestimates CL_{CR} thus not recommended, however CL_{24H} is an accurate method of determining renal function in paraplegia [9].

A study by Mirahmadi et al. investigated 58 male hospitalized patients with SCI/D and 22 ambulatory subjects, and compared their measured CL_{24H} by autoanalyzer method versus the predicted by CL_{CG} [10]. The authors found that the predicted CL_{CG} and measured CL_{24H} values closely matched in the ambulatory group while the predicted values consistently exceeded the measured values in SCI/D [10]. Between the two anatomical degrees of SCI/D, the paraplegic group had a markedly higher SCr (1.0 ± 0.4 mg/dL) and 24-hour urinary creatinine excretion (16 ± 9 mg/kg) compared to the tetraplegic group where the respective values were 0.8 ± 0.3 mg/dL and 11 ± 4.6 mg/kg [10]. The authors modified the original CG formula using a correction factor of 0.8 for paraplegics and 0.6 for tetraplegics to overcome significant overestimation by CL_{CG} [10]. The correction factors improved the accuracy and precision of the predicted CL_{CG} shown by the difference between the predicted and measured CL_{CR} approaching zero and the slope of a linear correlation between the predicted and measured values approaching one with decreased Y-intercept values ($p < 0.01$) [10].

b. **The MDRD equation (MDRD)**

4-Variable MDRD:

GFR (mL/min/1.73 m^2) = 175 x standardized SCr$^{-1.154}$ x age$^{-0.203}$ x 1.212 (if black) x 0.742 (if female)

A more recently developed MDRD has been widely used to estimate GFR in the nephrology arena. It is one of the two equations recommended by The National Kidney Disease Education Program for drug dosing [1].

The MDRD equation was derived from a study of a relatively young non- paraplegic population (mean age 51±13 years) with chronic kidney disease, primarily to stage kidney disease [11-12]. The original 6-variable MDRD formula integrates patient parameters including age, gender, race, blood urea nitrogen (BUN), SCr, and serum albumin [11-12]. The performance of this equation can be limited by variability among clinical laboratories in calibrating SCr assays [13]. Thus, the formula was re-expressed as the 4-variable MDRD equation based on standardized SCr assays as shown above [13]. Despite SCr calibration, the accuracy of the equation remains compromised at levels of GFR >60 mL/min/1.73 m^2 [12-14]. Nevertheless, MDRD stands useful for GFR <60 mL/min/1.73 m^2 in non- paraplegia and is endorsed by the National Kidney Disease Foundation for estimating GFR in CKD patients [1, 11-12].

Chikkalingaiah et al. compared the performance of the 4-variable MDRD and CG equations with CL_{24H} in 64 patients with chronic paraplegia of greater than 6 months duration and stages II-V CKD [15]. Precision and bias of MDRD and CG formulas were measured by combined root mean square error (CRMSE) calculated as the square root of [(mean difference of estimated GFR and measured CL_{24H})^2 + (SD of the difference)^2]. Respective CRMSE values for original MDRD and CG equations were 29 and 19.3 mL/min/1.73m^2. In order to improve the performance of the prediction equations, a correction factor of 0.7 for MDRD and 0.8 for CG were applied which resulted in a decrease in their CRMSE values to 11.4 and 13 mL/min/1.73m^2, respectively [15]. Accuracy of both prediction equations was evaluated by the percentage of patients who did not deviate >15%, 30%, or 50% from measured CL_{24H}. Respective percentages for MDRD were 12.5, 25, and 48.4 before the correction, and 25, 42, 68 after the correction [15]. Respective percentages for CG were 22, 37.5, and 58 before the correction, and 25, 50, 75 after the correction [15]. On the whole, the CG equation had less bias and was more precise and more accurate than the MDRD equation, however still overestimated GFR in subjects with chronic paraplegia with measured CL_{24H} < 90 mL/min/1.73m^2. Application of the correction factors markedly improved in the overall bias, precision, and accuracy of both MDRD and CG equations shown by both decreased CRMSE values and increased percentage of subjects in whom GFR did not deviate >15%, 30%, or 50% from measured CL_{24H} [15].

c. The CKD-EPI equation (CKD-EPI)

GFR (mL/min/1.73 m^2) = 141 x min $(SCr/\kappa, 1)^{\alpha}$ x max $(SCr/\kappa, 1)^{-1.209}$ x 0.993^{Age} x 1.018 [if female] x 1.159 [if black]

where κ is 0.7 for females and 0.9 for males, α is -0.329 for females and -0.411 for males, min indicates the minimum of SCr/κ or 1, & max indicates the maximum of SCr/κ or 1.

In order to overcome the known bias of the MDRD equation for GFR values of ≥60 mL/min/1.73 m^2, the researchers pooled the data from 26 studies to develop and validate a new equation, the CKD-EPI equation, to define dose modification across the GFR range in patients with and without CKD [14]. The data showed that the CKD-EPI equation was more precise and accurate compared to MDRD, especially at GFR > 60 mL/min/1.73 m^2, however it is not frequently used in current clinical practice when determining dosages of drugs that are primarily eliminated by the kidneys due to need for further validation. Furthermore, the sample population used to develop the CKD-EPI formula did not include paraplegia, thus its use in paraplegia may be misleading.

d. 24-Hour endogenous creatinine clearance (CL_{24H})

CL_{24H} (mL/min) = [urine creatinine x urine volume (mL)] / [SCr x time (hours) x 60]

Current literature reports that CL_{24H} better predicts renal function compared to CL_{CG} and MDRD in paraplegia, however this method is not routinely utilized for drug dosing due to the impracticability of collecting multiple urine samples as well as the propensity for error from serial collections [8, 16].

3. Evaluation of different methods of estimating CL_{CR} or GFR compared with patient-specific vancomycin and aminoglycoside (AG) clearance (CL_{DRUG}) in individuals with SCI/D

Data on the application of methods of estimating renal function compared with patient-specific CL_{DRUG} in paraplegia is scarce.

Lavezo et al. compared the pharmacokinetics of vancomycin in 14 SCI/D and 14 non-SCI/D control patients with their age, weight, pharmacokinetic parameters of total body clearance, volume of distribution, and mean predicted dosages matched. Demographic data between the groups differed only in mean SCr where the values were 0.8 ± 0.4 in the SCI/D group and 1.1 ± 0.3 in the able-bodied control group ($p=0.04$). The investigators obtained the pharmacokinetic parameters via two steady-state vancomycin serum concentrations by the Sawchuk and Zaske method [17] and found that compared to the control group, mean elimination rate constant was significantly smaller, therefore mean elimination half-life significantly longer in patients with SCI/D [18]. The authors concluded that patients with SCI/D may require longer dosing intervals of vancomycin compared to non-SCI/D [18].

In 2011, Lee and Dang published the results of a retrospective pharmacokinetic analysis of data on 141 patients with long-term SCI/D in the Veterans Affairs (VA) hospital with the largest inpatient SCI center in the VA system. The investigators evaluated frequently employed methods to estimate GFR (CL_{CG}, modified CG, CL_{24H}, MDRD, and CKD-EPI) against patient-specific drug clearance of vancomycin and AG (CL_{DRUG}) [16]. Table 3 shows that all methods overestimate CL_{DRUG} ($p <0.001$). The mean difference between CL_{DRUG} and MDRD is largest where overestimation by MDRD is more than two-fold. Almost 70% of the patients had overestimation of CL_{DRUG} by greater than 30 mL/min when using MDRD to predict empiric dosing for vancomycin and AG ($p < 0.001$) [16]. The authors modified the original CG equation by rounding SCr to 1 mg/dL for patients with SCr < 1 mg/dL while using the actual SCr for patients with SCr ≥ 1 mg/dL in attempts to account for low SCr in SCI/D and to overcome gross overestimation of renal function by CL_{CG} [16]. The investigators found that the modified CG equation (CL_M) better estimated CL_{DRUG} in SCI/D, compared with other frequently employed methods for predicting GFR. The mean difference between CL_{DRUG} and CL_M was smallest among the equations evaluated where overestimation by CL_M was approximately 40%. Almost 65% of the patients had prediction of CL_{DRUG} within 30 mL/min when using CL_M to estimate empiric dosing for vancomycin and AG ($p < 0.001$) [16]. Despite pronounced improvement by modification of CG, overestimation may not be clinically acceptable.

(N=141)	Mean ± S.D. (mL/min)	Difference from CL_{DRUG} (mL/min)	P-Value
CL_{DRUG}	49.77 ± 19.97	0	--
MDRD	119.76 ± 61.49	69.99	<0.001
CKD-EPI	90.71 ± 27.44	40.94	<0.001
CL_{24H}	85.16 ± 33.88	35.39	<0.001
CL_{CG}	91.24 ± 36.90	41.47	<0.001
CL_M	69.38 ± 13.49	19.61	<0.001

Abbreviations: GFR, glomerular filtration rate; CL_{DRUG}, actual drug clearance; MDRD, the Modification of Diet in Renal Disease equation; CKD-EPI, Chronic Kidney Disease Epidemiology Collaboration equation; CL_{24H}, 24-hour endogenous creatinine clearance; CL_{CG}, the Cockcroft-Gault formula; CL_M, modified Cockcroft-Gault formula; S.D., standard deviation. Published with permission of Lee [16].

Table 3. Evaluation of Different Methods to Estimate GFR

4. Estimation of renal function between the two anatomical degrees of SCI when compared with CL_{DRUG}

As previously mentioned, Mirahmadi et al. reported that both SCr and mean urinary creatinine excretion were markedly lower in paraplegics compared with ambulatory subjects [10]. The authors recommended an adjustment of the original CG equation by 20% for paraplegics to correct for reduction of muscle mass relative to the total body weight in such population [10].

Chikkalingaiah et al. found that both prediction equations (MDRD and CG) overestimated GFR in the paraplegic group with an overestimation by MDRD to a higher degree [15]. The fractional prediction error (FPE = (variable 1-variable 2) x 100/variable 1) for MDRD and CG were, respectively, 48.5% and 29.5% for paraplegic subjects, where an FPE greater than 20% was considered to be clinically unacceptable [15]. A correction factor of 0.7 for MDRD and 0.8 for CG proposed by the authors decreased the FPE to 3.9% and 3.6%, respectively, for the paraplegic group [15].

Lee and Dang sought to evaluate various methods to predict CL_{DRUG} for different anatomical degrees of SCI/D (Table 4) [16]. The mean difference between CL_{SCI} and CL_{DRUG} was not statistically significant when separated into paraplegia and tetraplegia [16]. Similar finding was noted for CL_M and CL_{24H} [16]. On the other hand, the mean differences between CL_{CG}, CKD-EPI, and MDRD and CL_{DRUG} were statistically significant between the two anatomical degrees of SCI where tetraplegics had a gross overestimation of CL_{DRUG} compared with paraplegics [16]. The investigators stated that such difference may have risen from rounding SCr up to 1 mg/dL for patients with SCr < 1 mg/dL and using a ratio of urine creatinine to SCr done in CL_M and CL_{24H}, respectively, contrary to using the actual SCr in the other equations [16].

Individuals with paraplegia have variable functionality and range of mobility and movement depending on the injury levels. Degree of paralysis of lower body and legs and upper body strength could affect muscle mass therefore potentially alter SCr and CL_{CR} or GFR. For example, one with high paraplegia (>T7) may have weaker upper body strength and balance compared to the one with low (T7-T12) paraplegia thus may have lower muscle mass and SCr resulting in a falsely low estimation of renal function compared to the low paraplegia. Unfortunately, there has yet been a study that assesses renal function between different anatomical levels or severity of injury in paraplegia.

	Mean Difference from CL_{DRUG} ± S.D. (mL/min)		p-Value
	Paraplegics (n = 52)	Tetraplegics (n = 89)	
CL_{SCI}	-3.11 ± 13.14	-5.39 ± 21.16	0.48
CL_M	21.04 ± 13.81	18.76 ± 22.26	0.5
CL_{24H}	32.60 ± 30.78	37.02 ± 35.29	0.45
CL_{CG}	27.26 ± 20.56	49.76 ± 38.55	<0.001
CKD-EPI	27.52 ± 25.50	48.77 ± 24.76	<0.001
MDRD	40.68 ± 40.71	50.64 ± 64.56	<0.001

Abbreviations: CL_{DRUG}, actual drug clearance; SCI, spinal cord injury; CL_{SCI}, spinal cord injury equation; CL_M, modified Cockcroft-Gault formula; CL_{24H}, 24-hour endogenous creatinine clearance; CL_{CG}, the Cockcroft-Gault formula; CKD-EPI, Chronic Kidney Disease Epidemiology Collaboration equation; MDRD, the Modification of Diet in Renal Disease equation; S.D., standard deviation. Published with permission of Lee [16].

Table 4. Evaluation of Methods to Predict CL_{DRUG} for Different Anatomical Degrees of SCI/D

5. The "Spinal Cord Injury Equation" (CL_{SCI})

Gross overestimation of CL_{DRUG} by the frequently employed methods for estimating GFR prompted the authors Lee and Dang to develop an alternative method of estimating CL_{DRUG} in SCI/D, the "spinal cord injury equation" (henceforth referred to as the CL_{SCI} equation):

$$CL_{SCI}\ (\text{mL/min}) = 2.3\ \text{X}\ CL_M^{\ 0.7}$$

where CL_{SCI} and CL_M denote, respectively, clearance values determined via use of the CL_{SCI} equation and the CL_M formula [16]. The CL_{SCI} equation yields a value along the *line of best fit* (the straight trend line depicting the line of least variability in all points on a scatterplot of data derived by regression analysis of two variables) between CL_M and patient-specific vancomycin clearance (CL_V) values [16].

Figures 1 and 2 depict, respectively, plots of actual drug clearance versus modified CG predicted drug clearance and linear regression plots of actual drug clearance versus predicted drug clearance using the CL_{SCI} equation [16]. The slope of a linear correlation between the predicted and measured CL_V values approach one, and the Y-intercept of a linear correlation between the predicted and measured CL_V values is minimum [16].

The CL_{SCI} equation was tested against other methods through a retrospective analysis of 87 hospitalized patients with long-term SCI/D [19]. The study population had similar baseline characteristics to the previous population by Lee and Dang, exclusively elderly, overweight, males with similar SCr. The authors used the Sheiner and Beal method [20] for determining predictive performance (precision and bias) to evaluate the predictive ability of the CL_{SCI} equation in estimating vancomycin clearance, relative to five alternative methods (CL_{CG}, modified CG, CL_{24H}, MDRD, and CKD-EPI). Compared with other equations, the CL_{SCI} equation was found to be less biased and more precise, with the smallest calculated mean prediction error (ME) and square root of the mean squared prediction error (RMSE) values ($p < 0.005$) (Table 5) [19]. Predictive performance of the CL_{SCI} relative to each of the other five methods was measured by change in ME (relative bias between two methods) and change in MSE (relative precision) (Table 6). Negative values for changes in ME and MSE indicate an advantage favoring the comparator; a greater negative value signifies a greater magnitude of error. The five alternative equations significantly overestimated CL_V, by 45-92% ($p < 0.05$) (Table 7) [19]. The CL_{SCI} equation underestimated CL_V by approximately 6%, however not to a significant degree ($p = 0.06$) [19]. The results of their finding were consistent with the previous study by Lee and Dang.

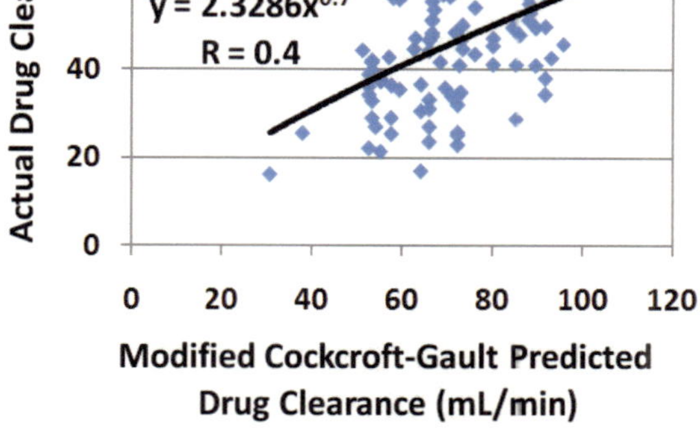

Figure 1. Plots of Actual Drug Clearance versus Modified Cockcroft–Gault Predicted Drug Clearance. Published with permission of Lee [16].

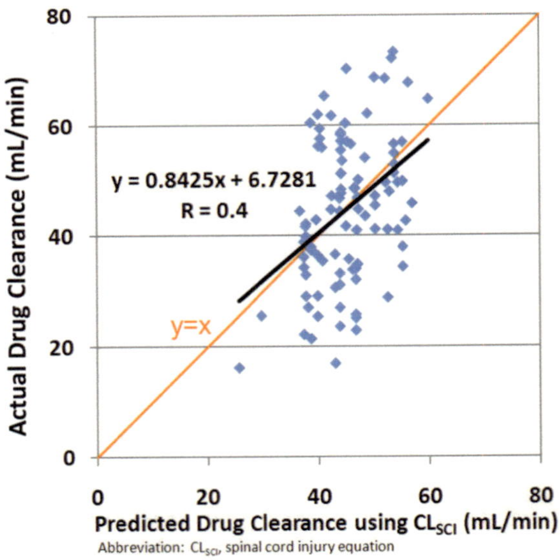

Figure 2. Linear Regression Plots of Actual Drug Clearance versus Predicted Drug Clearance Using the Spinal Cord Injury Equation. The red line, y=x, represents a line with a slope of 1 that indicates a perfectly one-to-one association between the actual and predicted drug clearance. Published with permission of Lee [16].

Parameter	CL_{SCI}	CL_M	CL_{24H}	CKD-EPI	CL_{CG}	MDRD
Bias						
ME (mL/min)	-3.1	21.5	32.5	33.0	44.5	47.5
95% CI (mL/min)	-6.3 to 0.1	17.8 to 25.1	26.2 to 38.8	27.7 to 38.4	36.2 to 52.7	31.2 to 55.8
Precision						
MSE (mL^2/min^2)	235.2	748.9	1925.2	1712.7	3450.1	3760.3
95% CI (mL^2/min^2)	168.9 to 301.4	562.7 to 935.2	1191.2 to 2659.2	1271.6 to 2153.8	2334.8 to 4565.3	2640.1 to 4880.5
RMSE (mL/min)	15.3	27.4	43.9	41.4	58.7	61.3
95% CI (mL/min)	13.0 to 17.4	23.7 to 30.6	34.5 to 51.6	35.7 to 46.4	48.3 to 67.6	51.4 to 69.9

Abbreviations: ME, mean error; CI, confidence interval; MSE, mean squared error; RMSE, root mean squared error; CL_{SCI}, spinal cord injury equation; CL_M, modified Cockcroft-Gault formula; CL_{24H}, 24-hour endogenous creatinine clearance; CKD-EPI, Long-term Kidney Disease Epidemiology Collaboration equation; CL_{CG}, the Cockcroft-Gault formula; MDRD, the Modification of Diet in Renal Disease equation. Published with permission of Lee [19].

Table 5. Absolute Predictive Performance of Vancomycin Clearance

	ΔME (CI) (mL/min)	ΔMSE (CI) (mL^2/min^2)
CL_{SCI} vs. CL_M	-24.5 (-26.8 TO -22.3)	-513.8 (-709.8 to -317.8)
CL_{SCI} vs. CL_{24H}	-35.5 (-42.6 TO -28.5)	-1690.0 (-2436.5 to -943.5)
CL_{SCI} vs. CKD-EPI	-36.1 (-41.3 TO -30.9)	-1477.5 (-1922.8 to -1032.3)
CL_{SCI} vs. CL_{CG}	-47.5 (-55.9 TO -39.1)	-3214.9 (-4331.1 to -2098.7)
CL_{SCI} vs. MDRD	-50.6 (-59.1 TO -42.1)	-3525.1 (-4645.0 to -2405.2)

Abbreviations: ΔME, the difference in mean errors; ΔMSE, the difference in mean squared errors; CI, confidence interval; CL_{SCI}, spinal cord injury equation; CL_M, modified Cockcroft-Gault formula; CL_{24H}, 24-hour endogenous creatinine clearance; CKD-EPI, Long-term Kidney Disease Epidemiology Collaboration equation; CL_{CG}, the Cockcroft-Gault formula; MDRD, the Modification of Diet in Renal Disease equation. Published with permission of Lee [19].

Table 6. Relative Predictive Performance of Vancomycin Clearance

N = 87	Mean ± S.D. (ml/min)	Difference from patient-specific CL_V (ml/min)	p-value
CL_{SCI}	45.2 ± 9.1	-3.1	0.06
CL_M	69.7 ± 19.7	21.5	< 0.05
CL_{24H}	82.8 ± 36.0	34.6	< 0.05
CKD-EPI	81.2 ± 30.4	33.0	< 0.05
CL_{CG}	92.7 ± 47.0	44.4	< 0.05
MDRD	95.7 ± 45.2	47.5	< 0.05

Abbreviations: CL_V, patient-specific vancomycin clearance ; S.D., standard deviation; CL_{SCI}, spinal cord injury equation; CL_M, modified Cockcroft-Gault formula; CL_{24H}, 24-hour endogenous creatinine clearance; CKD-EPI, Long-term Kidney Disease Epidemiology Collaboration equation; CL_{CG}, the Cockcroft-Gault formula; MDRD, the Modification of Diet in Renal Disease equation. Published with permission of Lee [19].

Table 7. Evaluation of Different Methods to Estimate CL_V

6. Conclusion

SCr determinations are used to estimate the dose of potentially toxic drugs eliminated primarily by the kidneys. Due to immobility and muscle atrophy, individuals with long-duration paraplegia have lower SCr levels relative to their CL_{CR}; this could lead to substantial overestimation of GFR resulting in higher than desired concentrations of medications that increase the risk of toxicity and/or ADRs, especially in persons with existing renal insufficiency. To date, there is no accepted standard method that can reliably predict renal function in paraplegia. Review of the current literature shows that the most widely used CG and MDRD equations overestimate GFR thus not recommended in paraplegia. Although CL_{24H} better predicts renal function compared to CL_{CG} and MDRD in paraplegia, unpracticality of collecting multiple urine samples as well as the propensity for error from serial collections make this method clinically unfeasible. Different authors have recommended different modification of existing methods. Until more studies become available, the following methods can serve as valuable tools in estimating CL_{DRUG} and renal function in individuals with paraplegia: 0.8 CG, 0.7 MDRD, or CL_{SCI} equations.

Acknowledgements

Supported in full by Grant # 2867 from the PVA Research Foundation.

Author details

Jennifer Pai Lee*

Address all correspondence to: jennifer.lee4332a@va.gov

Pharm.D., BCPS, Pharmacy, Veterans Affairs Long Beach Healthcare System, Long Beach, USA

References

[1] National Institutes of Diabetes and Digestive and Kidney Disease and National Kidney Disease Education Program. Chronic kidney disease and drug dosing: information for providers 2009. www.nkdep.nih.gov/professionals/drug-dosing-information.htm (accessed 10 May 2011).

[2] McKinely WO, Jackson AB, Cardenas DD, et al. Long-term medical complications after traumatic spinal cord injury: a regional model systems analysis. Archives of Physical Medicine and Rehabilitation 1999;80: 140-210.

[3] Rogers WH, Kazis LE, Miller DR, et al. Comparing the health status of VA and non-VA ambulatory patients: the veterans' health and medical outcomes studies. The Journal of Ambulatory Care Management 2004;27: 249–262.

[4] Kazis LE, Miller DR, Clark J, et al: Health-related quality of life in patients served by the Department of Veterans Affairs: results from the Veterans Health Study. Archives of Internal Medicine 1998;158: 626-632.

[5] Myers J, Lee M, Kiratli J: Cardiovascular disease in spinal cord injury: an overview of prevalence, risk, evaluation, and management. American Journal of Physical Medicine and Rehabilitation 2007;86: 142-152.

[6] Vaziri ND, Cesarior T, Mootoo K, et al. Bacterial infections in patients with chronic renal failure: occurrence with spinal cord injury. Archives of Internal Medicine 1982;142: 1273-1276.

[7] Fischer MJ, Krishnamoorthi VR, Smith BM, et al. Prevalence of chronic kidney disease in patients with spinal cord injuries/disorders. American Journal of Nephrology 2012;36: 542-548.

[8] Cockcroft DW, Gault MH. Prediction of Creatinine Clearance from Serum Creatinine. Nephron 1976; 16: 31-41.

[9] Macdiarmid SA, Mcintyre WJ, Anthony A, et al. Monitoring of renal function in patients with spinal cord injury. The British Journal of Urology 2000; 85: 1014-1018.

[10] Mirahmadi MK, Byrne C, Barton C, et al. Prediction of creatinine clearance from serum creatinine in spinal cord injury patients. Paraplegia 1983; 21(1) 23-29.

[11] Levey AS, Bosch JP, Lewis JB, et al. A more accurate method to estimate glomerular filtration rate from serum creatinine: a new prediction equation. Annals of Internal Medicine 1999; 130 (6) 461-70.

[12] Stevens LA, Coresh J, Feldman HI, et al. Evaluation of the modification of diet in renal disease study equation in a large diverse population. Journal of the American Society of Nephrology 2007; 18(10) 2749-57.

[13] Levey AS, Coresh J, Greene T, et al. Expressing the Modification of Diet in Renal Disease Study Equation for Estimating Glomerular Filtration Rate with Standardized Serum Creatinine Values. Clinical Chemistry 2007; 53(4) 766-772.

[14] Levey AS, Stevens LA, Schmid CH, et al. A New Equation to Estimate Glomerular Filtration Rate. Annals of Internal Medicine 2009; 150(9) 604-12.

[15] Chikkalingaiah KBM, Grant ND, Mangold TM et al. Performance of Simplified Modification of Diet in Renal Disease and Cockcroft-Gault Equations in Patients With Chronic Spinal Cord Injury and Chronic Kidney Disease. The American Journal of the Medical Sciences 2010; 339(2) 108-16.

[16] Lee JP, Dang AT. Evaluation of Methods to Estimate Glomerular Filtration Rate versus Actual Drug Clearance in Patients with Chronic Spinal Cord Injury. Spinal Cord. 2011; 1-6.

[17] Sawchuk RJ, Zaske DE, Cipolle RJ et al. Kinetic model for gentamicin dosing with the use of individual patient parameters. Clinical Pharmacology and Therapeutics 1977; 21: 362-369.

[18] Lavezo LA, Davis RL. Vancomycin pharmacokinetics in spinal cord injured patients: a comparison with age-matched, able-bodied controls. The Journal of Spinal Cord Medicine 1995; 16: 233-235.

[19] Lee JP, Wang YJ. Testing the Predictive Ability of the "Spinal Cord Injury Equation" in Estimating Vancomycin Clearance. American Journal of Health-System Pharmacy 2013 70(8) 669-674.

[20] Sheiner LB, Beal SL. Scientific Commentary—Some Suggestions for Measuring Predictive Performance. Journal of Pharmacokinetics and Biopharmaceutics 1981; 9:503-12.

Section 4

Research in Paraplegia

Chapter 10

Animal Models in Traumatic Spinal Cord Injury

Mahdi Sharif-Alhoseini and Vafa Rahimi-Movaghar

Additional information is available at the end of the chapter

http://dx.doi.org/10.5772/57189

1. Introduction

Traumatic spinal cord injury (SCI) causes high mortality, severe disability, expensive cure, extensive rehabilitation, and a high economic burden. There has been no definite treatment for SCI, but numerous studies including experimental modeling are being performed to assist resolving this fundamental problem.

The first reported SCI model was presented by Allen in 1911 where a mass was dropped from a prescribed height onto the dorsal surface of the canine dura. After that, the animal models of SCI from simple lamprey to non-human primates were used to develop pathophysiological knowledge on cell injury and repair process of spinal cord.

Currently, to choose an animal model, some factors are considered depending upon the proposed aim of the study. Transections and contusions of the spinal cord are the most commonly used methods for animal modeling of SCI. While transection models provide an idealized setting for studying spinal cord regeneration across a complete lesion, but transected spinal cords are rarely encountered in human SCI. In other words, most injured spinal cords maintain some tissue continuity across the area of injury. But contusion and compression models are more clinically relevant. These models can create graded injuries and characterized by hemorrhagic necrosis, ischemia, inflammation, and central cavitation. Besides, compression models contribute to simulate the persistent spinal canal occlusion that is common in human SCIs.

The ongoing development of SCI animal models reflects the need to review all types of them and gauge about their advantages or disadvantages. The purpose of this chapter is to review animal models in SCI from studies indexed in Medline.

2. Why animal models?

Animal model refers to the use of a living, non-human animal to simulate the human disease or injury, for better understanding the disease where it is practically or ethically difficult to use humans. It is used to learn more about a disease, its pathophysiologic changes, diagnosis and treatment. Animal models are often preferable for experimental disease or injury research because of their unlimited supply, ease of manipulation, the possibility to standardize the condition, the capability to use more invasive procedures to observe the effects of treatment, and no concern for the patients' safety [1, 2]. In fact, many potential therapies require testing for safety and efficacy in animals before it is possible to move to a clinical trial.

To serve as a useful model of a human condition, a modelled disease or injury not only must be similar in the etiology and function to the human equivalent but also has to offer advantages over direct clinical observation and experiment [2, 3].

On the other hand, spinal cord injury (SCI), as a fundamental problem in medicine, causes high mortality, severe disability, expensive cure, extensive rehabilitation, and a high economic burden. So far management of SCI is challenging and there has been no definite treatment for it. But numerous studies including experimental modeling are being performed to assist understanding the anatomical and biological consequences of injury and repair, and testing the efficacy and the risk-to-benefit ratio of a proposed therapy [3]. Animal models have been developed with the aim of recreating features of either complete or incomplete SCI to increase the knowledge about disease mechanisms and evolution of injury, and provides a clinically relevant platform for developing and evaluating therapies in SCI [4, 5]. Animal models have also some other benefits over their human equivalent; e.g. the specified tissue needed can be used and processed for histological purposes to investigate co-localization of proteins of interest, mRNA analysis (microarray) to give expression of proteins and protein analysis (western blotting) to give levels of protein [6].

3. History

Various methods for induction of experimental SCI have been used in the past. The first reported SCI model was presented by Allen in 1911 where a mass was dropped from a prescribed height onto the dorsal surface of the canine dura. He used a simple irrefutable logic that when a known weight dropped from a constant height shall produce same impact force on all occasions. Based on this concept, he prepared a metal tube with pores. A rod of 10 g was inserted into the tube and can be stopped at various heights using a pin inserted into the pores on the tube at regular intervals. By aiming the tube over a surgically exposed spinal cord and by withdrawing the pin holding the rod, a reproducible impact force would be created when the rod get dropped on the spinal cord. For unknown reasons, most data available concerning experimentally induced SCI are modifications of an injury model proposed by Allen [7].

In 1936, the load throw devices were used to make a spinal cord contusion [8]. In 1953, a model was created in which a dog had its spinal cord injured by an inflated balloon inside the spinal canal [9]. In 1976, Eidelberg created an SCI model in rats caused by direct epidural compression [10]. New techniques were developed and improved, e.g. spinal cord stabilization and precise distribution of strengths involved on impact, the use of mechanisms able to measure the strength to which an animal's spinal cord is exposed, as well as the invention of pneumatic impact mechanisms [11].

Because the weight-drop techniques deliver a single, rapid blow to the spinal cord, neither model simulates ongoing cord compression secondary to residual spinal column displacement. Thus, in 1978, Rivlin and Tator introduced a clip compression model of SCI in rats, in which the spinal cord was compressed for variable durations between the arms of a modified aneurysm clip [12]. This model demonstrated the relation between the severity of neurologic injury and the length of compression.

Afterwards, more technical devices such as Ohio State University's electromagnetic spinal cord injury device (OSU impactor) and New York University (NYU) impactor came into use. In 1987, the researchers at Ohio State University applied a computer feedback-controlled electromagnetic force to create contusion and concussion in the spinal cord of rats [13]. In this model, after laminectomy, the OSU impactor probe is slowly screwed down to the dural surface, which it contacts and displaces 30 micrometers with a force of approximately 3000 dynes. This is meant to provide a consistent starting point from which to initiate the injury. The system then is triggered, and the device rapidly impacts the cord for a predetermined amount of displacement before releasing [14]. Because the OSU impactor is actively withdrawn, there is no bouncing of the impactor back onto the cord, which is a probable basis of variation in a weight-drop technique. NYU impactor was at first described by Gruner in 1992 and then refined by a consortium of eight spinal cord laboratories in the United States called MASCIS (Multicenter Animal Spinal Cord Injury Study). The NYU-MASCIS weight-drop model standardizes grades of contusive spinal cord injury by dropping a 10g rod from specific heights of 6.25 (mild), 12.5 (moderate), 25 (severe) or 50 mm (very severe) upon the exposed dorsal surface of the spinal cord [15]. Usage of the recent impactors requires intense training, extensive maintenance and sophisticated software which give more room to exclude the post-operative animals being used for the experiments.

In addition to traumatic SCI, spinal cord ischemia remains an underappreciated clinical dilemma which mostly occurs after aortic problems. Therefore, experimental models of spinal cord ischemia have been developed in different animals with variable reproducibility [16-19].

In the last decades, transection has been favored to study approaches of nerve fiber regeneration and cell transplantation that are likely to be most appropriate to the subacute stage.

4. Level of SCI

The majority of reported human injuries occurs at the cervical level, often secondary to vertebral fracture, producing compression or contusion of the spinal cord [20]. Functional deficits after cervical injury are a result of damage to both white and gray matter. At this level, white matter disruption leads to spastic paralysis below the injury, sensory loss/chronic pain, cardiovascular, gastrointestinal, and sexual dysfunction. Motor neurons controlling the upper limb musculature reside there, and their loss induces flaccid paralysis [21]. But so far, thoracic SCI is the most commonly used location in animal models. Since gray matter loss at this spinal level causes less identifiable functional loss, thoracic SCI could contribute to isolate and study white matter deficits. In addition, high cervical levels can result in diaphragm dysfunction due to interruption of bulbospinal respiratory drive to phrenic motoneuron pools (C3–C5) [22, 23]. Thus thoracic SCI models are obviously reliable and easy to reproduce [24, 25].

However, due to differences in spinal cord diameter, the distance of injury from both the neuronal cell body and the original targets of innervations, the relative dedication of the cord to specific ascending and descending systems and their different termination sites, the degree of vascularization, the size of the sensory and motor neuron populations, the level of their importance in locomotion, and white/gray matter distribution, histological, behavioral, and therapeutic findings in the thoracic spinal cord, may not be so readily applicable to the cervical level [26].

On the other hand, rats do not use their hindlimbs as skilfully as their forelimbs. Also the hindlimb paw and digit use cannot be evaluated as carefully as the forelimb paws and digits. Thus, forelimb evaluation could superiorly assess the efficacy of potential therapies, especially in mild degrees of improvement. Therefore, some scientists tried to characterize cervical SCI in rats [26, 27]. In 2001, Soblosky et al. characterized a unilateral cervical contusion SCI model which allowed the contralateral side to serve as a within-subject control [24]. In this model, the injury did not cause overt bladder dysfunction, which significantly reduced the need for chronic intensive care after SCI. In 2005, this model has been further standardizes by Gensel et al. [21].

5. Injury paradigms

In general, experimental models can be naturally occurring (e.g. injured dogs in road traffic crashes), congenital disease (e.g. a spontaneous mutant), or induced (surgical, genetically engineered) that is similar to a human condition. SCI models are mostly created based on surgical methods which are determined by the experimental aims of a particular research. Every injury techniques concentrate on a special question, and hence each carries their own pros and cons:

- *Contusion:* If the pathophysiology of secondary injury is the main part of research interest, a contusion and/or compression model could be selected; because most human SCIs involve contusive or compressive injury [28]. Contusion is the oldest and most widely used for SCI models. The contusive models can create graded injuries and characterized by hemorrhagic necrosis, ischemia, inflammation, and central cavitation. It elicits both motor and sensory dysfunction, such as tactile allodynia, neuropathic pain, and thermal hyperalgesia.

Some devices exist to create contusion in a controlled way to limit the variation between animals and allow the comparison between results obtained in different laboratories. (Figure 1)

http://dx.doi.org/10.5772/57189

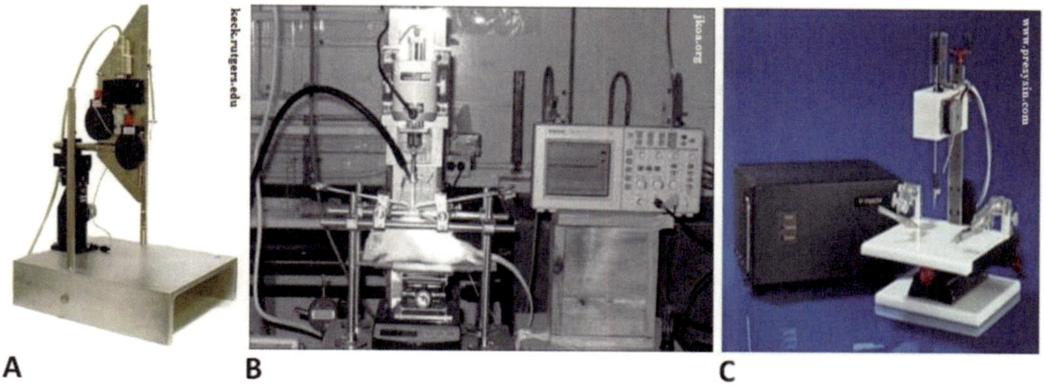

Figure 1. A: NYU Impactor. B: OSU Impactor. C: IH Impactor.

The most widely used device is the NYU impactor which concurrent recording of kinematic parameters of the impounded probe allows the validation of the injury process.

OSU impactor electromagnetically drives an impounder tip onto the cord until a desired displacement of the cord surface is reached. After a defined time, the tip is retracted and the pressure released [29]. This computer controlled contusion model consists of an animal trap that reproducibly delivers a defined weight to the exposed spinal cord, with a computer monitoring the dynamics of the impact [30].

In a similar way operates the only commercially available device, the Infinite Horizon (IH) impactor. A stepping motor applies a defined force to the cord. Once the force is reached, the impactor retracts [31].

The NYU impactor is rather easier to use, but the OSU impactor and IH impactor have more precision to produce lesions more reliably [32].

Hemicontusion: Hemicontusion or unilateral contusion is used in cervical spinal cord, because life-threatening adverse effects could occur in cervical contusion. Since motor dysfunction appears in the forelimbs, pain related behavior is difficult to estimate, and for this reason, cervical contusion is often utilized for motor functional analysis [21].

- *Compression:* Compression models contribute to simulate the persistent spinal canal occlusion that is common in human SCIs and investigate the effects of compression or the optimal timing of decompression. For this reason, a clip, balloon, spacer, or forceps compression model would be appropriate. (Figure 2)

Clip compression injury is similar to spinal contusion injury at the point of the injury caused by pressure to the spinal cord. Following laminectomy, a vascular clip is dorsoventrally closed over the entire cord. With this method, the spinal cord becomes ischemic and mimics common clinical injuries and outcomes. Compressive injury is induced with clips calibrated to exert a convinced force to induce mild, moderate or severe injury [33, 34].

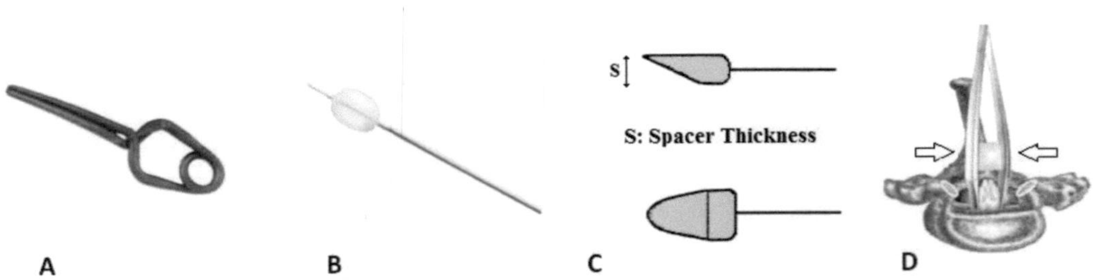

Figure 2. A: Aneurysm clips. B: Fogarty catheter. C: Spacer. D: Forceps [2].

The balloon-induced method has been used because it is a simple method that does not cause any damage to the surrounding structures. The volume of balloon inflation must be measured several times and used in combination with the size of the experimental animals when determining a sufficient amount of injury to inflict [35]. A Fogarty catheter is inserted into the dorsal epidural space through a small hole made in vertebral arch, advanced cranially to one or two higher spinal levels. Spinal cord damage is graded by increasing the volume of saline used to inflate the balloon.

To use a spacer, at first the average anteroposterior spinal canal diameter should be determined from the spines of animals of similar weight and age. This allowed for the determination of the spacer size needed to produce a precise degree of narrowing of the spinal canal diameter [36].

The calibrated forceps can produce a lateral compression injury by inserting on either side of the spinal cord and closing together to induce a central hemorrhagic necrosis and displacement of the centrally located, damaged tissue in cranial and caudal directions [2].

- *Transection:* The transected spinal cords are rarely encountered in human SCI, but transection models provide an idealized setting for studying hypotheses that concern regeneration, degeneration, tissue engineering strategies, or plasticity on an axonal level. These types of lesions are most usefully combined with neuroanatomical tract tracing and electrophysiological studies [32, 37]. Transection models are also increasingly used to model the effects of scaffolds, biomaterials, neurotrophic factors, and combinatorial therapies on axon regeneration after injury [6]. To allow for regeneration, sterile gel foams have been placed between the two ends of transected cords with variable degree of success [38]. Besides, if a device is to be implemented, a partial or complete transection model might be best suited for device placement. Many studies have reported bilateral muscle spasms, neuropathic pains, mechanical allodynia and thermal hyperalgesia at same, above, and/or below the level of the lesion following complete spinal transection model [38].

Spinal cord transection is performed after laminectomy with fine surgical scissors (iridectomy scissors) that allows the targeted interruption of a particular nerve fiber systems such as motor tracts (corticospinal tract, rubrospinal tract) or sensory tracts (dorsal columns), or even complete interruption of the spinal cord [32].

For certain applications, partial transection can be a viable alternative to complete transection. In other words, because the lesion that results from a complete transection creates such a hostile tissue environment, injury paradigms have been developed that decrease the physical damage to the cord and the consequential cavitation and physical separation. Thus researchers can selectively interrupt certain pathways with partial transections to hold a tissue bridge between the proximal and distal ends of the cord, and maintain tissue continuity [39]. A dorsal hemisection for selective transection of the corticospinal tract can be performed with some feedback from the change in color and texture between the white and gray matter, giving a sign of the entirety of the hemisection [2, 37]. But dorsal hemisection cannot be used rigorously to assess true axon regeneration [39]. Dorsolateral quadrant lesions are used to interrupt the rubrospinal tract, and lateral hemisections disrupt all tracts on one side but spare some or all tracts on the opposite side.

- *Photochemical model:* This model was developed by Watson et al. in 1986 [40] and was proven to be one of the most reliable and reproducible graded ischemic experimental models of SCI [41]. With the exposed spinal column intact, irradiation of the translucent dorsal surface induces excitation of the systemically injected dye (e.g. rose Bengal) in the spinal cord microvasculature. The resultant photochemical reaction leads to vascular stasis, hemorrhagic necrosis of the central grey matter, edematous pale-staining white matter tracts and vascular congestion. The main benefit of this technique is that the resulting injury does not induce mechanical trauma to the cord, because there is no need for laminectomy. On the other hand, an intravascular photochemical reaction occurs through the use of a dye that is activated by an argon ion laser to produce single oxygen molecules at the endothelial surface of spinal cord vessels. This leads to a severe platelet reaction, subsequent vessel occlusion, and parenchymal tissue infarction. Also, the degree of injury is hard to control [38].

- *Ischemic model:* Initial studies used the methods described by Lang-Lazdunski et al. [16]. This method uses an anterior sternotomy with temporary aortic occlusion created by aneurysm clips sited at the aortic arch plus left subclavian artery [42].

- *Excitotoxic model:* Following intraspinal or intrathecal injection of some excitotoxins (e.g. A-metabotropic receptor agonist quisqualic acid or other excitatory amino acids such as glutamate, N-methylasparate, and kainic acid), the cascade of events described following ischemic and traumatic SCI, including prominent inflammation, neuronal loss, astrocytic scaring, cavity formation, syringomyelia, long-lasting spontaneous pain, and mechanical allodynia occur. This model can correlate specific areas of tissue damage with behavioral changes. But almost all animals develop varying degrees of hypersensitivity to mechanical and thermal stimuli [38, 43].

- *Combination:* For some particular goals, a combination of models might be designed. For example, the early stages of an experimental study that explores axon regeneration may use transection paradigms to definitely reveal regenerated axons and recognize the most promising therapies, which can then be examined in contusion models [37].

6. Species of animals used

Rodents are the most common type of mammal employed in SCI experimental studies, and widespread research have been conducted using rats, mice, gerbils, guinea pigs, and hamsters [1]. Other animal experiments include cats, non-human primates, goats, pigs, and dogs [1, 4, 35, 44-49]. Of course, larger mammals such as cats, dogs, or pigs are also used but very rarely and are less experienced models based in SCI research, requiring expensive after care and housing as well as stringent ethical considerations [6, 37]. Other models include invertebrates, such as eels [50], whose unique regenerative capacities have been studied in efforts to apply novel strategies to human SCI.

- *Rat:* Rat models are most widely used to study SCI. They are inexpensive, friendly, easy to care for, and can be studied in large numbers. They have a well understood anatomy and few surgical infections. There are also well-established functional analysis techniques in rats. Early mortality of them is not costly [37, 38]. In addition, rats develop large fluid-filled cystic cavities at the injury site, similar to the human pathology. Therefore those are preferable for studies where mimicking the human pathology is important, including preclinical studies that focus on the efficacy of novel cellular and/or pharmacological therapies [51]. Rats can be used when the size is of less importance [52]. The corticospinal tract of rat is mostly dorsal. As two disadvantages of the rat models, the corticospinal tract lesions would not significantly create disability, and rats are quadrupeds not bipeds.

- *Mouse:* In SCI research, mouse models have also been implemented increasingly, but the small working size prohibits many surgical maneuvers and device implantations [37, 38]. The injury site in mice is densely packed with cells and actually decreases in size over time (that do not have a cyst). Thus to gain mechanistic insights into the basic cellular and molecular biology of SCI, mouse models may have more to offer [51, 53].

Among rodents, the majority of genetic studies, especially those involving disease, have employed mice, not only because their genomes are so similar to that of humans, but also because of their availability, ease of handling, high reproductive rates, and relatively low cost of use [30, 54, 55]. Using mice with a knockout of a target molecule has become the gold-standard for functional testing, and Cre-Lox technology along with increasing numbers of transgenic mice have provided greater temporo-spatial control of the knockout strategy that has proven invaluable for providing mechanistic insights into the cellular and molecular processes of axon regeneration [51].

- *Cat:* Use of cats can clarify the histopathologic features of acute and chronic stages of SCI. Their larger size allows implementation of more intensive therapeutic regimens, such as implantation of electrical stimulators, than is possible when smaller animal models are studied [52]. Cats have been a popular model for spinal cord electrophysiologists [56].

- *Pig:* Because of large size and greater likeness to human physiology, pig models are becoming more important as a preclinical model that is intermediate in size between rodents and humans [51].
- *Dog:* Dogs can be surveyed after naturally occurring SCIs e.g. following road traffic accidents or disc degenerations. The mechanisms of injury in clinical SCI in dogs are similar to those in human patients: vertebral fracture–luxation and disc extrusions – both of which produce the mixed contusion-compression lesion to the ventral aspect of the cord that is problematical to model in the laboratory [45]. To date, dogs have been used to study spinal cord injuries because neurological examinations could be carried out easily, and more detailed pathophysiological studies could be conducted [35, 46]. Compared to analysis of trials in human patients, dogs have the advantage that there is less of an ethical problem.
- *Non-human primate:* Non-human primate models are limited by extremely high costs related to the intensive animal care and ethically challenging, but may be imperative to prove safety and efficacy on a small scale prior to human experimentation, particularly for strategies involving device implantation [25]. Because of similar anatomy and pathology to human, a primate model could provide greater positive predictive value to human therapies, and lead to basic discoveries that might not be identified in rodent models [4].

7. Outcome assessments

- **Behavior**

Behavioral outcome in experimental SCI models is the most important factor for evaluating the extent of injury and treatment efficacy. It is directly related to the extent of neuronal damage in the gray matter at the injury site, the loss of ascending and descending axons in the white matter, and the reorganization of the remaining nervous system [57, 58]. Sedy et al. categorized the behavioral tests as: locomotor tests (testing the locomotor apparatus of the animal), motor tests (analyzing the strength, coordination and other abilities of the skeletal muscles), sensory tests (evaluating proprioception, touch, pain or temperature sensing), sensory–motor tests (testing the proper connection between the sensory and motor systems), autonomic tests (evaluating the function of the sympathetic and parasympathetic systems), and reflex-response based tests [58]. (Table 1)

Rahimi-Movaghar et al. showed usefulness of the tail-flick reflex in the prognosis of functional recovery in paraplegic rats [59]. Although there has been an abundant interest in locomotion in animal studies, the connection between locomotion and spinal cord integrity at the site of injury in the animal is not at all easy. In particular, behavioral measurements in the context of lateral or dorsal hemisection are even more difficult [2]. Table 2 shows recommended testing methods for SCI models.

Behavioral tests	Tests	Reflects	Lesion severity: Mild	Moderate	Severe	Pros	Cons
Locomotor tests	Primary open-field	Locomotion		■	■	Simple, cheap	Low sensitivity
	BBB	Locomotion	■	■	■	Simple, cheap	Subjective
	Open-field activity	Locomotion	■	■		Unique data	Depends on motivation
	Automated walkway	Locomotion	■	■		Precise	Equipment
	Footprint analysis	Motor coordination	■	■		Precise	Environment-dependent
	Kinematic analysis	Locomotion	■	■		Detailed	Equipment
	Thoracolumbar height	Weight support		■		Examines only one characteristic	Equipment
	Swim	Swimming ability	■	■		Spontaneous locomotion	Subjective
	Eshkol–Wachmann notation	Locomotion	■	■		Detailed	Requires training of scientist
Motor tests	Inclined plane	Muscle strength	■	■	■	Simple, cheap	Not standard among laboratories
	Limb hanging	Grasping	■	■		Unique data	Not for severe injuries
	Limb grip strength	Muscle strength	■	■		Precise	Equipment
	Forelimb asymmetry	Paw preference	■	■		Sensitive to chronic deficits	Not for severe injuries
	Rearing	Paw preference	■	■		Sensitive to selective limb use	Not for severe injuries
	Food pellet reaching	Motor coordination	■			Fine motor function test	Food deprivation
Sensory tests	Hot plate-based	Temperature	■	■	■	Simple	Risk of injury

Behavioral tests	Tests	Reflects	Lesion severity			Pros	Cons
			Mild	Moderate	Severe		
	Cold sensitivity-based	Temperature				Simple	False positivity
	Von Frey filaments	Mechanical allodynia				Simple	Low sensitivity
	Paw compression	Pain				Simple, cheap	High chance of mistakes
	Withdrawal reflexes	Reflex				Simple	Low sensitivity
Sensory–motor tests	Rope walk testing	Balance				Simple, cheap	Low sensitivity
	Narrow beam	Balance				Uncovers discrete changes	Requires training
	Grooming	Sensory–motor connection				Simple, cheap	Subjectivity
	Foot slip	Sensory–motor coordination				Uncovers discrete changes	Requires training
	Grid walking	Sensory–motor coordination				Uncovers discrete changes	False-positives or negatives
Reflex response-based tests	Toe spread reflex	Reflex				Simple, cheap	Low sensitivity
	Contact placing response	Reflex				Simple, cheap	False positivity
	Righting reflex	Reflex				Simple, cheap	Low sensitivity
Autonomic tests	Ex copula erection	Erection				Unique data	Subjectivity
	Non-contact erection	Erection				Unique data	Low sensitivity
	Mating	Erection				Unique data	Subjectivity
	Telemetric monitoring	Micturition erection				Precise	Equipment
	Autonomic dysreflexia	Autonomic dysreflexia				Unique data	Equipment

* Modified by: Mahdi Sharif-Alhoseini

Table 1. Main behavioral methods for testing SCI models* [58]

Level of injury		First choice	Second choice	Third choice
Cervical		Forelimb asymmetry	Footprint analysis	BBB
Thoracic	Compression	BBB	Hot plate	Inclined plane
	Contusion	BBB	Electrophysiology	Von Frey, Hot plate
	Transection	BBB	Electrophysiology	Kinematic analysis
	Hemisection	BBB	Electrophysiology	Hot plate, Von Frey
	Excitotoxic	Hot plate	Cold testing	Von Frey
	Ischemic	BBB	Electrophysiology	Inclined plane, Hot plate
Other		BBB	Electrophysiology	Hot plate, Grid walk

Table 2. Recommended testing methods for SCI models [58].

- **Electrophysiology**

Electrophysiological assessments via the evoked potentials are useful to survey the neural substrates underlying deficits and functional recovery. They are also used to examine neural pathway integrity [58, 60].

Somatosensory evoked potentials (SSEP) are valuable for the assessment of sensory spinal axon conduction. They involve electrical stimulation of the paws with electrodes temporarily inserted into them, and the recording of evoked potentials from electrodes previously implanted in the cranium over the somatosensory cortex [61].

Magnetically evoked inter-enlargement responses (MIER) are helpful for the evaluation of propriospinal conduction. The MIER procedure involves noninvasive magnetic stimulation at the animal's hip or knee and the recording of evoked potentials with EMG electrodes temporarily inserted into forelimb and masseter muscles [62].

Motor evoked potentials (MEP) assess supraspinal axon conduction with EMG electrodes temporarily inserted into hindlimb muscles [63]. The MEP offers a precious insight into the physiological status of motor tracts within the spinal cord and is appropriate to animal studies. It is seen as complementary to SSEP monitoring rather than an alternative for it [64].

All evoked potential methods take a few minutes and cause only slight pain and distress and so could be done without anesthesia. But there are the restricted information content, and the need for rigorous electrophysiological interpretation of the resulting signals [64].

Electromyography (EMG): EMG can be elicited both by intramedullary manipulation and rapidly applied transaxial spinal cord compression. Presumably, rapid deformation of spinal motor tracts generates descending volleys which can bring to firing threshold lumbar motor neurons [65]. It can also be used to survey autonomic dysreflexia [66].

- **Neuroimaging**

Functional magnetic resonance imaging(fMRI): fMRI is an accurate but challenging technique which could measure the anatomic functional/metabolic correlates of sensory-motor activities

[67]. It should be done under anesthesia and mechanically ventilation [58]. After the stimulation of the limb electrodes, a signal in the somatosensory cortex and/or subcortical sensory areas can be recorded. This method makes it possible to distinguish between the recovery of sensory and motor function [68].

Magnetic Resonance Imaging (MRI): MRI findings of parenchymal hemorrhage/contusion, edema, and spinal cord disruption in acute and subacute SCI may contribute to the understanding of severity of injury and prognosis for neurological improvement [67].

MRI-Diffusion Weighted Imaging (MRI-DWI): It is an MRI-based imaging modality that determines the free diffusion of water molecules, enabling the recognition of imaging information beyond the resolution of conventional MRI methods [69]. MRI-DWI can be utilized to measure response to various cellular therapy interventions after experimental SCI [67].

Computerized Tomography (CT): The assessment of the bone loss following SCI in an animal model could be done by high-resolution CT images [70].

- **Neuroanatomical tracing**

Recently, several studies used neuroanatomical tracing procedures to study axonal remodeling after cell transplantation in experimental SCI models [71-76].

- **Histology**

Histological outcome measures, including sparing at the lesion epicenter, sparing throughout the extent of the lesion, quantification of myelin loss rostral and caudal to the lesion, and motor neuron counts, are demonstrated via staining sections of the spinal cord [21].

Hematoxylin and Eosin (H&E) is useful as a general structural stain in most tissues. But the high lipid content of nervous tissue makes it less suited to H&E than most others.

Cresyl violet stains both neurons and glia. It bonds well with acidic parts of cells such as ribosomes, nuclei and nucleoli and demonstrates the nissl substance. It stains cell bodies a blue/violet.

Luxol Fast Blue gives particularly good delineation of nerve tracts in the CNS. It is probably one of the most popular stains for the demonstration of normal myelin.

Osmium tetroxide is both a stain and a fixative. While it's primarily used these days as a fixative in electron microscopy, since it binds to lipids strongly, it's particularly well suited to reveal the details of myelin in nerves.

Eriochrome cyanine (EC) staining protocol for differentiation of white matter and cell bodies is used to calculate the amount of spared tissue in sections of injured cords.

8. Considerations

To choose an animal model, the proposed aim of the study must precisely be noted. The researchers involved in scientific work with animals should know the ethical standards in animal experiments and investigate what animals are appropriate for each area of study in their models. Reproducible experimental SCI requires suitable training, animal care, experience with animal spine surgery, and proper surgical equipment. A standard housing environment with ad libitum access to food and water is a necessity for animal experiments. Pre-training and habituation of animals are important. When a behavioral testing is planned, animals must be trained inadequate sessions pre-operatively. Anesthetizing, surgery, and/or sacrificing have to been performed based on confirmed methods, attentively. All animals should be inspected regularly for wound healing, weight loss, dehydration, infection, autophagia and any discomfort [77]. Animal models, particularly complete SCI ones, need to serious care including preparation of supportive fluids, analgesia, and antibiotics, and also continuous bladder and bowel care. Appropriate veterinary care was provided as needed. All behavioral, histological, etc. analysis should be precisely selected before beginning a study and conducted by personnel blind to groups of study.

9. Conclusion and future perspectives

Animal models of SCI have confirmed to be helpful for the development of experimental therapies, and certainly will continue to play an essential role in the studies related to SCI. They give researchers an opportunity to discover the characteristic pattern of cell death and sparing, and measurement of any neuroprotection, regeneration, collateral sprouting, demyelination, and recovery of locomotor or other deficits. All injury paradigms are useful, but differ in the information that can be gained. The contusion models better simulate the biomechanics and neuropathology of human injury. The transection models, either completely or partially, are valuable for investigating the anatomic regeneration. The conclusions of rodent studies should examine in other animal models to survey their biological responses. In parallel, controlling and monitoring the injury mechanism within the surgical field, and evaluation of behavioral and histological outcomes have to be enhanced by applying technological improvements. Finally, more experimental studies should be designed to quantify neuronal damage after ischemic SCI.

Author details

Mahdi Sharif-Alhoseini[1] and Vafa Rahimi-Movaghar[1,2*]

*Address all correspondence to: v_rahimi@sina.tums.ac.ir, v_rahimi@yahoo.com

1 Sina Trauma and Surgery Research Center, Tehran University of Medical Sciences, Tehran, Iran

2 Research Centre for Neural Repair, University of Tehran, Tehran, Iran

References

[1] Simmons D. The use of animal models in studying genetic disease: transgenesis and induced mutation. Nature Education 2008;1(1).

[2] Blight AR. Animal models of spinal cord injury. Topics in Spinal Cord Injury Rehabilitation 2000;6(2) 1-13.

[3] Blight AR, Tuszynski MH. Clinical trials in spinal cord injury. J Neurotrauma 2006;23(3-4) 586-93.

[4] Nout Y, Rosenzweig E, Brock J, Strand S, Moseanko R, Hawbecker S, et al. Animal Models of Neurologic Disorders: A Nonhuman Primate Model of Spinal Cord Injury. Neurotherapeutics 2012;9(2) 380-92.

[5] Rahimi-Movaghar V, Rasouli MR, Smith H, Vaccaro AR. An evidence-based spinal cord injury decompression in experimental animals and human studies. In: Berkovsky TC. (ed.) Handbook of Spinal Cord Injuries: Types, Treatments, and Prognosis. NewYork: NOVA; 2009. p635-63

[6] Kundi S, Bicknell R, Ahmed Z. Spinal cord injury: Current mammalian models. American Journal of Neuroscience 2013;4(1) 1.

[7] Vijayaprakash K, Sridharan N. An experimental spinal cord injury rat model using customized impact device: A cost-effective approach. J Pharmacol Pharmacother 2013;4(3) 211-3.

[8] Amako T. Surgery of spinal injuries due to impact: II experimental study. J Jap Surg Soc 1936;37 1843-74.

[9] Tarlov I, Klinger H, Vitale S. Spinal cord compression studies: I. experimental techniques to produce acute and gradual compression. Archives of Neurology and Psychiatry 1953;70(6) 813.

[10] Eidelberg E, Staten E, Watkins J, McGraw D, McFadden C. A model of spinal cord injury. Surgical neurology 1976;6(1) 35.

[11] Braga-Silva J, Gehlen D, Roman JA, Machado DC, Costa JCd, Faúndez M, et al. Experimental model of spinal cord injury in rats with a device for local therapeutic agents access. Acta Ortopédica Brasileira 2007;15(3) 155-7.

[12] Rivlin AS, Tator CH. Effect of duration of acute spinal cord compression in a new acute cord injury model in the rat. Surg Neurol 197810(1) 38-43.

[13] Bresnahan JC, Beattie MS, Todd FD, 3rd, Noyes DH. A behavioral and anatomical analysis of spinal cord injury produced by a feedback-controlled impaction device. Exp Neurol 1987;95(3) 548-70.

[14] Kwon BK, Oxland TR, Tetzlaff W. Animal models used in spinal cord regeneration research. Spine (Phila Pa 1976) 2002;27(14) 1504-10.

[15] Agrawal G, Kerr C, Thakor NV, All AH. Characterization of Graded MASCIS Contusion Spinal Cord Injury using Somatosensory Evoked Potentials. Spine 2010;35(11) 1122.

[16] Lang-Lazdunski L, Matsushita K, Hirt L, Waeber C, Vonsattel J-PG, Moskowitz MA. Spinal Cord Ischemia: Development of a Model in the Mouse. Stroke 2000;31(1) 208-13.

[17] Gaviria M, Haton H, Sandillon F, Privat A. A mouse model of acute ischemic spinal cord injury. J Neurotrauma 2002;19(2) 205-21.

[18] Nouri M, Rasouli M, Shafiei S, Tavasoly A, Dehpour AR, Rahimi-Movaghar V. Does abdominal aorta clamping, as a method of spinal ischemia in rats, really work? Surg Neurol 2006;66(3) 332-3.

[19] Rasouli MR, Rahimi-Movaghar V, Vaccaro AR. Re: Usul H, Arslan E, Cansever T, et al. Effects of clotrimazole on experimental spinal cord ischemia/reperfusion injury in rats. Spine (Phila Pa 1976) 2009;34(17) 1884.

[20] Rahimi-Movaghar V, Sayyah MK, Akbari H, Khorramirouz R, Rasouli MR, Moradi-Lakeh M, et al. Epidemiology of Traumatic Spinal Cord Injury in Developing Countries: A Systematic Review. Neuroepidemiology 2013;41(2) 65-85.

[21] Gensel JC, Tovar CA, Hamers FP, Deibert RJ, Beattie MS, Bresnahan JC. Behavioral and histological characterization of unilateral cervical spinal cord contusion injury in rats. J Neurotrauma 2006 Jan;23(1) 36-54.

[22] Lane MA, Fuller DD, White TE, Reier PJ. Respiratory neuroplasticity and cervical spinal cord injury: translational perspectives. Trends in Neurosciences 2008;31(10) 538-47.

[23] Goshgarian HG, Koistinen JM, Schmidt ER. Cell death and changes in the retrograde transport of horseradish peroxidase in rubrospinal neurons following spinal cord hemisection in the adult rat. J Comp Neurol 1983;214(3) 251-7.

[24] Soblosky JS, Song J-H, Dinh DH. Graded unilateral cervical spinal cord injury in the rat: evaluation of forelimb recovery and histological effects. Behavioural Brain Research 2001;119(1) 1-13.

[25] Rahimi-Movaghar V. Clinical trials for the treatment of spinal cord injury: cervical and lumbar enlargements versus thoracic area. Brain 2009;132(7) e115.

[26] Pearse DD, Lo TP, Jr., Cho KS, Lynch MP, Garg MS, Marcillo AE, et al. Histopathological and behavioral characterization of a novel cervical spinal cord displacement contusion injury in the rat. J Neurotrauma 2005;22(6) 680-702.

[27] Ohta K, Fujimura Y, Nakamura M, Watanabe M, Yato Y. Experimental study on MRI evaluation of the course of cervical spinal cord injury. Spinal Cord 1999;37(8) 580-4.

[28] Nobunaga AI, Go BK, Karunas RB. Recent demographic and injury trends in people served by the model spinal cord injury care systems. Archives of Physical Medicine and Rehabilitation 1999;80(11) 1372-82.

[29] Jakeman LB, Guan Z, Wei P, Ponnappan R, Dzwonczyk R, Popovich PG, et al. Traumatic spinal cord injury produced by controlled contusion in mouse. J Neurotrauma 2000;17(4) 299-319.

[30] Stokes BT, Jakeman LB. Experimental modelling of human spinal cord injury: a model that crosses the species barrier and mimics the spectrum of human cytopathology. Spinal Cord 2002;40(3) 101-9.

[31] Scheff SW, Rabchevsky AG, Fugaccia I, Main JA, Lumpp JE, Jr. Experimental modeling of spinal cord injury: characterization of a force-defined injury device. J Neurotrauma 2003;20(2) 179-93.

[32] Brösamle C, Huber AB. Cracking the black box–and putting it back together again: Animal models of spinal cord injury. Drug Discovery Today: Disease Models 2007;3(4) 341-7.

[33] Rahimi-Movaghar V, Yazdi A, Karimi M, Mohammadi M, Firouzi M, Zanjani LO, et al. Effect of decompression on complete spinal cord injury in rats. Int J Neurosci 2008;118(10) 1359-73.

[34] Jazayeri SB, Firouzi M, Abdollah Zadegan S, Saeedi N, Pirouz E, Nategh M, et al. The effect of timing of decompression on neurologic recovery and histopathologic findings after spinal cord compression in a rat model. Acta Med Iran 2013;51(7) 431-7.

[35] Lim JH, Jung CS, Byeon YE, Kim WH, Yoon JH, Kang KS, et al. Establishment of a canine spinal cord injury model induced by epidural balloon compression. J Vet Sci 2007;8(1) 89-94.

[36] Dimar JRI, Glassman SD, Raque GH, Zhang YP, Shields CB. The Influence of Spinal Canal Narrowing and Timing of Decompression on Neurologic Recovery After Spinal Cord Contusion in a Rat Model. Spine 1999;24(16) 1623.

[37] Talac R, Friedman JA, Moore MJ, Lu L, Jabbari E, Windebank AJ, et al. Animal models of spinal cord injury for evaluation of tissue engineering treatment strategies. Biomaterials 2004;25(9) 1505-10.

[38] Nakae A, Nakai K, Yano K, Hosokawa K, Shibata M, Mashimo T. The animal model of spinal cord injury as an experimental pain model. J Biomed Biotechnol 2011; doi: 10.1155/2011/939023

[39] Steward O, Zheng B, Tessier-Lavigne M. False resurrections: Distinguishing regenerated from spared axons in the injured central nervous system. The Journal of Comparative Neurology 2003;459(1) 1-8.

[40] Watson BD, Prado R, Dietrich WD, Ginsberg MD, Green BA. Photochemically induced spinal cord injury in the rat. Brain Res 1986;367(1-2) 296-300.

[41] Piao MS, Lee JK, Jang JW, Kim SH, Kim HS. A mouse model of photochemically induced spinal cord injury. J Korean Neurosurg Soc 2009;46(5) 479-83.

[42] Awad H, Ankeny DP, Guan Z, Wei P, McTigue DM, Popovich PG. A mouse model of ischemic spinal cord injury with delayed paralysis caused by aortic cross-clamping. Anesthesiology 2010;113(4) 880-91.

[43] Yezierski RP, Liu S, Ruenes GL, Kajander KJ, Brewer KL. Excitotoxic spinal cord injury: behavioral and morphological characteristics of a central pain model. PAIN 1998;75(1) 141-55.

[44] Zheng YH, Fang Z, Cao P, Zheng T, Sun CH, Lu J, et al. A model of acute compression spinal cord injury by a mini-invasive expandable balloon in goats. Zhonghua Yi Xue Za Zhi 2012;92(23) 1591-5. [In Chinese]

[45] Jeffery N, Smith P, Lakatos A, Ibanez C, Ito D, Franklin R. Clinical canine spinal cord injury provides an opportunity to examine the issues in translating laboratory techniques into practical therapy. Spinal Cord 2006;44(10) 584-93.

[46] Fukuda S, Nakamura T, Kishigami Y, Endo K, Azuma T, Fujikawa T, et al. New canine spinal cord injury model free from laminectomy. Brain Res Protoc 2005;14 171-80.

[47] Moon L, Bunge MB. From animal models to humans: strategies for promoting CNS axon regeneration and recovery of limb function after spinal cord injury. Journal of Neurologic Physical Therapy 2005;29(2) 55-69.

[48] Lemon RN, Griffiths J. Comparing the function of the corticospinal system in different species: organizational differences for motor specialization? Muscle & nerve 2005;32(3) 261-79.

[49] Courtine G, Bunge MB, Fawcett JW, Grossman RG, Kaas JH, Lemon R, et al. Can experiments in nonhuman primates expedite the translation of treatments for spinal cord injury in humans? Nat Med 2007;13(5) 561-6.

[50] Doyle LMF, Stafford PP, Roberts BL. Recovery of locomotion correlated with axonal regeneration after a complete spinal transection in the eel. Neuroscience 2001;107(1) 169-79.

[51] Lee D-H, Lee J. Animal models of axon regeneration after spinal cord injury. Neurosci Bull 2013;29(4) 436-44.

[52] Khan T, Havey RM, Sayers ST, Patwardhan A, King WW. Animal models of spinal cord contusion injuries. Comparative Medicine 1999;49(2) 161-72.

[53] Metz GA, Curt A, van de Meent H, Klusman I, Schwab ME, Dietz V. Validation of the weight-drop contusion model in rats: a comparative study of human spinal cord injury. J Neurotrauma 2000;17(1) 1-17.

[54] Jakeman L, Ma M, Stokes B. Considering the Use of Transgenic Mice in Spinal Cord Injury Research. New York: Prominent Press; 2001.

[55] Jakeman L, Ma M, Stokes B. Considering the use of transgenic animals in spinal cord injury research. In: Marwah J, Dixon E, Banik NL. (ed.) Traumatic CNS Injury. Prominent Press; 2001. p180–201.

[56] Rossignol S, Bouyer L, Langlet C, Barthélemy D, Chau C, Giroux N, et al. Determinants of locomotor recovery after spinal injury in the cat. In: Shigemi Mori DGS, Mario W. (ed.) Progress in Brain Research. Elsevier; 2004. p163-72.

[57] Basso DM. Behavioral testing after spinal cord injury: congruities, complexities, and controversies. J Neurotrauma 2004;21(4) 395-404.

[58] Šedý J, Urdzíková L, Jendelová P, Syková E. Methods for behavioral testing of spinal cord injured rats. Neuroscience & Biobehavioral Reviews 2008;32(3) 550-80.

[59] Rahimi-Movaghar V, Yazdi A, Mohammadi M. Usefulness of the tail-flick reflex in the prognosis of functional recovery in paraplegic rats. Surgical neurology 2008;70(3) 323-5.

[60] Onifer SM, Rabchevsky AG, Scheff SW. Rat Models of Traumatic Spinal Cord Injury to Assess Motor Recovery. ILAR Journal 2007;48(4) 385-95.

[61] Onifer SM, Zhang YP, Burke DA, Brooks DL, Decker JA, McClure NJ, et al. Adult rat forelimb dysfunction after dorsal cervical spinal cord injury. Experimental Neurology 2005;192(1) 25-38.

[62] Beaumont E, Onifer SM, Reed WR, Magnuson DSK. Magnetically evoked inter-enlargement response: An assessment of ascending propriospinal fibers following spinal cord injury. Experimental Neurology 2006;201(2) 428-40.

[63] Linden RD, Zhang YP, Burke DA, Hunt MA, Harpring JE, Shields CB. Magnetic motor evoked potential monitoring in the rat. J Neurosurg 1999;91(2 Suppl) 205-10.

[64] Blight AR. Motor evoked potentials in CNS trauma. Cent Nerv Syst Trauma 1986;3(3) 207-14.

[65] Skinner SA, Transfeldt EE. Electromyography in the detection of mechanically induced spinal motor tract injury: observations in diverse porcine models. Journal of Neurosurgery: Spine 2009;11(3) 369-74.

[66] Rivas DA, Chancellor MB, Huang B, Salzman SK. Autonomic dysreflexia in a rat model spinal cord injury and the effect of pharmacologic agents. Neurourol Urodyn 1995;14(2) 141-52.

[67] Lammertse D, Dungan D, Dreisbach J, Falci S, Flanders A, Marino R, et al. Neuroimaging in traumatic spinal cord injury: an evidence-based review for clinical practice and research. J Spinal Cord Med 2007;30(3) 205-14.

[68] Hofstetter CP, Schweinhardt P, Klason T, Olson L, Spenger C. Numb rats walk - a behavioural and fMRI comparison of mild and moderate spinal cord injury. Eur J Neurosci 2003;18(11) 3061-8.

[69] Schwartz ED, Hackney DB. Diffusion-weighted MRI and the evaluation of spinal cord axonal integrity following injury and treatment. Experimental Neurology 2003;184(2) 570-89.

[70] Voor MJ, Brown EH, Xu Q, Waddell SW, Burden RL, Jr., Burke DA, et al. Bone loss following spinal cord injury in a rat model. J Neurotrauma 2012;29(8) 1676-82.

[71] Wu Y, Satkunendrarajah K, Teng Y, Chow DS, Buttigieg J, Fehlings MG. Delayed post-injury administration of riluzole is neuroprotective in a preclinical rodent model of cervical spinal cord injury. J Neurotrauma 2013;30(6) 441-52.

[72] Seitz A, Aglow E, Heber-Katz E. Recovery from spinal cord injury: a new transection model in the C57Bl/6 mouse. J Neurosci Res 2002;67(3) 337-45.

[73] Pal R, Gopinath C, Rao NM, Banerjee P, Krishnamoorthy V, Venkataramana NK, et al. Functional recovery after transplantation of bone marrow-derived human mesenchymal stromal cells in a rat model of spinal cord injury. Cytotherapy 2010;12(6) 792-806.

[74] Martin D, Robe P, Franzen R, Delree P, Schoenen J, Stevenaert A, et al. Effects of Schwann cell transplantation in a contusion model of rat spinal cord injury. J Neurosci Res 1996;45(5) 588-97.

[75] Hodgetts SI, Simmons PJ, Plant GW. Human mesenchymal precursor cells (Stro-1(+)) from spinal cord injury patients improve functional recovery and tissue sparing in an acute spinal cord injury rat model. Cell Transplant 2013;22(3) 393-412.

[76] Abematsu M, Tsujimura K, Yamano M, Saito M, Kohno K, Kohyama J, et al. Neurons derived from transplanted neural stem cells restore disrupted neuronal circuitry in a mouse model of spinal cord injury. J Clin Invest 2010;120(9) 3255-66.

[77] Rahimi-Movaghar V, Yazdi A, Saadat S. Saturated Picric Acid Prevents Autophagia and Self-Mutilation in Laboratory Rats. Acta Medica Iranica 2008;46(4) 283-6.

Chapter 11

Mesenchymal Stem Cells in Spinal Cord Injury

N.K. Venkataramanaa and Rakhi Pal

Additional information is available at the end of the chapter

http://dx.doi.org/10.5772/58323

1. Introduction

Spinal cord injury is the most devastating neural injury associated with road traffic accidents or fall from height. Due to the compact arrangement of nerve fibers injury often leads to significant deficits. In addition the cellular components of the spinal cord are highly susceptible to injury. Together with the brain the ability of self-repair in comparison to other tissues of the body is poor.[1]. Recently it is noted that the tissue response of the spinal cord to injury is distinctly different from that of brain. The structure, cellular arrangement, vascularity, blood spinal cord barrier, and lack of exposure to inflammatory cells are some of the limiting factors for repair. Added to it receptor and membrane specializations that allow chemical and electrical neuro transmission is prone to major ionic shifts. Though regeneration of spinal cord in teleost fishes and urodele amphibians is established, no adult mammal is able to regenerate. Hence, any insult can result in permanent and significant loss of body function. The therapies currently practiced (surgery, drugs, rehabilitation), are grossly inadequate. The available surgical treatment could only achieve prevention of further injury, maintain and support blood flow, relieve the compression and secure stabilization of spine for early mobilization and rehabilitation. Thus any new treatment for spinal cord injury that enables recovery of function is the need of the hour and could be a significant advancement in clinical care. Biological therapies are now being developed to augment the endogenous repair capabilities. They are aimed at preservation of tissue, promotion of cell survival, activation of neuronal regrowth, reduction in growth inhibition, scarring and cavitation, promotion of myelin repair thus enhancing neuronal circuits.

We have studied and evaluated such applications to attempt spinal cord regeneration. Adult human mesenchymal stem cells were the obvious choice due to their self-renewal property, ease of availability, hypo-immunogenic property, non-teratogenicity, multi-potentiality with high genetic stability.

2. Incidence

More than half of all spinal cord injuries occur in the cervical area; and a third of them affect thoracic region. And the rest afflicts lumbar region. Most of the affected ones are young, in their teens or twenties.. The leading causes of acute spinal cord injury include vehicular accidents-41%, violence-22%, falls-21% and sports-8% [2]. Population studies shows the incidence that vary between 2-20%. The official figure is 12% majority being, due to trauma. The total number of people suffering a spinal cord injury in the US alone is 200,000; and 11,000 being added annually. The United Kingdom had over 700 new spinal cord injuries in 2004 (according to the International Campaign for Cures of Spinal Cord Injury).

Spinal cord injury (SCI) is the third most prevalent disease in our country after diabetes and myocardial infarction. More than 12% of the Indian population suffers from the complications associated with spinal cord injury and at least 10,000 are being affected annually [3]. Majority are in the age group 21-36 years, the most productive years of life and 10-12% of severe head injuries are associated with spinal injury. Awareness of this fact is important to protect spine during pre hospital care. The clinical dictum is to suspect spinal injury in all high speed injuries.. Penetrating injuries are relatively rare.

3. Pathophysiology

The biological response to spinal cord injury is customarily categorized into 3 phases that follows a distinct but somewhat overlapping temporal sequence: acute or primary (seconds to minutes after the injury), secondary or sub-acute (minutes to weeks after the injury), and chronic (months to years after the injury) [4] Table 1. Primary injury is due to direct impact, damaging the neurons, cell membranes, disrupting blood supply, and destabilizing the spinal column. Secondary damage soon follows causing oedema, inflammation and free radical production. A series of molecular changes then produce a cascading effect with liberation of toxins compounding the primary injury. This can continue for few days to even up to six months. [5,6,7] Diverse type of cells and molecules from nervous, immune and vascular system are known to be involved in each phase. Most of the involved cells reside within the spinal cord; also some other cells are recruited through the circulatory system [8]. Hypotension and hypoxia can induce secondary permanent damage.

The onset of acute phase begins within seconds after an insult to spinal cord injury and is marked by both local and systemic events. Cascade of sequential pathological changes can occur during this phase. Local events such as cord compression, release and accumulation of various neurotransmitters such as catecholamines and excitotoxic amino acids to a toxic level enough to kill neural cells have been postulated to occur within seconds of injury [8]. Soon after trauma, hypotension, shock, low cardiac output and respiratory failure and hypoxia occur due to autonomic system failure. Between 15 to 30 minutes of post trauma, edema in white matter and hemorrhage in gray matter have been reported. Electron microscopic studies

http://dx.doi.org/10.5772/58323

Primary events (0-2 hrs)	Secondary events (1-6 hrs)	Spinal shock (12 hrs –3 weeks)	Post spinal shock Reflexes reappear
Mechanical compression of neural elements by bone fragments, disc material, and ligaments, laceration, shear and distraction	1. Toxic metabolites 2. Electrolyte loss 3. Hypoperfusion of gray matter 4. Loss of autoregulation and microcirculation 5. Vasospasm, thrombosis and hemorrhage. 6. Accumulation of neurotransmitters : like Glutamate leading to excitotoxicity 7. Elevated calcium levels 8. Cell membrane disruption and loss of cell integrity 9. Cytotoxicity/free radicals/apoptosis/ prostaglandin release and lipid peroxidation 10. Demyelination 11. Edema 12. Invasion of glial cells and activation of resident microglial cell population.	1. Neurogenic shock. 2. Respiratory distress. 3. Impaired autonomic functions. 4. Quadriplegia. 5 Anesthesia below affected level. 6. Delayed gastric emptying. 7. Paralytic ileus	1. Superficial abdominal reflex 2. Criemasteric reflex 3. Bulbocavernous reflex 4. Withdrawal reflex 5. Beevar sign etc

Table 1. Illustrates the different phases of spinal cord injury and the cascade of events associated with it.

revealed accumulation of intra-and extracellular fluids in the intercellular space. Ischemia or local anemia has been reported within first few hours after severe trauma using angiographic methods. A major reduction in spinal cord blood flow and lack of perfusion has been observed. This ischemic zone encompasses a large portion of gray matter and surrounding white matter. The main reasons postulated for ischemia are vasospasm (due to vasoconstrictors and vasoactive amines), thrombosis, and platelet aggregation and hemorrhage [9]. By 4th hour, axonal degeneration followed by vesicular disruption in myelin sheaths and ischemia becomes evident. In other patients who do survive the initial injury, hyperaemia and other vascular changes become prominent in 12 to 24 hours. These reactions are mediated through prostaglandins, catecholamines and other agents [10]. At the end of 24 hours, necrosis starts and remains active for another 24 hours which triggers the inflammatory response and disruption of cell membranes resulting in release of intracellular contents of neurons and endothelial cells lining them. This progressive, coagulative and patchy necrosis generally occupies the previous hemorrhagic region and develops infarcts. Increased intracellular calcium influences enzymes, such as phospholipases and phosphatases, to promote the breakdown of the cell membrane. This results in liberation of free fatty acids, which are converted to prostaglandins which further increases the constriction of the blood vessels (vasospasm), which in turn contributes to final cell death [11].

The secondary mechanisms are still ill understood. In literature(shows) there are approximately 25 well established secondary injury mechanisms are described [12, 13]. Secondary phase sets in minutes and lasts from days to months. Some classical examples of secondary injury mechanisms are continuation of events from the acute phase as outlined by Charles. They are vasospasm, cell death from direct insult, ischemia, edema, derangements in ionic homeostasis and accumulation of neurotransmitters. In addition some novel features, marks the secondary phase such as free-radical production, lipid peroxidation, nitrous oxide excess, conduction block, excess noradrenaline, energy failure and decreased ATP, immune cells invasion and release of cytokines, inflammatory mediated cell death, neurite growth-inhibitory factors (Nogo-A, Rho-A, oligodendrocyte myelin glycoprotein (OMgp) myelin-associated, glycoprotein (MAG), and chondroitin sulfate proteoglycans, central chromatolysis,). vertebral compression / column instability, demyelination of surviving axons, initiation of central cavitation, astroglial scar launch, plasma membrane compromise /permeability, mitochondrial malfunctions and activation of death signals causing apoptosis [8] are the remaining..

The third phase (chronic phase), along with the events in secondary phase, such as demyelination, apoptosis, central cavitation, glial scar formation, is marked by the emergence of new types of pathologies both at micro and macro level [8]. At microlevel, death of oligodendrocytes, susceptible to Reactive Oxygen Species (ROS), loss of electrical impulse conduction by axons due to demyelination and altered neurocircuits and alteration of ion channels and receptors occur [9]. At macrolevel, formation of the glial scar represents an attempt by Glial cells to contain the injury site and promote healing. In addition to reactive astrocytes, scar formation also involves oligodendrocyte precursor cells, microglia, and macrophages. The pathobiology of glial scar is due to reactive gliosis and extra cellular matrix (ECM) remodeling [8]. These changes during reactive astrogliosis have the potential to alter astrocyte activities both through gain and loss of functions that could be beneficial as well as detrimental to surrounding neural and non-neural cells [16, 17, and 18].

More than a quarter of spinal cord injured patients develop cavities which eventually lead to Syringomyelia [19]. Pathogenesis of post traumatic syrinx is not clear. Widely accepted theory recognized two steps in the pathogenesis, namely formation of cavity followed by its enlargement and extension. Microscopic examination demonstrated gliosis, which is an astrocytic response to adjacent tissue damage, appears as high MRI signals around the syrinx. [20]. The intial cystic lesion results from multiple factors like mechanical damage, local ischemia [19], arterial and venous obstruction, liquifaction of hematoma, by lysosomal and other intracellular enzymes [21].

Beside, chronic phase also initiates number of neuroprotective and regenerative responses.But they are insufficient for regeneration of the nerve root by Schwann cells or oligodendrocytes. Some compensation by spared neurons (sprouting) often with inappropriate connectivity.

Finally the reactive astrogliosis itself hinders the axonal regrowth and the functional recovery of the injured spinal cord [22].

3.1. Impediments for regeneration

Cord tissue comprises of several components with variable sensitivity to injury.[1].Injury often causes cavitation of epicenter due to cell death, ischemia, mechanical injury, exitotoxicity and neuro inflammation. This cavity can enlarge extending the injury up and down. In addition it becomes a physical barrier for regeneration and cell transmission and cell migration. Body attempts to contain the injury and promote healing resulting in gliosis. This astrocytic gliosis becomes an impediment to the growth of axon described by Raymon Y Cajal in 1928 [1]. These gliotic cells also secrete inhibitory molecules for the axonal growth and connectivity. Inflammation slows down the initial angiogenesis response and oligodendrocytes (secrete Nogo molecules), glycoproteins Semaphoring 4D and Epherin B3,also have been shown to have inhibitory role.[21,22,23]

4. Tools for assessing spinal cord injury and repair

4.1. Molecular, genetic, and in vitro tools

Techniques now have been developed that allow researchers to isolate and grow populations of neurons to investigate the effects of specific proteins and molecules on neuronal injury and repair. Neurons can be grown in isolation or with glial cells such as oligodendrocytes or Schwann cells to study the processes of axonal outgrowth and myelination using DNA or protein analysis. Furthermore, the elucidation of the signaling pathways responsible for this switch in response may lead to the discovery of a strategy for enhancing axon regeneration.

Often, in vitro assays are tested along with animal models which allow better understanding of the effects detected in vitro and to be validated in a more complex system. The best studied example includes chondroitin sulfate proteoglycans, a potent inhibitor of neurite outgrowth in *in vitro* experiments. Analysis with animal models demonstrated that the levels of these proteoglycans are enhanced, or up-regulated, during central nervous system (CNS) injury and led to the development of a strategy to break down these substances and promote the regrowth of axons in the intact rat spinal cord after an injury [21].

4.2. Animal models for spinal cord injury

No single animal model has dominated for research in this area. Two broad classes of models have accounted for the great majority of studies. Both involve surgical exposure of the cord. Most commonly used models are transection or partial injuries for detailed studies of regeneration and experimental contusion and compression. Allen's weight drop model, the oldest method in use and produced by dropping a known weight onto the dorsal side of the exposed spinal cord. This is mainly to address the early processes of injury. Besides the above mentioned category, microlesion formation and transgenic models, [25] Photochemical SCI model, excitotoxic spinal cord injury have also been developed in recent years [26].

During the last two decades, various researchers have shown interest in developing variety of animal models based on the above two categories, that mimic different attributes associated with spinal cord injuries. Depending upon the purpose of the study and the specific aspect of the injury to be investigated, researchers determine which animal model most closely replicates the injury in humans. Commonly used animal models for the investigation includes [8] Primates – to test the safety and efficacy of the therapy, [9] Cat – to examine and define spinal cord circuitry, [10] Mouse and rat – mainly used for the investigations of molecular, genetic and anatomical response to injury and to modify genes to test the effect of restoration or loss of function.

The kind of inquiries currently in focus can be addressed with rodent models, for which the maximum number of biological reagents and tools are available. In time, there may be a need to examine the conclusions of rodent studies in other models, to deal with questions of species differences (biological responses, chromosomal arrangements, genetic variability and the spatial arrangement of the nerve tracts) and mechanical scale (animal size, limited number of animals for experimentation) and ethics [9].

5. Assessing SCI and repair mechanisms

5.1. Conventional treatment strategies

Treatment for Spinal cord injury starts at the site of accident or trauma. Manual spine immobilization or using cervical collar and spine board, followed by administration of analgesics to reduce pain is an established practice to achieve comfort to the patient. Careful monitoring of airway, respiration, and arterial pressure is essential. Hypotension, hypoxia are deleterious and should be avoided at all cost. From the scene of trauma, the patient is moved to the medical center and assessed further with neurological status and clinical level of injury. Base line clinical status is established and documented. In parallel other systemic injuries were also evaluated. ASIA impairment scale modified BENZEL scale and FRANKEL scales are commonly used to evaluate progress. MRI is the gold standard in imaging to delineate the anatomy of injury. In addition, size and extent of cord contusion, hemorrhage and edema have prognostic significance. Throughout its mandatory to avoid secondary insults to spinal cord. Several drugs have been tried with no demonstrable benefit. There is no role for steroids and Methylprednisolone. All attempts of direct surgical repair of spinal cord have failed.

5.2. Experimental strategies

Almost every aspect of the management of SCI is controversial, due to lack of good-quality evidence. Currently all the modes of the experimental therapy falls into any of the following categories: neuroprotection, repair/regeneration, enhancing the plasticity and replace/assist function. The details of all can be found at ICORD website (http://icord.org/).

5.3. Neuroprotection (randomized clinical trials)

Clinical trials should augment the neurological recovery data with outcome measures designed to assess the functional significance of the neurological recovery. To date more than 70 clinical trials have been done on functional recovery of Spinal Cord Injury with drugs and other therapeutic intervention (http://clinicaltrials.gov/). Of those, drugs which have direct application in treatment regimen for SCI and the reason for their pitfalls are discussed here.

1. Pharmacological therapy

The first and extensive studied drug is Methyl prednisolone sodium succinate (MPSS), an anti inflammatory corticosteroid exerting its function as antioxidant, enhancer of spinal cord blood flow, by reducing calcium influx, posttraumatic axonal die back and attenuating lipid peroxidation. The drawback of this drug is that it did not rescue neurons from cell death and [16] its high rates of adverse events such as the occurrence of pulmonary and gastrointestinal complications and others. [8, 9, 15].

A noncompetitive N-methyl-d-aspartate receptor antagonist, gacyclidine (GK-11), showed promise as a neuroprotective agent as evidenced by walking recovery, motor performance, attenuation of spinal cord damage, reducing apoptosis of oligodendrocytes via inhibition of proNGF production in microglia [18] etc, in rat model. However, this agent is no longer being pursued for SCI [11] and the use of minocycline following contusion of cord requires further investigation before clinical trials are implemented [17].

Minocycline, an antibiotic and anti-inflammatory substance facilitated overall motor recovery and attenuated mechanical hyperalgesia in a rat model [8], but did not increase the survival of the preganglionic parasympathetic neurons (PPNs) [20].

2. GM-1(Sygen), a ganglioside found in the neuronal cell membranes, was found to promote recovery in a number of animal models. In human trials it resulted in statistically significant improvement in ASIA motor score but failed to demonstrate a significant difference in its primary outcome measure, a 2-point improvement on the modified Benzel walking scale [8, 9].

3. Erythropoietin, a potent cytokine [25], and its analogues have been thoroughly investigated [26] and shown to protect neuronal cell in vitro from apoptosis and also suppress the up-regulated expression of TGF-β [27, 25] reduces the inflammation, and restores the vascular integrity [21].

4. Immunomodulatory treatment

Inflammatory processes that occur at the injury site of the spinal cord are both beneficial and harmful. Phagocytic macrophages have been indicated in secondary destruction of neural tissue post SCI [28; 29] but are not sufficient as compared with peripheral nerve injury. Rapalino *et al.*, [30], has demonstrated that implantation of activated macrophages in the site of injury in adult injured rats results in partial recovery. On the contrary, Popovich *et al.*, [31] suggested that depletion of macrophages may result in preservation of myelinated axons and functional recovery following injury. A phase I clinical trial demonstrated the safety of autologous macrophage transplantation into the damaged spinal cord within 14 days of injury.

5. Neurotrophic factors: Neurotrophic factors have been documented to improve cell survival and axonal regeneration and various approaches have been developed to deliver these factors to the site of injury. Stem cells from different sources like bone marrow [32, 33, adipose tissue, dental pulp [34], Wharton's jelly, olfactory ensheathing cells [35], neural stem cells [36] and embryonic stem cells [37] when transplanted *in vivo* have shown significant recovery.

6. In a controlled double-blinded study, 20 patients receiving thyrotrophin releasing hormone treatment showed significantly higher motor, sensory, and Sunnybrook scores than placebo treatment. But because of patients lost to subsequent follow-up, data were not highly informative [18]. Another study in rats treated with thyrotropin-releasing hormone showed significant improvement in Neural Scores 14 days post-injury, but there were no significant differences in morphometric parameters between saline-and TRH-treated rats [19]. TRH has disadvantages, including its analeptic, endocrine, and autonomic effects, but a new generation of TRH analogs has been developed that have the protective effects of TRH without its adverse effects [20].

6. Repair and regeneration

A variety of promising substances have been tested in animal models, but few have had potential application to human spinal cord injury (SCI) patients. This category of treatment includes both the pharmacological intervention using FDA approved drugs and cell transplantation. (The latter will be discussed in detail in the forthcoming titles). Several drugs were tested for their efficacy in restoring spinal cord function as evidenced by multiple preclinical studies. Some of the Drugs such as Cethrin [47-50], rolipram [41-45], ATI-355 [45-51], chondroitinase [51-56] and riluzole [57-64] were thoroughly reviewed which are not limited to neuroprotection, axonal regeneration, motor neuron recovery, reduction in muscle spasms, enhanced sprouting of corticospinal axons, improved behavioral outcome and corticospinal plasticity, recovery of forelimb function, inhibition of apoptosis and suppression of glial scar formation with varying degree of success. The major drawback of the pharmacological intervention is their side effects and direct application in human trials.

6.1. Plasticity enhancement and rehabilitation

An inability to perform self-care activities is considered a "burden of care" by the medical community. The individual with acute SCI faces many challenges with the resumption of self-care tasks. Hence considerable efforts have been taken by the therapist in order to guide the

http://dx.doi.org/10.5772/58323

patient move their upper limb and lower limb and support their body weight after a spinal trauma. Upon discharge from a hospital setting, family members, other caregivers, or both share the burden of care. Medical insurance programs have required reliable data on which to determine benefits, including coverage of durable medical equipment, treatment, and care giving assistance. Task specific training i.e., activities of daily living (ADL) which include self feeding, bathing, bowel and bladder maintenance, dressing, hygiene maintenance, computer usage etc., plays a central role for the patient to be independent. Other techniques such as body weight support and treadmill training using upper and lower limb orthosis and knee orthosis, have shown recovery in maintaining the body gait and postures. Tilt table standing, robot-aided gait training, electric stimulated wheel chairs are also used in recent days for posture maintenance. Recreation and leisure skill development such as reading, writing, painting, exercises, All-Terrain Vehicles (ATVs) (cycling, fishing, horseback riding, climbing, diving, etc) arm ergometry and Nautilus-type machines. Although these techniques are considered to be promising, less is known about their mechanism and efficacy on the functional recovery. Hence a deeper understanding of the underlying mechanism for adaptation and plasticity after spinal cord injury is needed to improve rehabilitation regimes [65-81].

6.2. Non pharmacological intervention for the treatment of SCI

Functional electrical stimulation (FES) is the technique of applying safe levels of electric current to activate the damaged or disabled nervous system. Although no absolute contraindications exist for the use of externally applied FES, a patient with a cardiac demand pacemaker or an automatic implanted defibrillator should be approached with extreme caution. Some of the relative contraindications for FES include patients with cardiac arrhythmias, congestive heart failure, pregnancy, electrode sensitivity, and patients with healing wound(s) that could be stressed during stimulation (i.e., muscle stimulation would adversely move healing tissues). As with any implant in the body, individuals with implanted FES systems need to obtain antibiotic prophylaxis when undergoing invasive procedures such as oral surgery. Functional uses for FES after SCI include applications in standing, walking, hand grasp (and release), bladder, bowel, and sexual function, respiratory assist, and electro ejaculation for fertility. [82-88]. Functional magnetic stimulation (FMS) can be defined as a technology that applies a time varying magnetic field to produce useful bodily function. There were no significant side effects of magnetic stimulation that were reported. However safety consideration such as magnetic effect, electric effect and power dissipation should be kept in mind during stimulation. A few reports have shown that repetitive transcranial magnetic stimulation may result in increased seizure activities [89-94].

Hypothermia, CSF Drainage, durotomy and subarachnoid perfusion, Functional electrical stimulation, Electromagnetic stimulation, hyperbaric oxygen were tried with some success. But none of them reached to the level of functional therapeutic options.

6.3. Replace or assist function

Over the past 2 decades, advances in understanding the pathophysiology of spinal cord injury (SCI) have stimulated the recent emergence of therapeutic strategies. Functional repair of the injured central nervous system (CNS) is one of the greatest challenges addressed by neurobiologists. The rapidly growing field of stem cell biology offers a promising future for cell replacement and neural regeneration therapies. Stem cells have seen its good days with success in Parkinson disease and Huntington's disease and hold a long history of research on the possible use of progenitor cells in the treatment of SCI. The application of cell-based therapies to SCI is a natural expansion of research in other fields, such as cancer, diabetes, and heart diseases.

Spinal Cord Injury and Stem cells: Some Cellular transplantation strategies

Spinal cord injury though uncommon leads to profound lifelong disability and systemic effects. So far no single therapy have proved its efficacy,.therefore combination therapies might hold the future design. In order to repair the injured spinal cord, it is essential to reduce secondary damage and promote regeneration. Several biological agents such as proteins, antibodies, enzymes and cells were used to achieve this goal..

The adult spinal cord has an endogenous progenitor cell pool said to have been located, in the ependymal region around the central canal. [95-97]. While others believe their presence throughout the spinal cord [98]. The response of these endogenous cells post injury is insufficient and does not bring about adequate recovery following SCI [95-97]; probably due to the insufficient cell numbers, microenvironment at the injury site, and presence of tissue debris. Neural inflammation, immune mediated destruction and loss of vascularity also becomes major hindrance. There could be an imbalance between the degree of repair vs damage. Cell transplant strategies have the potential of reducing such secondary damage and promoting regeneration by replacement of dead cells and production of Neurotrophic factors promoting regeneration [99-101].

Oligodendrocytes and astrocytes are the major supportive cells within the central nervous system and are responsible for myelination of axons, so it is believed that replacement of this cell population will support the frame work in regenerative processes.

Immature glial cells have been shown to reduce the inhibitory properties of the lesion epicentre and promote axonal growth [102]. Immature oligodendrocytes provide remyelination after injury [103], whereas immature astrocytes promote axonal growth and survival after injury [104]. A recent study supports the idea of ensuring both of these cell types, astroglial, are replaced, since oligodendrocytes precursors failed to remyelinate the spinal cord in the absence of astrocytes.

Cao *et al.,* [99] has demonstrated that after the transplantation of stem cells into lesioned adult rat spinal cord most of these transplanted cells have differentiated into astrocytes and no neurons or oligodendrocytes were observed. This indicates that it would be essential to transplant a progenitor cell population capable of trans-differentiating into a mixed lineage *in vivo* or should be able to secrete neurotrophic factors *in vivo*. Studies have elucidated that MSCs do have the capacity to Trans-differentiate into the astroglial lineage and also secrete cytokines which may be essential for regeneration in spinal cord injury.

6.4. Proposed scope of using stem cells / regenerative medicine

Type of stem cells	Species	Injury type	Site of injection	Results	Salient features	Reference
BM MSC						
Transgenically labeled BMMSC (autologous) and lineage restricted neural precursor (LRNP) (2x106 cells)	Inbred Fisher-344 rats	Partial cervical hemisection injury	Intravenously, Intraventricularly, Intrathecally and Lumbar puncture	Intravenous route – least efficient. Intrathecally and intraventricular administration shows enhanced cell migration and grafting	Axonal growth was observed around the transplanted cells. Grafted LRNP cells differentiation into mature neurons, their survival and integration within the host spinal Cord might lead to functional recovery.	Ajay bakshi et al
BMSCs and GCSF	Male Wistar rats	Compression lesion	Intravenously (BMSCs) and subcutaneously (GCSF)	Higher BBB scores and better recovery of hind limb sensitivity	Significant increases in the spared volume of white matter due to the synchronized action of various factors released by MSCs	Lucia Urdzíková et al
Bone-marrow-derived mesenchymal stem cell (autologous and allogenic)	Adult Beagle dogs		Intrathecal	Improved neurological signs in pelvic limbs Significant high Olby scores	Recovery may be due to the synchronized action of various factors as evidenced by high rate of mRNA expression for neurotrophic factors.	Dong-In Jung et al

Type of stem cells	Species	Injury type	Site of injection	Results	Salient features	Reference
LA MSC						
Adipose-derived stem cells (allogenic)	Adult mixed-breed dogs	Epidural balloon compression	Injured site	Nerve conduction velocity was significantly improved GFAP, Tuj-1 and NF160 were observed	Neuronal transdifferentiati on Survived MSCs produces large amounts of bFGF and VEGFR 3 which aid the recovery	
Cotransplantation of Mouse Neural Stem Cells (mNSCs) With Adipose Tissue-Derived Mesenchymal Stem Cells	Adult Male Sprague-Dawley rats	Clip compression	Epicenter of the injured spinal cord	AT-MSCs inhibited the apoptosis of mNSCs mNSCs transplanted with AT-MSCs showed better survival rates	Biomolecular substances secreted by ATMSCs improve mNSC survival and inhibit mNSC apoptosis, mainly VEGF	Jin Soo Oh et al
WJ MSC						
Human Umbilical Cord-Derived Schwann-Like Cell Combined with Neurotrophin-3	Adult Female SD rats	Transection	Lesion site	NT-3 administration significantly promoted the survival of the grafted cells Improved motor function and promotes neurite outgrowth	GDNF, BDNF, NT-3 and bFGF provided neurotrophic support	Guo Yan-Wu et al
Human umbilical cord mesenchymal stem cells	Female Sprague-Dawley rats	Weight drop method (contusion)	At the dorsal spinal cord 2 mm rostrally and 2 mm caudally to the injury site	Significant Recovery of hindlimb locomotor function Increased length of neurofilament-positive fibers and increased numbers of growth cone-like structures	Transplanted cells survived, migrated over short distances, and produced large amounts of glial cell line-derived neurotrophic	Hu SL et al

Type of stem cells	Species	Injury type	Site of injection	Results	Salient features	Reference
				Fewer reactive astrocytes were observed	factor and neurotrophin-3.	
Human umbilical cord mesenchymal stem cells	Adult Female Sprague-Dawley rats	Transection	Lesion site	Promotion of regrowth of injured corticospinal fibers change in the distribution of astrocytes in spinal cords reduction in the activation of microglia	Production of large amounts of human neutrophil-activating protein-2, NT-3, bFGF, glucocorticoid induced TNF-receptor, and VEGFR 3 in host spinal cord, may have helped in spinal cord repair.	Chang-Ching Yang et al
GLIAL CELLS						
Multineurotrophin-Expressing Glial-Restricted Precursor Cells	Adult Female Fischer 344 rats	Contusion	Lesion site	Improved transcranial magnetic motor-evoked potential responses Improved Electrophysiological and locomotor functional recovery	Grafted GRPs formed normal-appearing myelin sheaths around the axons in the ventrolateral funiculus (VLF) of spinal cord and restores the conduction.	Qilin Cao et al
NSC/ NSPC						
poly(lactide-co-glycolide) (PLGA) polymer seeded with human neural stem cells	African green monkey	Hemisection	Lesion site	Enhanced hindlimb motor neuron performance	Major mechanism of action of implanted cells may be due to trophic support rather than	Pritchard et al

Type of stem cells	Species	Injury type	Site of injection	Results	Salient features	Reference
					neuronal replacement	
Spinal cord-derived NSPCs and BMSCs	Adult male rat	Clip compression	Lesion site	No functional improvement was seen in either transplant group. But significant inverse corelation between the functional scores and the number of transplanted astrocytes was observed	Differentiation of NSPCs into astrocytes and oligodendrocytes promoting remyelination, and potential axonal guidance	Parr et al
Neural stem cells	Marmoset	Contusion	Lesion site	Recovery of motor function was observed mainly in the hindlimbs Significantly higher spontaneous movement	Grafted human NSCs survived and differentiated into neurons astrocytes and oligodendrocytes and restores motor function	Iwanami et al
Epidermal Neural Crest Stem Cell (EPI-NCSC)	Wild type C57BL6/J and C57BL/6-TgN (ACTbEGFP) 1Osb	Contusion	Intraspinal	Differentiated into gabaergic neurons and myelinating oligodendrocytes	combination of pertinent functions including cell replacement, neuroprotection, angiogenesis and modulation of scar formation	Sieber
Spinal cord-derived neural stem/ progenitor cells (NSPCS) and Bone Marrow-derived	Rat	Compression	Lumbar puncture	Expression of oligodendrocyte markers	wide dissemination of cells in the subarachnoid	Mothe et al

Type of stem cells	Species	Injury type	Site of injection	Results	Salient features	Reference
mesenchymal stromal cells (BMSCS)					space of the spinal cord	
Immortalized human NSC line over expressing VEGF (F3.VEGF cells)	Adult Sprague–Dawley female rats	Contusion	2 mm rostral and 2 mm caudal from the lesion epicenter	Elevated the amount of VEGF in the injured spinal cord tissue and increased phosphorylation of VEGFR flk-1 Enhanced cellular proliferation and tissue sparing	VEGF increased the number of early proliferating cells that differentiated into mature oligodendrocytes	Kim et al
Poly(lactic-co-glycolic acid) (PLGA) seeded with neural stem cell (NSC)	Adult dog	Hemisection	Lesion site	Grafted NSC survived the implantation procedure and showed migratory behavior	Ectopic expression of a therapeutic neurotrophin-3 gene was observed	Kim et al
hESC derived PROGENITOR CELLS						
hESC-derived oligodendrocyte progenitors (OPC) and/or motoneuron progenitors (MP)	Adult rats	Complete transection	Site of injury	Locomotor function was significantly enhanced OPC and MP survived, migrated, and differentiated into mature oligodendrocytes and neurons	The recoveries can be attributed to the reconnection of the axons above and below the lesion site	SLAVEN ERCEG et al (
hESC derived Oligodendrocyte Progenitor Cells	Female Sprague Dawley adult rats	Contusion	Lesion site	Transplanted cells survived, redistributed over short distances, and differentiated into oligodendrocytes	Widespread oligodendrocyte remyelination throughout the white matter	Keirstead et al

Table 2. Provides a list of preclinical animal studies conducted for spinal cord injury

6.4.1. Current status of cell replacement therapy

During the last 2 decades, the search for new therapies has been revolutionized by the discovery of stem cells, which has inspired scientists and clinicians to search for stem cell–based reparative approaches to many diseases. The adult spinal cord harbors endogenous stem/progenitor cells, collectively referred to as neural progenitor cells (NPCs) that might be responsible for normal turnover of the cells. However, the proliferative activity of endogenous NPCs is too limited to support significant self-repair after SCI. Thus, various cellular transplantation strategies have been adopted in models of SCI.

Current goals of cell replacement approach are broadly classified into two broad types: 1) regeneration and 2) repair. Alternatively the cell transplanted may promote protection to the endogenous cells from further damage.

A summary of cell therapy approaches has been listed in Table 2 mentioned above.

6.4.2. Different cell types proposed to have therapeutic potential

Human Embryonic Stem Cell derived progenitor cells

Cocultures of hESC derived ologodendrocytes with or without motor neuron progenitors have been used for the treatment of SCI by different researchers with different injury models [14, 17]. The functional recovery concluded by both study is in vivo differentiation of the transplanted cells into oligodendrocytes and neurons promoting remyelination and axonal regrowth.

Adult derived stem cells

Bone marrow derived stem cells

In a hemisection model of rats, Bakshi et al has shown that BMSC co-transplanted with that of neural progenitors shows better cell migration and grafting when injected intraventricularly or intrathecally. However, intravenous route shows the least cell migration to the site of injury. Alternatively, Urdzíková and his team reported that when BMSCs were transplanted intravenously with GCSF in subcutaneous region, spared white matter increases in size and enhanced recovery of hind limb sensitivity was observed. A canine model of injury using both auto and allogeneic BMSCs transplanted intrathecally shows improvement in neurological signs. But the mechanism of recovery observed was the synchronized action of the growth factors released by the grafted cells [11].

Strangely no functional recovery was observed in rat model of SCI wherein a co culture of Spinal cord-derived NSPCs and BMSCs were transplanted at the lesion site. Alternatively a reverse correlation was observed between the functional scores and number of astrocytes transplanted [25]. But the same group of cells when injected via LP shows potent oligodendrocyte marker [21].

Adipose tissue derived stem cells

In 2009, Hak-Hyun Ryu and his colleagues reported the use of adipose derived stem cells on a canine model of SCI using compression method. ADMSCs show better recovery by significant increase in nerve conduction, neuronal transdifferentiation and production of bFGF and VEGFR3 in large quantity. In yet another study [2] using rat as animal model of SCI, transplanted ADMSC and Mouse Neural Stem Cells (mNSCs) and observed that ADMSC protect mNSCs from apoptosis and increases the survival rates by secreting biomolecular substances, preferably VEGF in various conditions like hypoxia, oxidative stress and combined injury.

Human umbilical cord mesenchymal stem cells

In two trans-section and one contusion injury model of rats studied using Human umbilical cord mesenchymal stem cells had revealed that the grafted cells survived, migrated and produced large amount of GDNF, BDNF, NT-3, bFGF [9] glial cell line-derived neurotrophic factor, [13] neutrophil-activating protein-2, glucocorticoid induced TNF-receptor, and VEGFR 3 [16].

Glial precursor cells

Improved transcranial magnetic motor-evoked potential responses and improved electrophysiological and locomotor functional recovery was observed in rat contusion model of spinal trauma using Multi-neurotrophin-expressing glial-restricted precursor cells. The reason behind the functional recovery in restoring conduction was proposed to be formation of myelin sheath around the axons by the grafted cells [12].

Neural stem cells and Neural progenitor cells

Various animal injury models were studied for the transplantation of NSC/NPC. This include primates and rodents model. NSC in PLGA scaffold was tested in African Green Monkey using hemisection and Pritchard concluded the regulatory mechanism as the signaling by various factors released by NSCs [10]. In a contusion model of injury using marmoset, Iwanami et al [18] reported the differentiation of NSPCs into astrocytes and oligodendrocytes which promotes remyelination and promotes functional recovery. In another contusion injury model, the efficacy of EPI-NSC in restoring function was due to differentiation of grafted cells into Gaba-ergic neurons and myelinating oligodendrocytes resulting in neuroprotection, angiogenesis and scar modulation [18].

Expression of a therapeutic neurotrophin-3 gene, which leads to the recovery, was observed when PLGA coated with NSC was grafted in a canine hemisection model [20]. While others [25] observed no functional improvements in either groups transplanted with spinal cord-derived NSPCs and BMSCs on rats at the lesion site, Mothe et al observed recovery by injecting the cells via LP. Differentiation of SC derived NSPC into astrocytes and oligodendrocytes were observed by both the teams. Elevated amount of VEGF in the injured spinal cord tissue and increased phosphorylation of VEGFR flk-1 enhanced cellular proliferation and tissue sparing and increase in the density of blood vessels was the result reported by Kim et al using immortalized human NSC line over expressing VEGF (F3.VEGF cells) in a contusion model of injury in rats [15].

6.5. Clinical trials for SCI

Cell transplantation therapies have become a major focus in pre-clinical research as a promising strategy for the treatment of spinal cord injury. Various types of stem cells such as bone marrow stromal cells (BMSCs), adipose tissue Mesenchymal stem cells (ADMSCs), Schwann cells, olfactory ensheathing cells (OECs), neural stem cells or progenitor cells have been reported for their potential to form myelin, promote axonal regrowth and guidance, bridging the site of injury.

More than a dozen of clinical trials have been registered in the official website of clinical trials (http://www.clinicaltrials.gov). A brief listing of the selected trials is given below.

The results obtained are as follows:

S. No	NCT study number	Title/ Brief summary	Study type/ phase	Study status
1	NCT01325103	To evaluate autologous bone marrow stem cells transplantation as a safe and potentially beneficial treatment for patients with spinal cord injury	Interventional, Phase I	Active, not recruiting
2	NCT01490242	Phase I/II, multicenter, prospective, non-randomized, open label study to evaluate the safety/efficacy of autologous bone marrow-derived stem cell transplantation in spinal cord injury patients.	Interventional, Phase I / II	Recruiting
3	NCT01393977	To study the efficacy difference between Rehabilitation Therapy and Umbilical Cord Derived Mesenchymal Stem Cells transplantation	Interventional, Phase II	Recruiting
4	NCT01328860	1. To see if Bone Marrow Cell harvest and transplantation are safe in children and 2. To determine if late functional outcome is improved following Bone Marrow Cell transplantation.	Interventional, Phase I	Recruiting
5	NCT01446640	A phase I/II trial designed to establish the safety and efficacy of intravenous combined with intrathecal administration of autologous bone marrow derived mesenchymal stem cells	Interventional, Phase I / II	Recruiting
6	NCT01162915	A Phase I, single-center trial to assess the safety and tolerability of an intrathecal infusion (lumbar puncture) of autologous, ex vivo expanded bone marrow-derived mesenchymal stem cells	Interventional, Phase I	Active, not recruiting
7	NCT01321333	A Phase I/II Study of the Safety and Preliminary Efficacy of Intramedullary Spinal Cord Transplantation of Human Central Nervous System (CNS) Stem Cells	Interventional, Phase I / II	Recruiting

http://dx.doi.org/10.5772/58323

S. No	NCT study number	Title/ Brief summary	Study type/ phase	Study status
		(HuCNS-SC®) in Subjects With Thoracic (T2-T11) Spinal Cord Trauma		
8	NCT01186679	Surgical Transplantation of Autologous Bone Marrow Stem Cells With Glial Scar Resection for Patients of Chronic Spinal Cord Injury and Intra-thecal Injection for Acute and Subacute Injury	Interventional, Phase I / II	Completed
9	NCT01274975	To assess the safety of intravenous autologous adipose derived mesenchymal stem cells transplant in spinal cord injury patients.	Interventional, Phase I	Completed
10	NCT00816803	To assess the safety of autologous bone marrow derived cell transplant in chronic spinal cord injury patients.	Interventional, Phase I / II	Completed
11	NCT01217008	To evaluate the safety of GRNOPC1 administered at a single time-point between 7 and 14 days post spinal cord injury	Interventional, Phase I	Active, not recruiting
12	NCT01231893	Assessment of the safety and feasibility of transplantation of autologous olfactory ensheathing glia and olfactory fibroblasts obtained from the olfactory mucosa in patients with complete spinal cord injury.	Interventional, Phase I	Recruiting

In an article published, Wolfram Tetzlaff et al has reviewed in detail, all the types of cells being used in the treatment of spinal cord injury from the available pre-clinical literature. Their review shows that rodent stem cells have been most extensively studied for SCI. Limited studies have been done on human stem cells. Majority of trials are with bone marrow stromal cells. Also reported was, while chronic treatments were rare and often failed to yield functional benefits, all the preclinical studies conducted, was in acute and subacute stage [8].

Also Fehlings et al [9] in his recently reviewed article has shown the efficacies and limitations of every type of cells, either alone or in various combinations as registered for trial studies, in use and has demonstrated the potential use of other promising candidate stem cells evaluated in pre-clinical studies but are not yet in Clinical Trials. Also they have made recommendations for the conduct and evaluation of pre-clinical studies and clinical trials of cell therapies for SCI [9].

However no clinical intervention is risk free and we require understanding more on the pathophysiology of SCI and the clinical potential of stem cells to translate the use of the same as a therapeutic agent.

NPCs/OPCs:

Geron conducted a Phase 1 clinical trial in the United States in October 2010, to evaluate the safety of human embryonic stem cell-based product candidate, GRNOPC1, in patients with thoracic spinal cord injuries. Accordingly, GRNOPC1, an investigational product for treatment of Spinal Cord Injury, is a population of living cells containing oligodendrocyte progenitor cells (OPC).

HUMSCs:

WJCs can undergo repeated freeze–thaw cycles without a significant loss of viability, mesodermal differentiation potential, and without accumulating karyotypic abnormalities and thus represent a potential for the treatment of the neurodegenerative disorders including SCI. Two studies so far have examined the use of WJCs in SCI models, but were poorly conceived and designed.

6.6. Ongoing clinical trials for spinal cord injury using stem cells

Based on the encouraging preclinical animal results, Sarel et al, has conducted a phase II clinical trial of a cell therapy for patients with acute spinal cord injury using monocytes isolated from peripheral blood of human donors. They were able to stimulate by co-incubation with skin tissue, producing a distinct cellular phenotype which is said to be associated with wound healing. These features of skin-co incubated macrophages suggest possible mechanisms by which they may support an immune response that promotes neuronal cell survival and repair.

Jones *et al.*, 2004 [105] observed the long-term outcomes after complete spinal cord injury followed by subsequent treatment with a therapy consisting of autologous incubated macrophages that have been pre-incubated with autologous skin and injected into the lesion site. The study so far has been conducted on 14 patients. Recovery of clinically significant neurological function has been observed in several subjects after treatment, whereas untreated patients with complete SCI rarely recover significant function.

Auerbach *et al.*, 2004 [106], has conducted open-label, non-randomized trials to assess the safety of autologous macrophages in 16 patients with acute complete spinal cord injury. The macrophages were prepared from monocytes isolated from patient blood and co-incubated with autologous skin tissue. The cells were then injected into the spinal cord parenchyma within 14 days of injury. The study shows that administration of autologous macrophages has a favorable benefit to risk ratio for the treatment of patients with acute, complete spinal cord injury.

Keirstead *et al.*, 2005 [107] have shown human embryonic stem cells differentiate into oligodendrocytes in high purity and showed regeneration of the spinal cord in rat. On the basis of this study Geron Inc is currently conducting a FDA approved phase-I clinical trial.

Moviglia *et al.*, 2006, [108] demonstrated a case report of two patients who were administered BM-MSCs co cultured with an autologous pure population of T cells, intravenously 48 hours prior to transplantation of trans-differentiated NCS. This was followed up with 6 months of neuro-rehabilitation. The authors conclude that *in vitro* cultures of MSCs and anti CNS T cells can induce transdifferentiation of MSCs into neural stem cells.

Kang *et al.*, 2005 [109] transplanted human umbilical cord cells into a 37 year old female with T11/T12 complete injury and have observed recovery but have not ruled out the fact that the laminectomy itself may have released compressed areas of the spinal cord and brought about recovery.

Zhou *et al.*, 2004 differentiated BM-MSCs into neural stem cells and transplanted them into SCI patients. 3 patients reported adverse events of intracranial infection requirement treatment. This study has not mentioned the baseline status of the patients, neither the details of the follow-up study conducted nor the details of the intervention.

Deda *et al.*, 2009 [110], reported that autologous hematopoietic progenitor stem cells are an effective and safe method for treatment of chronic SCI. In this study autologous hematopoietic progenitor stem cells were injected at the site of injury and three weeks post transplantation the patients have demonstrated improved sensory and motor functions.

7. Our experience

Realizing the unmet medical need in producing reasonable clinical recovery in spinal cord injury we have designed a preclinical experimental animal study. We developed a rodent model of spinal cord contusion injury and transplanted bone marrow derieved mesenchymal stem cells both at the site of injury and into the CSF using lumbar puncture technique. The results were very encouraging [111]. Motivated by this an initial pilot study was conducted on 10 patients with chronic spinal cord injury. The initial results showed only partial sensory improvement. Only 2 patients showed minimal motor improvement but not clinically useful. Surprisingly 4 of them showed reasonable improvement in bladder function. This fact has triggered further interest in us to pursue this and try different methods to improvise the clinical results. Though an attempt was made to quantify the recovery, none of the existing methods were satisfactory.

But this study has raised several questions like a)Timing of intervention) Route of cell administration c)Dosage of cells D)Type of cell e) Number and interval of doses f)Autologous vs allogenic MSC g) problems of chronic injury h)Method of monitoring, evaluation and quantifying the results.

In our further study we attempted to address some of these questions: 1) route-Intrathecal, direct at the site of injury, Direct delivery into the cord during surgery 2) excision of scar 3) scaffold to bridge the damaged ends of the cord 4) number of injections 5) number of cells 6) Cell type – mesenchymal autologous, allogenic & mononuclear 7) source-bone marrow,adipose and Wharton jelly 8) additional systemic injections. 100 volunteers with clinically complete cord injury were recruited. Clinical, MRI and tractography were done at baseline and at periodic intervals to monitor the course of events post stem cell infusion.

8. Study plan

The objective of this study was to demonstrate the safety and feasibility of various stem cells as a possible therapeutic strategy for Spinal cord injury. For this, 52 volunteers were recruited and grouped into 4, on the basis of stem cells they received for the treatment. Group 1 received autologous bone marrow derived mononuclear cells (BMMNCs) for transplantation, group 2 were infused with autologous bone marrow derived Mesenchymal stem cells (BMMSCs), while group 3 were transplanted with different allogeneic stem cells (subgroup 1: Bone Marrow derived Mesenchymal cells, subgroup 2: Wharton's Jelly derived Mesenchymal stem cells (WJMSCs) and subgroup 3: Adipose Tissue derived Mesenchymal cells (ADMSCs). Also, in this study, we demonstrated, delivery of stem cells via 3 different routes (laminectomy, lumbar puncture, site of injury guided by CT scan and intravenous delivery) were safe and feasible and do not cause any infections and adverse reactions post transplantation.

a. Regulatory approval, Informed consent:

As per national guidelines, approval from institutional ethics committee (IEC) was taken and informed consent was obtained from every patient who participated in the study. Any deviations, drop-outs and adverse events were documented and the IEC informed.

b. Patient selection:

Patients were enrolled for this study as per the inclusion and exclusion criteria designed by and adapted in a pilot clinical study [1]. The inclusion Criteria in the study was as follows

i. the patients could be of either sex,

ii. must be between the ages 18 and 55 years,

iii. the level of spinal injury between C4 and T10 level (neurologic),

iv. (SCI was clinically complete and categorized as per the American Spinal Injury Association (ASIA) impairment scale.

Exclusion criteria for the study was

i. Difficulty in assessing the size and location of the injury multiple sites of injury,

ii. gun shot or penetrating injuries,

iii. serious pre-existing medical conditions, disease or impairment that precluded adequate neurologic examination

iv. Respiratory insufficiency requiring support.

v. if he/she is enrolled in any other clinical trial

vi. Not able to understand and comply with follow up

vii. Diagnosed with infections like HIV, HCV,CMV and VDRL.

viii. Fixed deformities.

c. Screening of the patients:

Before enrollment each patient was screened for HIV: Human Immunodeficiency Virus; HBV: Hepatitis B Virus; HCV: Hepatitis C Virus; CMV: Cytomegalovirus; and VDRL: Venereal Disease Research Laboratory, by a nationally certified testing laboratory.

d. Isolation and propagation of stem cells:

i. Autologous Bone Marrow derived Mesenchymal Stem Cells:

Patients willing to undergo autologous cell transplantation were screened 7 days before the aspiration for infectious disease mentioned above. Thereafter, BM-derived MSC were isolated and expanded using a method reported previously [1].

Briefly, 60 ml BM was aspirated aseptically from the iliac crest of each patient under aseptic conditions. The BM was diluted (1:1) with Knockout Dulbecco's modified Eagle's medium (KO-DMEM) and centrifuged at 1800 r.p.m. for 10 min to remove anticoagulants. The supernatant was discarded and the BM washed once with culture medium. Mononuclear cells (MNC) were isolated by layering onto a lymphoprep (Axis Shield, Norway) density gradient. The MNC present in the buffy coat were washed again with culture medium. The mononuclear fractions containing MSC were plated at a density of 1000 cells/cm2 onto T-75cm2 flasks and cultured in KO-DMEM. The media were supplemented with 10% fetal bovine serum (FBS), 200 mM Glutamax and Pen-Strep. The cultures were maintained at 370C in a humidified 5% CO2 atmosphere for 2 days. The non-adherent cells were removed after 48 h of culture and replenished with fresh medium. Subsequently, the medium was replenished every 5th day until the required number of cells obtained. Once confluent, the culture flasks were washed with Dulbecco`s Phosphate Buffered Saline (DPBS) and harvested using 0.25% Trypsin-EDTA solution and re-plated in 5 cell stacks (Corning, USA) for further expansion till the required number of cells obtained. On the day of transplantation the cells were harvested and suspended in saline solution, packed in sterile container and given for the transplantation procedure.

ii. Autologous Bone Marrow derived Mononuclear cells (MNCs):

All the patients were examined by a designated medically qualified staff member to establish their eligibility for bone marrow aspiration. Briefly, 60 ml BM was aspirated aseptically from the iliac crest of each patient under aseptic conditions. The BM was diluted (1:1) with Knockout Dulbecco's modified Eagle's medium (KO-DMEM) and centrifuged at 1800 r.p.m. for 10 min to remove anticoagulants. The supernatant was discarded and the BM washed once with culture medium. Mononuclear cells (MNC) were isolated by layering the bone marrow samples onto a lymphoprep (Axis Shield, Norway) density gradient. The MNC present in the buffy coat were washed again with culture medium and then with saline for 2-3 times, resuspended in the same and given for infusion.

9. Scaffolds

Scaffolds are basically structures to support and connect the cut ends of spinal cord. They are used after scar excision or otherwise in chronic injuries to bridge the healthy ends. The stem cells are deposited over the membrane. It helps to hold the cells in place, and grows along using this as support.We have used Gelfoam as well as a special biological membrane, which is inert and biocompatible made out of Chitosin. It is a thin and transparent glucosamine polymer. Stem cells have grown in sheets over this membrane in our invitro studies.

In acute phase, the chemical changes resulted out of injury presumably attracts stem cells even after remote injection whereas in chronic injuries there are additional problems.

1. Scar intervenes ends of normal cords 2.In severe injuries there is thinning and atrophy causing anatomical discontinuity. 3. Due to ongoing degeneration there is a functional void between the two ends, with or without an abnormal cord intervening. The main purpose of scaffolds is to bridge this gap and create continuity for the cells to reach both ends.

10. Screening of potential donors for bone marrow aspiration

Potential voluntary donors were interviewed, counseled and examined by the investigator or a designated medically qualified staff member to establish their eligibility for bone marrow aspiration. Donors were informed with full description about the nature and purpose of the aspiration and written consent were obtained from them before proceeding with study. Some of the inclusion criteria include (i) the donor must be healthy (ii) may be of either sex (iii) must be between 18-30 years of age (iv) able to understand the voluntary donation program, and ready to provide voluntary written informed consent. The donors were excluded if (i) diagnosed with a past history of illness such as autoimmune disorders, tuberculosis, malaria and any other infection, any illness which precludes the use of general anesthesia, history of malignancy, diabetes, hypertension, significant heart disease, genetic or chromosomal disorders, history of any inherited disorders, hemoglobin less than 10, and pregnant women. Also, at the time of obtaining informed consent they were screened for infection with human immunodeficiency virus (HIV), hepatitis B (HBV), hepatitis C (HCV), cytomegalovirus (CMV), and syphilis (VDRL) and excluded, if found positive.

11. Allogeneic BM-MSCs

As per the donor selection criteria, donors were recruited and bone marrow samples were aspirated from the iliac crest of the donors and further processed for the isolation of mononuclear fraction using Lymphoprep (Axis Shield, Norway) density gradient. Thus obtained fraction was seeded in T-75cm^2 and cultured at 37°C in 5% CO_2 atmosphere. The non-adherent cells were removed after 48 hours by replacing the medium and the adherent cells were grown for additional 4 or 5 days till it reached 80-85% confluency. On confluency, confluence, adherent cells were detached by treatment with a Trypsin-EDTA solution and re-plated at a density of 1000 cells/cm² in 5 cell stacks and cultured in the same condition for 14-16. The cell stacks were checked regularly and replenished with medium on every 5th day. The cells were then harvested at 80-90% confluency and cryopreserved in 10% Dimethyl Sulfoxide (DMSO, Sigma-Aldrich) and 85% Plasmalyte (Baxter, USA) and 5% Human Serum Albumin (HSA, Baxter) in liquid nitrogen till further use.

12. Adipose tissue derived mesenchymal stem cells

The use of lipoaspirate as a source for stem cells with multipotent differentiation potential offers a far less invasive procedure for cell sampling than the aspiration of bone marrow (BM), and numbers of stem cells obtained are reportedly higher in lipoaspirate than its BM counterpart. Lipoaspirate, an otherwise disposable byproduct of cosmetic surgery, has been shown to contain a putative population of stem cells, termed adipose-derived stem cells (ADSCs) that share many similarities to marrow stromal cells (MSCs) from BM, including multilineage differentiation capacity. Furthermore, these cells also show high colony-forming unit frequencies as well as an apparent pluripotent ability to differentiate to cells of a neuronal phenotype [9, 10].

This protocol describes the preparation of MSCs from human lipoaspirate obtained from cosmetic surgery. Briefly, the liposuctioned fat first washed thoroughly in phosphate-buffered saline (PBS) with antibiotic solution (Penstrep, 2X), until the bottom layer containing blood cells contaminant was clear, before being subjected to enzymatic digestion using collagenase type I (0.2%, diluted in KO-DMEM) for 45-60 minutes at 37°C in shaking condition, in order to obtain a soupy single-cell suspension. After digestion, the action of collagenase was neutralized by the addition of FBS. The suspension was then mixed well and passed through 40 µm cell strainer before being subjected to centrifugation at 1400 rpm for 10 minutes. After centrifugation, cell pellet, termed as stromal vascular fraction (SVF) is resuspended in KO-DMEM and seeded in a T-75cm² flask at a density of 1,000 cells/cm². The non-adherent cells were removed after 48 h of culture and replenished with fresh medium. Subsequently, the medium was replenished every 4th day and the cells were harvested at 80% confluency and replated in 5 cell stacks to obtain the sufficient number of cells required for the infusion. The plates were checked for confluence every day and the cells are fed with fresh medium. After the cell stacks were confluent enough, the cells were harvested using Trypsin-EDTA solution and cryopreserved in liquid nitrogen till further use.

13. Wharton's Jelly derived mesenchymal stem cells

Studies have demonstrated the multipotent properties of mesenchymal stromal cells isolated from the inner matrix of the Wharton's Jelly derived from the umbilical cord. These cells have also been demonstrated to differentiate into neuronal lineage and supporting glia [11, 12]. Based on these studies, in the current trial we have attempted to understand the therapeutic potential of WJ-MSCs in spinal cord injury.

After appropriate informed consent, a clean, healthy, straight clamped umbilical cord approximately 10 cms in length was collected in sterile normal saline bottle and transported to the laboratory. Briefly, the umbilical cord was washed with normal saline followed by DPBS (with 0.2% of Penstrep solution) wash for 3-4 times. This was followed by quick dip in 100% ethanol and was cleared off in DPBS. The tissue was washed free of contaminating blood with normal saline throughout the process and cut into 2-5 mm^3 pieces. Using sterile scalpel and forceps the cord was dissected, unfolded and the exposed arteries and vein were removed and discarded. The cord was then scrapped gently with scalpel to obtain the viscous, jelly like substance. The obtained suspension was passed through a 100 mm cell strainer to obtain single-cell suspension. The resultant suspension was then diluted with saline to reduce the viscosity of the suspension. Cells were centrifuged at 1400 rpm for 10 minutes at 37°C and the pellet was resuspended in KO-DMEM supplemented with FBS (10%), Glutamax (1%) , Penstrep (0.5%), FGF-2 (1ng/ml) and cultured in T-75cm^2 flasks at 370 C in 5% CO_2 until confluent (80-85%). Upon confluency, the cells were harvested from the flasks and transferred to 5 cell stacks at a seeding density of 1000 cells/cm^2 for 10-12 days in order to obtain the required number of cells for the transplantation. The harvested cells were processed and frozen in cryobags in liquid nitrogen till use.

14. Characterization

1. Immunophenotype:

This is a technique used to study the expression of cell surface antigens on the MSCs using flow cytometry. Briefly, the cells were dissociated with 0.25% Trypsin-EDTA and resuspended in wash buffer at a concentration of 1 × 10^6 cells/ml. 200 μL cell suspensions were incubated in the dark for 15 min at 4°C with saturating concentrations of phycoerythrin (PE) conjugated antibodies. The following markers were analyzed: CD34-PE, CD45-PE, CD73-PE, CD105-PE, CD166-PE, and CD90-PE (BD Pharmingen, San Diego, CA, USA). Flow cytometry was performed on a 5HT Guava instrument. Appropriate isotype-matched controls were used to set the instrument parameters. Cell viability was measured using 7-amino actinomycin D (7-AAD). Cells were identified by light scatter for 10,000 gated events and analyzed.

2. Multipotent differentiation assay

The mesenchymal properties of human stem cells isolated from various sources as described above, were investigated using specific differentiation kits for the three different lineages i.e., osteogenic, adipogenic and chondrogenic (as per ISCT criteria).

Briefly, *Osteoblast differentiation* was induced by culturing human MSCs in KO-DMEM supplemented with 10% FBS (Hyclone), 200 26mM Glutamax (Invitrogen), 10^{-8} M dexa methasone (Sigma-Aldrich), 30 μgm/ml ascorbic acid (Sigma-Aldrich) and 10 mM β-glycerophosphate (Sigma-Aldrich Chemical Private Limited, Bangalore, Karnataka, India) for 3 weeks. Fresh medium was replenished every 3 days. Calcium accumulation was assessed by von Kossa staining. The differentiated cells were washed with PBS and fixed with 10% formalin for 30 min. The fixed cells were incubated with 5% $AgNO_3$ for 60 min under ultraviolet (UV) light and then treated with 2.5% sodium thiosulphate for 5 min. Images were captured using an Nikon Eclipse 90i microscope (Nikon Corporation, Towa Optics, New Delhi, India; www.nikon.com) and Image-Pro Express soft ware (Media Cybernetics Inc., Silver Spring, MD, USA; www. mediacy.com).

To induce *adipogenic differentiation*, human MSCs were cultured for 21 days in KO-DMEM supplemented with 10% FBS, 200 mM Glutamax, 1 μm dexamethasone, 0.5 mM isobutylmethylxanthine, 1 μg/ml insulin and 100 μm indomethacin (from Sigma-Aldrich). Inducing factors were fixed in 10% formalin for 20 min and 200 μl Oil Red O staining solution added and incubated for 10 min at room temperature. The cells were rinsed five times with distilled water. The images were captured using Nikon Eclipse 90i microscope (Nikon) and Image-Pro Express software (Media Cybernetics).

For *chondrogenic differentiation*, human MSCs were cultured for 21 days using Chondrogenesis differentiation kit (Life Technologies, USA) as per the manufacturer's recommendations and stained with Safranin O as specified. The images were captured using Nikon Eclipse 90i microscope (Nikon Corporation, Towa Optics, New Delhi, India).

14.1. Karyotyping

A standard G-banding protocol was performed by analyzing more than 200 cells per sample and reported according to the International System for Human Cytogenetic Nomenclature (ISCN). If the cells did not fall under the set standard of the above mentioned tests, they would not be released to the patient for transplantation was discarded appropriately.

14.2. Quality control testing

Based on the ISCT guidelines, certain quality control tests were performed on the end product before transplantation. These include Mycoplasma (using RT-PCR based method), Endotoxin testing by Limulus Amebocyte Lysate (LAL) method and cell surface markers like CD73, CD90, CD105, CD166, CD34, and CD45 via flow cytometry. The positive markers (CD73, CD90, CD105 and CD166) should be greater than 95% positive, while the negative markers (CD34 and CD45) must be less than 2% positive. 7-AAD (7-amino actinomycin D) was also analyzed via flow cytometry to determine the cell viability.

14.3. Processing of cells for transplantation

As described above, the cells were harvested and processed for transplantation. Briefly, the total cell count was calculated using a standard hemocytometer. The cells were washed several times with normal saline solution and finally resuspended in saline containing 0.2% human serum albumin. All the syringes and bottles were appropriately labeled. These were packaged in a sterile container and dispatched in a transportation container maintained at 22°C to the hospital for transplantation via the shortest route.

14.4. Route of administration

1. Intrathecal administration through Lumbar Puncture (LP) method:. The pateinet was positioned in lateral decubitous position and the part prepared. Under aseptic conditions lumbar puncture was performed at lowest possible level usually L4-5 or L5-S1 levels. Once clear CSF was obtained the cells were delivered into the intra thecal space gently. The procedure was repeated as per the protocol.

2. Intra Venous – Regular intravenous infusion of cells in 50 ml saline administered into the peripheral veins of the hand.

3. At the site of injury-either by laminectomy or image guidance

Laminectomy-was performed where ever decompression was indicated with or without stabilization. Surgical technique includes prone position and exposure of lamina at appropriate level under general anesthesia. Dura was opened and injured cord was inspected.

Scar excision-In chronic injuries with glial scar or neuroma the intervening tissue was removed gently till healthy appearing tissue was seen under high magnification. Cavity was decompressed. The cells were injected into the ends of the cord tissue through an insulin syringe. If the edges are apart a scaffold or gelfoam was used to bridge the gap. Dura was closed water tight. If the cord was oedematous (acute injury) doroplasty was performed. Additional cells were delivered into intra thecal space and Laminectomy was closed using standard technique.

Image guidance method-In chronic complete injuries CT guided technique was used to deliver the cells directly at the site of injury.

Clinical assessment was performed on all patients based on the parameters of the ASIA impairment scale (American Spinal Injury Association). This was considered as the primary measurable outcome of the clinical study.

A	Complete: No motor or sensory function is preserved in the sacral segments S4-S5.
B	Incomplete: Sensory but not motor function is preserved below the neurological level and Includes the sacral segments S4-S5.
C	Incomplete: Motor function is preserved below the neurological level, and more than half of key muscles below the neurological level have a muscle grade less than 3.
D	Incomplete: Motor function is preserved below the neurological level, and at least half of key muscles below the neurological level have a muscle grade of 3 or more.
E	Normal: Motor and sensory functions are normal.

Table 3. ASIA impairment scale

http://dx.doi.org/10.5772/58323

14.5. Follow up schedule

At every follow-up, the patients were assessed clinically using the ASIA scale rating system and with the Barthel's index (BI) for degree of independence and patient rating. MRI was performed to observe structural changes, if any.

15. Isolation and identification of mononuclear cells and mesenchymal stem cells

15.1. Autologous BM derived MNCs

BM samples were aspirated from the patients (n=9) after getting proper consent and the samples were processed in cGMP compliant clean room facility for the isolation of the MNCs following the standardized protocol as described above. CD34 expression was analyzed using PE conjugated CD34 antibody in flow cytometer and cell count was performed prior to transplantation.

15.2. Autologous bone marrow derived MSCs

BM samples obtained from the patients (n=11) after getting proper consent were processed in cGMP compliant clean room facility for the isolation propagation and expansion following the standardized protocol as described above. Flow cytometry analysis revealed that cell samples with positive markers are >95% and <2% of negative markers with >90% viability with 7AAD staining indicating the cells were mesenchymal in nature. Multipotent characteristics, as determined by Oil Red O stain, Von Kossa stain and Safranin O stain, respectively indicates the cell samples undergo adipogenic, osteogenic and chondrogenic differentiation. Karyotypes of all the cell samples were normal and no abnormalities/aberrations were found after ex vivo propagation figure. Endotoxin test using LAL method and Mycoplasma test using RT-PCR were found to be negative indicating the cells were safe for transplantation.

15.3. Allogenic BM derived MSCs

BM samples obtained from the donors after appropriate informed consent and the samples were processed in cGMP compliant clean room facility for the isolation, propagation and expansion. Stem cells thus extracted are cryopreserved as master cell bank (MCB) in liquid nitrogen. From MCB, working cell banks (WCB) were raised in tissue culture plates until required number of cells obtained for the infusion. The cells were then harvested and frozen as investigational product (IP) until use. Prior to transplantation the cells were thawed and processed further. The cell samples were found to express positive markers >95% and <2% for negative markers, with >95% viability, when stained with 7AAD as determined by flow cytometry indicating the Mesenchymal nature of the processed cells. Multipotent characteristics, as determined by Oil Red O stain, Von Kossa stain and Safranin O stain, respectively, indicating the cell samples undergo adipogenic, osteogenic and chondrogenic differentiation. Karyotype of all the cell samples was normal and no abnormalities/aberrations were found after ex vivo propagation figure. End product testing such as endotoxin test using LAL method and Mycoplasma test using RT-PCR were found to be negative indicating the cells were safe.

15.4. Adipose tissue derived MSCs

Mesenchymal stem cells isolated from fat samples received in a sterile container after liposuction were expanded in above mentioned conditions until the cells were confluent. Post confluent, the cells were harvested and stored frozen in liquid nitrogen as MCB, from which WCB were raised. IP were cultured on appropriate tissue culture plates on request. Prior to transplantation, in process test and end process test were done. Flow cytometric analysis showed that the cells express the surface markers with >95% for positive markers (fig) and <2% for negative markers (fig) with >90%% viabilty. The cells were found to undergo adipogenic, osteogenic and chondrogenic differentiation as determined by Oil Red O stain, Von Kossa stain and Safranin O stain, respectively. All the samples showed normal karyotypes and no abnormalities/aberrations were noted after ex vivo propagation. A representative ideogram is illustrated in Figure. The cell samples tested for endotoxin using LAL method and Mycoplasma test using RT-PCR were found to be negative indicating the cells were safe to be infused.

15.5. Wharton's Jelly derived MSCs

Umbilical cords obtained postpartum in a sterile container were processed according to the standard protocol described earlier. The cells were further up-scaled and expanded in order to provide the required number of cells for the patient. The cultured cells were found to show normal spindle shaped phenotype when observed (fig). Flow cytometric analysis showed that the cells were positive with >95% for positive markers and <2% for negative markers (fig) with >90% viability. The cells were found to undergo adipogenic, osteogenic and chondrogenic differentiation as determined by Oil Red O stain, Von Kossa stain and Safranin O stain, respectively. All the samples showed normal karyotypes and no abnormalities/aberrations were noted after ex vivo propagation by standard G banding method. A representative ideogram is illustrated in Figure. The cell samples tested for endotoxin using LAL method and Mycoplasma test using RT-PCR were found to be negative indicating the cells were safe for the transplantation.

16. Clinical assessment

16.1. Clinical examination and ASIA scale scoring

Clinical assessment was performed on all patients based on the parameters of the ASIA impairment scale. This was considered as the primary measurable outcome of the clinical study.

http://dx.doi.org/10.5772/58323

16.2. Results

As per the inclusion and exclusion criteria mentioned above, 52 volunteers were recruited for this study. This includes 8 females and 44 males between the age group 17 and 66 years. Duration of injury varied between 15 days after injury to 20 years. All the patients were divided into 4 groups based on the type of cells received. The details of the patients recruited for this study are given in Tables below.

Case No.	Age	Sex	Level of injury	Duration of injury	No. of injection	Route of infusion
1	23	M	D11-D12	0 month	1	Laminectomy + IV
2	31	M	D4, C6-7	7 months	1	Laminectomy + IV
3	23	M	D11	4 months	1	Laminectomy + IV
4	26	F	C5-C6	1 year	1	Laminectomy + IV
5	21	M	C4-C5	1 year	1	Laminectomy + IV
6	26	F	C5-C6	1 year	1	Laminectomy + IV
7	53	M	C6-C7	3 years	1	Laminectomy + IV
8	23	M	C5-C6	3 years	1	Laminectomy + IV
9	31	M	C6-C7	4 years	1	Laminectomy + IV

Table 4. Group 1-Autologous Bone Marrow derived mononuclear cells (BMMNCs; n=9).

Case No.	Age	Sex	Level of injury	Duration of injury	No. of injection	Route of infusion
1	59	F	D3-D5	7 years	1	CT Guided
2	34	M	C7	6 years	1	CT Guided
3	56	M	D4	14 years	1	CT Guided
4	54	M	D5-D6	2 years	1	CT Guided
5	49	M	D6	4 years	1	CT Guided
6	26	M	D12	2 years	1	CT Guided
7	23	M	C4-C6	1 years	1	CT Guided
8	31	M	L1	4 years	1	CT Guided
9	42	M	D12	3 years	1	CT Guided
10	28	M	C5-C6	3 years	1	CT Guided
11	28	M	D5-D6	5 years	1	CT Guided

Table 5. Group 2-Autologous Bone Marrow derived Mesenchymal stem cells (BMMSCs; n=11)

Table 6: Group 3-Allogeneic BMMSCs or Adipose tissue derived MSCs (ADMSCs) or Wharton's jelly derived MSCs (WJMSCs) (n=26)

Case No.	**Age**	**Sex**	**Level of injury**	**Duration of injury**	**No. of injection**	**Route of infusion**
1	19	F	D4-D6	1 year	1	CT Guided
2	36	F	D10	1 month	3	Intrathecal
3	27	M	T12-L1	1 year	1	CT Guided
4	36	M	C6-C7	2 months	1	Laminectomy + IV
5	26	M	D3	3 months	1	Laminectomy + IV
6	46	M	C3-C4	0 month	1	Laminectomy + IV
7	29	M	Partial	1 year	3	Intrathecal
8	45	M	C1-L1	1 year	1	Laminectomy + IV
9	50	F	C2	1 year	1	Laminectomy + IV
10	46	F	Dorsal SCI	1 year	3	Intrathecal
11	25	M	D9-D10	1 year	3	Intrathecal
12	29	F	D4	1 year	3	Intrathecal
13	27	M	SCI	10 months	1	Laminectomy + IV
14	26	M	C7-T1	3 years	3	Intrathecal
15	27	M	Cervical	6 months	3	Intrathecal
16	51	M	D4-D6	20 years	3	Intrathecal

(a)

Case No.	Age	Sex	Level of injury	Duration of injury	No. of injection	Route Of infusion
1	23	M	Cervical	2 years	3	Intrathecal
2	54	M	Thoracic	1 year	3	Intrathecal
3	54	M	C4-C5	6 months	3	Intrathecal
4	31	M	C2-D4	1 year	3	Intrathecal

(b)

Case No.	Age	Sex	Level of injury	Duration of injury	No. of injection	Route Of infusion
1	47	M	Cervical	8 months	3	Intrathecal
2	37	M	D12	4 years	3	Intrathecal
3	42	M	Thoracic		3	Intrathecal
4	35	M	C3-C4	0 month	3	Intrathecal
5	27	M	C5-C6	6 years	3	Intrathecal
6	37	M	Thoracic	13 years	3	Intrathecal

(c)

Table 6. (a): Subgroup 1: BMMSCs, (b): Subgroup 2: WJMSCs, (c): Sub group 3: ADMSCs

On an average, 2 million cells /kg bodyweight were transplanted via 3 different routes i.e., laminectomy, lumbar puncture, and intravenous injections. All the patients stood the procedure well, there were no postoperative complications and were discharged within a week's time from the hospital, indicating that there were no immediate cytotoxic effects due to implantation of various cell types (as mentioned above) and the procedures were safe.

The ASIA rating scale did not reveal any significant changes or further worsening or deterioration in neurological or functional level pre and post stem cells therapy.

Of the total patient recruited for the study, 9 patients have shown notable clinical and functional recovery. While follow-up, one patient (G3C2; Table 4a) whose baseline report was as follows: Motor – Upper limb-5/5, Lower limb-2/5, Sensory – Loss of sensation at D 10 and below for all modalities, reported to be able to stand and walk with support and does swimming.

Another patient (G4C3; Table 5], at baseline with power at shoulder-grade 3/5, Power at elbow joint-3/5 in flexion and extension and hand grip-2/5, lower limbs-grade 0/5 with generalized wasting in all limbs and spasticity in both the lower limbs, anesthesia below C6 dermatomes and exaggerated deep tendon reflexes in lower limbs, has shown minimal recovery.

Slight improvement in Upper Limb sensation after the first dose, was reported by one patient (G1C5; Table 2). However at times, the patient had painful sensations.

Post therapy one patient (G4C4; Table 5) was able to feel the bladder fullness from 3rd month of transplantation. In subsequent follow-up, the imbalance while sitting on the wheel chair has partially improved. Also, improvement in touch and pain sensation up-to the right knee on the right side and up to the upper thigh in the left side were noted. Bladder sensations have improved to some extent.

Additionally two patients (G4C5; Table 5 and G3C4; Table 4c) has shown improvement in sensation and able to sit with support.

Two patients (G3C1 and G3C3; Table 4c &4b) were able to walk with the aid of walker post therapy. But however, the latter patient had a fall and is now back to baseline.

One patient (G3C5; Table 4c) has regained some sensation in abdomen and lower back area and below feet. The patient can now feel stretching sensation in toes when performing exercises and becoming more aware of bowel movements.

Out of the 52 patients treated, only 3 patients reported pain after infusion. And two patients were lost to follow-up.

Barthel's Index Score

Barthel's index (BI) was performed on all patients, pre-and post-transplantation of the cells. No significant improvement or appreciable changes were observed in the patients with long history of injury. However, patients with less than 6 months of injury have shown improvement in the scores.

Magnetic resonance imaging (MRI) of the spinal cord before and after stem cell infusion:

No change was observed in MRI findings at baseline and post-stem cell transplantation. Also, no adverse effects of transplantation were detected on the MRI post transplantation. Further, no changes in cystic regions or syringomyelia, and no further external compression of the cord or formation of tumor-like masses in and around the injection site or along the cord, were visualized.

17. Discussion

Spinal cord essentially is a conduit integrating relay and transmission of signals and the functions of the body (motor, sensory and autonomic) with the higher centers (brain brainstem & cerebellum). SCI can be devastating with lifelong disability due to its complex architecture and compounding consequences that follows an injury. Disruption of such local integrative networks interrupts ascending and descending input and outputs resulting in dysfunction of motor, sensory, autonomic and dysregulation of various reflexes in the body. Majority are in the age range of 16-35. Damage to the spinal cord progresses rapidly in stages. In the last two decades, researchers have made their efforts to understand this complex pathobiology from several animal studies [6]. Ischemia,Scarring, cavitation, wallarian degeneration, axonal die back, excitotoxins, inflammation and several complex cellular and molecular changes are known to influence recovery of such injury. Several medical (pharmacological and others) and surgical attempts did not influence any substantial positive outcomes. Hence the attention was turned towards neurotrophic factors and cell based treatments. As a result spontaneous neurological recovery has been reported only in 6-13% of patients with only 2% gaining any functional recovery. [113-116].

Cell death is often rapid after SCI. The adult spinal cord harbors endogenous stem/progenitor cells, collectively referred to as Neural Progenitor Cells (NPCs) that might be responsible for normal turnover of the cells and repair process. Several studies have confirmed that new cells are born around the central canal from the ependymal precursors [1].However, the proliferative activity of endogenous NPCs is too limited and grossly inadequate to support spontaneous repair after SCI. Hence various cell transplantation strategies have been adopted in models of SCI such as embryonic stem cells, Wharton's jelly, adult neural stem cells, bone marrow and adipose tissue derived Mesenchymal stem cells [13]. They are currently being studied as potential sources of neurons, glial cells or neurotrophic factors. Transplantation of these cells to create or regenerate spinal cord as an alternative therapy has generated lot of interest. This study clearly documents the feasibility of such cell replacement strategies [14].

Several studies have reported several protocols different timings and type of cells [117-120]. We have studied autologous BMMNCs, BMMSCs (autologous and allogenic), WJMSCs and ADMSCs (allogenic) have been used to study their therapeutic potential in spinal cord injury. Those who received autologous BMMNCs showed only minimal improvement. The reason may be due to variations in age; extent, duration of injury; and variance in cell quantity and quality.

Nevertheless, autologous BMMSCs had shown good improvement, the concern with the transplantation is the availability of cells in time and other problems as mentioned above.

Recently, allogenic MSCs from sources like Bone marrow, Adipose tissue and Wharton's jelly shown to have attracted many, to use it as source for treatment and conducting trials on them.

The advantages of allogenic cells over autologous cells for transplantation may be that, they are readily available with defined cell quality and quantity. This makes allogenic stem cells, a good choice to make extensive research on the feasibility in other therapeutic interventions. In addition it offers an opportunity to use the cells as early as possible. It has been the observation that early intervention within few days has yielded marginally better results suggesting an optimal temporal window for cell mediated therapy. [121]. several studies have indicated better results with early intervention and acute injury. [122, 123, 121]. The preclinical literature also has suggested that there is an earlier window for the optimization of cell therapies [125, 124]. Now its well known that these cells do HOME at the required site. Homing could be mediated by the ongoing cell reactions, products of cell death or inflammation or some chemo attractants. We believe timing of delivery of cells is crucial for these cells to impregnate in large numbers.In delayed or chronic injuries cell reach may be poor and once gliosis sets in cell penetration may be difficult. In addition spinalcord –csf barrier doesn't allow cell migration into the parenchyma.

The strategy to cord injury is twofold-Initial control of damage and minimizing secondary deleterious effects, and later promotion of recovery. Cell therapy can play a role in both provided they were given at the right time.. However there is no sufficient data to indicate the exact time of maximizing the benefit. In general those who are likely to be benefited must be treated before the molecular mechanisms cause the irreparable damage. [5] The drawback of our study is timing could not be controlled since they were inducted as and when they came to our clinical service. In addition its difficult to have clinical controls.

A canine study from South Korea 2009 used autologous and allogenic cells. Though autologous BM-MSCs had better results than allogenic both showed better results compared to controls [126]

Literature shows several routes of administration like intra arterial, intravenous, intra thecal and direct injections to the injured cord. Intra thecal injection was most frequently used method. [121]. Our study also demonstrates that administration of MSCs via multiple routes such as laminectomy, lumbar puncture and intravenous delivery, are feasible and safe. Though direct injection into the cord appears logical,the apprehension of enhancing the injury always exists. In our opinion it is invasive and should be reserved for those where decompression or stabilization is indicated and most suitable in chronic complete inuries.. Saberi et al [119] reported no serious adverse effect after intraparenchymal injections. They also reported transient low grade fever with nausea, vomiting and headache. But we did not encounter such complications in our series. The use of scaffold is complimentary and may have positive influence. [110]. In chronic injuries widening of anatomical gap between the functional tissues of the cord is a challenge and a possible reason for poor outcomes. Degeneration makes this anatomical and functional gap wider with time. Often this gap gets replaced by glial scar which becomes a physical barrier preventing cellular penetration,regeneration and migration. Scaffolds can act as an anatomical substrate on which these cells can grow and connect the physiological ends.

It appears that the cytokines and bio active molecules secreted by these cells play a significant role in acute as well as sub acute phases. Therefore it is essential to retain the cells at the required area in sufficient numbers. We have included only complete injuries so as to remove the bias of spontaneous recovery. Based on our results and the positive role of anatomical continuity we feel partial injuries shall definitely benefit more. Cell therapy can augment the spontaneous recovery either by promotion or reducing the derogatory inhibitory influences.

In our findings delivery through lumbar puncture is simple and equally effective [111-112]. But cell survival in CSF and their functionality need to be enhanced. Retaining large number of cells at the site of injury is also a challenge. We did not encounter any adverse reaction or infection. After lumbar puncture majority had low pressure headaches which were treated with fluid therapy and analgesics effectively. Kishk et al reported neuropathic pain in 56% of their patients following intrathecal injection which was not noticed in our series.

Though the results of animal experiments are enticing the overall translation into clinical benefit is minimal and quite disappointing. Irrespective of site of injury, route of administration and type of cell the clinical recovery is very minimal and only less than 1/3rd showed signs of recovery. Useful functional recovery was seen only in 7-9%. This is rather disappointing. Therefore it appears that even cell therapy has its limitations. But there has been definite evidence of clinical recovery in few and are useful to understand the role of cell therapy. It appears we are somewhere closer to some success yet needs understanding to augment these benefits. Young age, focal segmental injury and early intervention seem to benefit or compliment recovery. Though all our patients expressed subjective well being, ability to sit for longer periods and actively participation in physical excercises following cell therapy could be mediated by cytokines and growth factors. In addition trunk muscles just above the site of injury showed definite clinical improvement. This could explain the need of anatomical integrity for recovery and also their enhanced ability to sit longer. In the distal segment sensory, long tracts and bladder have shown signs of recovery in many, but few had clinically useful benefit. Motor recovery is the most difficult to achieve. Possibly due to loss of trophic influence from higher centers, vascularity which leads to loss of anterior horn cells. Presently available imaging and electro physiological methods are not sensitive enough to detect or monitor regeneration in spinal cord. Those who recovered could be potential partial injuries (anatomical continuity) although behaved as complete injuries clinically.. This could be the possible reason of useful clinical recovery observed in our study. Presently we feel role of cell therapy is only complimentary. MSCs are known for immunomodulation and once administered in the right time may help in minimiging neural inflammation and immune mediated damage. Early intervention might reduce gliosis and promote recovery through secretion of cytokines, bioactive molecules and growth factors. These cells also known for angiogenesis hence benefit by revascularization of spinal cord. Lastly the role of effective activation native progenitor cells to come the rescue of adequate repair needs further exploration. Preservation and promotion of recovery of ant horn cells and reestablishing neuronal functional circuits should be the focus.

Going forward, SCI appears to be the most difficult clinical challenge today. Our understanding of its pathobiology is not complete. The challenges are local (site of injury), peripheral (body below the site of injury) and central (higher centers). The future strategy need to target all the three. Augmenting central influences; sustaining muscles with proper neurotization, rehabilitation, promoting recovery and regeneration at the site seems to be the goal. Several methods and mechanisms alone or in combination need to put in place.Rehabilitation does play a significant role in those with clinical recovery. We speculate that combination of rehab and regeneration may be better. The local neuronal circuits within the segments of the cord must be sustained to retain the integrity of the reflex arc. This appears complex and needs further experimental and clinical data to understand the underlying mechanisms.

18. Conclusion

In conclusion, the surge of research activities in the cell therapies for SCI has yielded only mixed results. While the pre clinical studies are quite promising it is difficult to reproduce similar results in the clinical scenario.. Knowing the mechanisms involved stem cells seems to have specific role and prospects for future studies. Future direction should focus on enhancing the benefits of cell therapy by combination of methods systematically addressing the challenges involved. Our study documents safety and influence on recovery to some extent paves the way for further preclinical and clinical studies with proper design. Such larger clinical studies only can overcome the present diversity in methods and outcomes.

Acknowledgements

The author acknowledges the assistance provided by the neurosurgery team, clinical research team at BGS Global Hospital and by the research team from ANSA.

Author details

N.K. Venkataramanaa[1] and Rakhi Pal[2]

1 Department of Neurosurgery. BGS Global Hospital, Kengeri, Bangalore, India

2 Advanced Neuroscience Allies Research Foundation, India

The authors state that there is no conflict of interest.

References

[1] James Guest: Principles of Translation of Biologic Therapies in Spinal Cord Injury Youmans Neurological Surgery, 6th Edition, Chapter 267, Volume 3; 2011.

[2] Barnett SC, Riddell JS. Olfactory ensheathing cells (OECs) and the treatment of CNS injury: advantages and possible caveats. J Anat. 2004 Jan;204(1):57-67. Review.

[3] Singh R, Sharma SC, Mittal R, Sharma A. Traumatic spinal cord injuries in Haryana: An epidemiological study. Indian journal of community medicine. 2003; XXV111(4): 184-86.

[4] Gregory W. J. Hawryluk, James Rowland, Brian K. Kwon and Michael G. Fehlings. (2008). Protection and repair of the injured spinal cord: a review of completed, ongoing, and planned clinical trials for acute spinal cord injury. Neurosurg Focus 25 (5):E14.

[5] Anjan Kumar Das, Renjitha Gopurappilly & Ishwar Parhar: Current Status & Prospective Application of Stemcell – Based Therapies for Spinal Cord Injury. Current Stem Cell Research & Therapy, Vol.6,No.1,6,00,2011.

[6] Schultz SS: Adult stemcell application in Spinal cord injury. Curr Drug Targets 6:63-73; 2006.

[7] Totoiu MO, Kierstead HS. Spinal Cord Injury is accompanied by chronic progressive demyelination. J Comp Neurol;486;373-83, 2005.

[8] Gerlinde A.S. Metz, Armin Curt, Henk Van De Meent, Isabel Klusman, Martin E. Schwab, Volker Dietz (2000). Validation of the Weight-Drop Contusion Model in Rats: A Comparative Study of Human Spinal Cord Injury. Journal of Neurotrauma. 17(1): 1-17.

[9] Fehlings, Michael G.; Rao, Sanjay C.; Tator, Charles H.; Skaf, Ghassan; Arnold, Paul; Benzel, Edward; Dickman, Curtis; Cuddy, Brian; Green, Barth; Hitchon, Patrick; Northrup, Bruce; Sonntag, Volker; Wagner, Frank; Wilberger, Jack (1999) The Optimal Radiologic Method for Assessing Spinal Canal Compromise and Cord Compression in Patients With Cervical Spinal Cord Injury: Part II: Results of a Multicenter Study. Spine, 24(6):605-613.

[10] Manuel Gaviria, Alain Privat, Pierre D'arbigny, Jean-Marc Kamenka, Henri Haton, and Freddy Ohanna (2000) Neuroprotective Effects of Gacyclidine After Experimental Photochemical Spinal Cord Lesion in Adult Rats: Dose-Window and Time-Window Effects. Journal of Neurotrauma. Vol. 17, No. 1: 19-30

[11] Pitts LH, Ross A, Chase GA, Faden AI. (1995) Treatment with thyrotropin-releasing hormone (TRH) in patients with traumatic spinal cord injuries. J Neurotrauma. 12(3): 235-43.

[12] Takami K, Hashimoto T, Shino A, Fukuda N. (1991). Effect of thyrotropin-releasing hormone (TRH) in experimental spinal cord injury: a quantitative histopathologic study. Jpn J Pharmacol. 57(3):405-17.

[13] Natasha Olby (1999). Current Concepts in the Management of Acute Spinal Cord Injury. J Vet Intern Med 13:399–407

[14] Cho DC, Cheong JH, Yang MS, Hwang SJ, Kim JM, Kim CH. (2011). The effect of minocycline on motor neuron recovery and neuropathic pain in rat model of spinal cord injury. J Korean Neurosurg Soc. 49:83-91.

[15] Ricardo Vieira Botelho, Jefferson Walter Daniel, José Luis Rom eo Boulosa, Benedicto Oscar Colli, Ronald de Lucena Farias, Osmar José Santos Mor aes, Wilson Eloy Pimenta Jr., Carlos Henrique Ribeiro, Francisco Ricardo Bor ges Ribeiro, Mario Augusto Taricco, Marcio Vinhal de Carvalho, Wanderley Marques Bernardo (2010) Effectiveness of methylprednisolone in acute spinal cord injury – a systematic review of randomized controlled trials. Rev Assoc Med Bras 56(6): 729-37.

[16] Jin-Moo Lee, Ping Yan, Qingli Xiao, Shawei Chen, Kuang-Yung Lee, Chung Y. Hsu, and Jan Xu. (2008) Methylprednisolone protects oligodendrocytes but not neurons following spinal cord. J Neurosci. 28(12): 3141–3149.

[17] Alberto Pinzon, Alexander Marcillo, Ada Quintana, Sarah Stamler, Mary Bartlett Bunge, Helen M. Bramlett, and W. Dalton Dietrich (2008) A Re-assessment of Minocycline as a Neuroprotective Agent in a Rat Spinal Cord Contusion Model. Brain Res. 3; 1243: 146–151

[18] Tae Y. Yune, Jee Y. Lee, Gil Y. Jung, Sun J. Kim, Mei H. Jiang, Young C. Kim, Young J. Oh, George J. Markelonis, and Tae H. Oh. (2007) Minocycline Alleviates Death of oligodendrocytes by Inhibiting Pro-Nerve Growth Factor Production in Microglia after Spinal Cord Injury. Journal of Neuroscience, 27(29):7751–7761.

[19] FANG Xiang-qian, FANG Mei, FAN Shun-wu and GU Chuan-long. (2009) Protection of erythropoietin on experimental spinal cord injury by reducing the expression of thrombospondin-1 and transforming growth factor-β. Chinese Medical Journal. 122(14):1631-1635

[20] Thao X. Hoang, Mahnaz Akhavan, Jun Wu, and Leif A. Havton. (2008) Minocycline Protects Motor but not Autonomic Neurons after Cauda Equina Injury. Exp Brain Res. 189(1): 71–77.

[21] Georgios K. Matis Theodossios A. Birbilis. (2009) Erythropoietin in spinal cord injury. Eur Spine J 18:314–323.

[22] Schwab NE. Nogo and axon regeneration. Curr Opin Nerobiol:1118-24,2004.

[23] Schwab ME, Repairing the Injured Spinal Cord. Science:295:1029-31,2002

[24] Liu BP, Fournier A, GrandPre T, Strittmatter SM, Myeliin –associated Glycoprotein as a functional ligand for the Nogo-66 receptor.Science;297:1190-03; 2002.

[25] Murat Celik, Necati G kmen, Serhat Erbayraktar, Mustafa Akhisaroglu, Selman Konakc, Cagnur Ulukus, Sermin Genc, Kursad Genc, Emel Sagiroglu, Anthony Cerami and Michael Brines. (2002) Erythropoietin prevents motor neuron apoptosis and neurologic disability in experimental spinal cord ischemic injury. PNAS vol. 99 no. 42258–2263.

[26] Carelli S, Marfia G, Di Giulio AM, Ghilardi G, Gorio A. (2011) Erythropoietin: recent developments in the treatment of spinal cord injury. Neurol Res Int.

[27] Dergham P, Ellezam B, Essagian C, Avedissian H, Lubell WD, McKerracher L. (2002) Rho signaling pathway targeted to promote spinal cord repair. J Neurosci. 22(15): 6570-7.

[28] Blight AR. Computer simulation of action potentials and afterpotentials in mammalian myelinated axons: the case for a lower resistance myelin sheath. Neuroscience. 1985 May;15(1):13-31.

[29] Blight AR. Macrophages and inflammatory damage in spinal cord injury. J Neurotrauma. 1992 Mar;9 Suppl 1:S83-91. Review.

[30] Rapalino O, Lazarov-Spiegler O, Agranov E, Velan GJ, Yoles E, Fraidakis M, Solomon A, Gepstein R, Katz A, Belkin M, Hadani M, Schwartz M. Implantation of stimulated homologous macrophages results in partial recovery of paraplegic rats. Nat Med. 1998 Jul;4(7):814-21.

[31] Popovich PG, Guan Z, Wei P, Huitinga I, van Rooijen N, Stokes BT. Depletion of hematogenous macrophages promotes partial hindlimb recovery and neuroanatomical repair after experimental spinal cord injury. Exp Neurol. 1999 Aug;158(2):351-65.

[32] Chopp M, Zhang XH, Li Y, Wang L, Chen J, Lu D, Lu M, Rosenblum M. Spinal cord injury in rat: treatment with bone marrow stromal cell transplantation. Neuroreport. 2000 Sep 11;11(13):3001-5.

[33] Ankeny DP, McTigue DM, Jakeman LB. One marrow transplants provide tissue protection and directional guidance for axons after contusive spinal cord injury in rats. Exp Neurol. 2004 Nov;190(1):17-31.

[34] Nosrat IV, Widenfalk J, Olson L, Nosrat CA. Dental pulp cells produce neurotrophic factors, interact with trigeminal neurons *in vitro*, and rescue motoneurons after spinal cord injury. Dev Biol. 2001 Oct 1;238(1):120-32.

[35] Lipson AC, Widenfalk J, Lindqvist E, Ebendal T, Olson Neurotrophic properties of olfactory ensheathing glia.LExp Neurol. 2003 Apr;180(2):167-71.

[36] Umezawa A, Ogawa S. Cardiomyocytes can be generated from marrow stromal cells *in vitro*. J Clin Invest 1999 103: 697-705.

[37] McDonald JW, Belegu V. Demyelination and remyelination after spinal cord injury. J Neurotrauma. 2006 Mar-Apr;23(3-4):345-59. Review.

[38] Fournier AE, Takizawa BT, Strittmatter SM. (2003) Rho kinase inhibition enhances axonal regeneration in the injured CNS. J Neurosci. 23(4):1416-23.

[39] Sung JK, Miao L, Calvert JW, Huang L, Louis Harkey H, Zhang JH. (2003) A possible role of RhoA/Rho-kinase in experimental spinal cord injury in rat. Brain Res. 959(1): 29-38.

http://dx.doi.org/10.5772/58323

[40] Fehlings MG, Theodore N, Harrop J, Maurais G, Kuntz C, Shaffrey CI, Kwon BK, Chapman J, Yee A, Tighe A, McKerracher L. (2011) A phase I/IIa clinical trial of a recombinant Rho protein antagonist in acute spinal cord injury. J Neurotrauma. 28(5): 787-96.

[41] Beaumont E, Whitaker CM, Burke DA, Hetman M, Onifer SM. (2009) Effects of rolipram on adult rat oligodendrocytes and functional recovery after contusive cervical spinal cord injury. Neuroscience. 163(4):985-90.

[42] Satkunendrarajah Kajana, and Harry G Goshgarian. (2009) Systemic administration of rolipram increases medullary and spinal cAMP and activates a latent respiratory motor pathway after high cervical spinal cord injury. Spinal Cord Med. 32(2):175-82.

[43] Whitaker CM, Beaumont E, Wells MJ, Magnuson DS, Hetman M, Onifer SM. (2008) Rolipram attenuates acute oligodendrocyte death in the adult rat ventrolateral funiculus following contusive cervical spinal cord injury. Neurosci Lett. 438(2):200-4.

[44] Nikulina E, Tidwell JL, Dai HN, Bregman BS, Filbin MT. (2004) The phosphodiesterase inhibitor rolipram delivered after a spinal cord lesion promotes axonal regeneration and functional recovery. Proc Natl Acad Sci 101(23):8786-90.

[45] Gonzenbach RR, Zoerner B, Schnell L, Weinmann O, Mir AK, Schwab ME. (2011) Delayed Anti-Nogo-A Antibody Application after Spinal Cord Injury Shows Progressive Loss of Responsiveness. J Neurotrauma.

[46] Maier IC, Ichiyama RM, Courtine G, Schnell L, Lavrov I, Edgerton VR, Schwab ME. (2009) Differential effects of anti-Nogo-A antibody treatment and treadmill training in rats with incomplete spinal cord injury. Brain. 132(Pt 6):1426-40.

[47] Gonzenbach RR, Gasser P, Zörner B, Hochreutener E, Dietz V, Schwab ME. (2010) Nogo-A antibodies and training reduce muscle spasms in spinal cord-injured rats. Ann Neurol. 68(1):48-57.

[48] Freund P, Wannier T, Schmidlin E, Bloch J, Mir A, Schwab ME, Rouiller EM. (2007) Anti-Nogo-A antibody treatment enhances sprouting of corticospinal axons rostral to a unilateral cervical spinal cord lesion in adult macaque monkey. J Comp Neurol. 502(4): 644-59.

[49] Liebscher T, Schnell L, Schnell D, Scholl J, Schneider R, Gullo M, Fouad K, Mir A, Rausch M, Kindler D, Hamers FP, Schwab ME. (2005) Nogo-A antibody improves regeneration and locomotion of spinal cord-injured rats. Ann Neurol. 58(5):706-19.

[50] Wiessner C, Bareyre FM, Allegrini PR, Mir AK, Frentzel S, Zurini M, Schnell L, Oertle T, Schwab ME. Anti-Nogo-A antibody infusion 24 hours after experimental stroke improved behavioral outcome and corticospinal plasticity in normotensive and spontaneously hypertensive rats. J Cereb Blood Flow Metab. 23(2):154-65.

[51] Bukhari N, Torres L, Robinson JK, Tsirka SE. (2011) Axonal regrowth after spinal cord injury via chondroitinase and the tissue plasminogen activator (tPA)/plasmin system. J Neurosci. 31(42):14931-43.

[52] Zhao RR, Muir EM, Alves JN, Rickman H, Allan AY, Kwok JC, Roet KC, Verhaagen J, Schneider BL, Bensadoun JC, Ahmed SG, Yáñez-Muñoz RJ, Keynes RJ, Fawcett JW, Rogers JH. (2011) Lentiviral vectors express chondroitinase ABC in cortical projections and promote sprouting of injured corticospinal axons. J Neurosci Methods. 201(1):228-38.

[53] Wang D, Ichiyama RM, Zhao R, Andrews MR, Fawcett JW. (2011) Chondroitinase combined with rehabilitation promotes recovery of forelimb function in rats with chronic spinal cord injury. J Neurosci. 31(25):9332-44.

[54] Zhang C, Yao C, He XJ, Li HP. (2010). Repair of subacute spinal cord crush injury by bone marrow stromal cell transplantation and chondroitinase ABC microinjection in adult rats. Nan Fang Yi Ke Da Xue Xue Bao. 30(9):2030-5

[55] Karimi-Abdolrezaee S, Eftekharpour E, Wang J, Schut D, Fehlings MG. (2010) Synergistic effects of transplanted adult neural stem/progenitor cells, chondroitinase, and growth factors promote functional repair and plasticity of the chronically injured spinal cord. J Neurosci. 30(5):1657-76.

[56] Tom VJ, Kadakia R, Santi L, Houlé JD. (2009) Administration of chondroitinase ABC rostral or caudal to a spinal cord injury site promotes anatomical but not functional plasticity. J Neurotrauma. 26(12):2323-33.

[57] Duschau-Wicke A, Caprez A, Riener R. (2011) Patient-cooperative control increases active participation of individuals with SCI during robot-aided gait training. J Neuroeng Rehabil. 10;7:43.

[58] Gregory W. J. Hawryluk, James Rowland, Brian K. Kwon, and Michael G. Fehlings. (2008) Protection and repair of the injured spinal cord: a review of completed, ongoing, and planned clinical trials for acute spinal cord injury. Neurosurg Focus 25 (5):E14.

[59] Lang-Lazdunski L, Heurteaux C, Mignon A, Mantz J, Widmann C, Desmonts J, Lazdunski M. (2000) Ischemic spinal cord injury induced by aortic cross-clamping: prevention by riluzole. Eur J Cardiothorac Surg. 18(2):174-81.

[60] Schuster JE, Fu R, Siddique T, Heckman CJ. (2012) Effect of prolonged riluzole exposure on cultured motoneurons in a mouse model of ALS. J Neurophysiol. 107(1): 484-92.

[61] Simard JM, Tsymbalyuk O, Keledjian K, Ivanov A, Ivanova S, Gerzanich V. (2011) Comparative effects of glibenclamide and riluzole in a rat model of severe cervical spinal cord injury. Exp Neurol.

[62] Pintér S, Gloviczki B, Szabó A, Márton G, Nógrádi A. J Neurotrauma. (2010) Increased survival and reinnervation of cervical motoneurons by riluzole after avulsion of the C7 ventral root. 27(12):2273-82.

[63] Kitzman PH. (2009) Effectiveness of riluzole in suppressing spasticity in the spinal cord injured rat. Neurosci Lett. 455(2):150-3.

[64] Nógrádi A, Szabó A, Pintér S, Vrbová G. (2007) Delayed riluzole treatment is able to rescue injured rat spinal motoneurons. Neuroscience. 144(2):431-8.

[65] Faghri PD, Glaser RM, Figoni SF. (1992) Functional electrical stimulation leg cycle ergometer exercise: training effects on cardiorespiratory responses of spinal cord injured subjects at rest and during submaximal exercise. Arch Phys Med Rehabil. 73:1085–1093.

[66] Hicks AL, Martin KA, Ditor DS, et al. (2003) Long-term exercise training in persons with spinal cord injury: effects on strength, arm ergometry performance, and psychological well-being. Spinal Cord. 41:34–43.

[67] Astorino TA, Tyerman N, Wong K, Harness E. (2008) Efficacy of a new rehabilitative device for individuals with spinal cord injury. J Spinal Cord Med. 31(5):586-91.

[68] Nash MS. (2005) Exercise as a health-promoting activity following spinal cord injury. J Neurol Phys Ther. 29(2):87-103, 106.

[69] Hagglund KJ, Clark MJ, Mokelke EK, Stout BJ. (2004) The current state of personal assistance services: implications for policy and future research. NeuroRehabilitation. 19(2):115-20.

[70] Adams MM, Hicks AL. (2011) Comparison of the effects of body-weight-supported treadmill training and tilt-table standing on spasticity in individuals with chronic spinal cord injury. J Spinal Cord Med. 34(5):488-94

[71] Stevens S, Morgan DW. (2010) Underwater treadmill training in adults with incomplete spinal cord injuries. J Rehabil Res Dev. 47(7): vii-x.

[72] Epifanov VA. (1980). Effect of physical exercises on the hemodynamic state in patients with an injury of the cervical spine and spinal cord. Vopr Kurortol Fizioter Lech Fiz Kult. (3):54-7.

[73] Rayegani SM, Shojaee H, Sedighipour L, Soroush MR, Baghbani M, Amirani OB. (2010) The effect of electrical passive cycling on spasticity in war veterans with spinal cord injury. Front Neurol. 2:39.

[74] Galvez JA, Budovitch A, Harkema SJ, Reinkensmeyer DJ. (2011)Trainer variability during step training after spinal cord injury: Implications for robotic gait-training device design. J Rehabil Res Dev 48(2):147-60

[75] Liu G, Keeler BE, Zhukareva V, Houlé JD. (2010) Cycling exercise affects the expression of apoptosis-associated micro RNAs after spinal cord injury in rats. Exp Neurol. 226(1): 200-6

[76] Johnston TE, Smith BT, Oladeji O, Betz RR, Lauer RT. (2008) Outcomes of a home cycling program using functional electrical stimulation or passive motion for children with spinal cord injury: a case series. J Spinal Cord Med 31(2):215-21.

[77] Hetz SP, Latimer AE, Buchholz AC, Martin Ginis KA; SHAPE-SCI Research Group. (2009) Increased participation in activities of daily living is associated with lower cholesterol levels in people with spinal cord injury. Arch Phys Med Rehabil. 90(10): 1755-9.

[78] Chafetz RS, Mulcahey MJ, Betz RR, Anderson C, Vogel LC, Gaughan JP, Odel MA, Flanagan A, McDonald CM. (2007) Impact of prophylactic thoraco-lumbosacral orthosis bracing on functional activities and activities of daily living in the pediatric spinal cord injury population. J Spinal Cord Med. 30 Suppl 1:S178-83

[79] Liem NR, McColl MA, King W, Smith KM. (2004) Aging with a spinal cord injury: factors associated with the need for more help with activities of daily living. Arch Phys Med Rehabil. 85(10):1567-77

[80] Watson AH, Kanny EM, White DM, Anson DK. (1995) Use of standardized activities of daily living rating scales in spinal cord injury and disease services. Am J Occup Ther. 49(3):229-34.

[81] Vernon W Lin, Diana D Cardenas, Nancy C Cutter, Frederick S Frost, Margaret C Hammond, Laurie B Lindblom, Inder Perkash, FACS, Robert Waters, and Robert M Woolsey. (2003) Spinal Cord Medicine: Principles and Practice. New York: Demos Medical Publishing; Pg 635-731.

[82] Chen D, Philip M, Philip PA, Monga TN. (1990) Cardiac pacemaker inhibition by transcutaneous electrical nerve stimulation. Arch Phys Med Rehabil 71:27–30.

[83] Segreti J. (1999) Is antibiotic prophylaxis necessary for preventing prosthetic device infection? Infect Dis Clin North Am 13(4): 871–877.

[84] Kahn NN, Feldman SP, Bauman WA. (2010) Lower-extremity functional electrical stimulation decreases platelet aggregation and blood coagulation in persons with chronic spinal cord injury: a pilot study. J Spinal Cord Med. 33(2):150-8

[85] Do AH, Wang PT, King CE, Abiri A, Nenadic Z. (2011) Brain-computer interface controlled functional electrical stimulation system for ankle movement. J Neuroeng Rehabil. 8:49.

[86] Gater DR Jr, Dolbow D, Tsui B, Gorgey AS. (2011) Functional electrical stimulation therapies after spinal cord injury. NeuroRehabilitation 28(3):231-48

[87] Hamid S, Hayek R. (2008) Role of electrical stimulation for rehabilitation and regeneration after spinal cord injury: an overview. Eur Spine J. 17(9):1256-69.

[88] Thrasher TA, Popovic MR. (2008) Functional electrical stimulation of walking: function, exercise and rehabilitation. Ann Readapt Med Phys. 51(6):452-60.

[89] Ahmed Z, Wieraszko A. (2008) Combined effects of acrobatic exercise and magnetic stimulation on the functional recovery after spinal cord lesions. J Neurotrauma. 25(10): 1257-69.

[90] Tsai PY, Wang CP, Chiu FY, Tsai YA, Chang YC, Chuang TY. (2009) Efficacy of functional magnetic stimulation in neurogenic bowel dysfunction after spinal cord injury. J Rehabil Med; 41(1):41-7

[91] Krause P, Straube A. (2003) Repetitive magnetic and functional electrical stimulation reduce spastic tone increase in patients with spinal cord injury. Suppl Clin Neurophysiol; 56:220-5.

[92] Lin VW, Nino-Murcia M, Frost F, Wolfe V, Hsiao I, Perkash I. (2001) Functional magnetic stimulation of the colon in persons with spinal cord injury. Arch Phys Med Rehabil; 82(2):167-73

[93] Lin VW, Hsiao IN, Zhu E, Perkash I. (2001) Functional magnetic stimulation for conditioning of expiratory muscles in patients with spinal cord injury. Arch Phys Med Rehabil. 82(2):162-6.

[94] Classen J, Witte OW. (1995) Epileptic seizures triggered directly by focal transcranial magnetic stimulation. Electroencephalography Clin Neurophysiology; 94:19–25.

[95] Beattie MS, Bresnahan JC, Komon J, Tovar CA, Van Meter M, Anderson DK, Faden AI, Hsu CY, Noble LJ, Salzman S, Young W.Endogenous repair after spinal cord contusion injuries in the rat. Exp Neurol. 1997 Dec;148(2):453-63.

[96] Mothe AJ, Tator CH. Proliferation, migration, and differentiation of endogenous ependymal region stem/progenitor cells following minimal spinal cord injury in the adult rat. Neuroscience. 2005;131(1):177-87.

[97] Namiki J, Tator CH.Cell proliferation and nestin expression in the ependyma of the adult rat spinal cord after injury. J Neuropathol Exp Neurol. 1999 May;58(5):489-98

[98] Horner PJ, Gage FH. Regenerating the damaged central nervous system. Nature. 2000 Oct 26;407(6807):963-70.

[99] Cao X, Tang C, Luo Y. Effects of nerve growth factor on N-methyl-D-asparate receptor 1 after spinal cord injury in rats. Chin J Traumatol. 2002 Aug;5(4):228-31.

[100] Koike M, Uchiyama Y, Toyama Y, Okano H. Transplantation of *in vitro*-expanded fetal neural progenitor cells results in neurogenesis and functional recovery after spinal cord contusion injury in adult rats. J Neurosci Res. 2002 Sep 15;69(6):925-33.

[101] Yan Y, Yang D, Zarnowska ED, Du Z, Werbel B, Valliere C, Pearce RA, Thomson JA, Zhang SC. Directed differentiation of dopaminergic neuronal subtypes from human embryonic stem cells. Stem Cells. 2005 Jun-Jul;23(6):781-90

[102] Houlé JD, Reier PJ. Transplantation of fetal spinal cord tissue into the chronically injured adult rat spinal cord. J Comp Neurol. 1988 Mar 22;269(4):535-47.

[103] Ankeny DP, McTigue DM, Jakeman LB. one marrow transplants provide tissue protection and directional guidance for axons after contusive spinal cord injury in rats. Exp Neurol. 2004 Nov;190(1):17-31.

[104] Fitch MT, Doller, C, Combs CK, Landreth GE, Silver J. Cellular and molecular mechanism of glial scarring and progressive cavitation: *in vivo* and *in vitro* analysis of inflammation-induced secondary injury after CNS trauma. 1999 J. Neurosci., 19(19), 8182-8198.

[105] Jones DG, Anderson ER, Galvin KA. Spinal cord regeneration: moving tentatively towards new perspectives. NeuroRehabilitation. 2003 18(4):339-51.

[106] Knoller N, Auerbach G, Fulga V, Zelig G, Attias J, Bakimer R, et al. Clinical experience using incubated autologous macrophages as a treatment for complete spinal cord injury: phase I study results. 2005 J Neurosurg Spine. Sep; 3(3):173-81.

[107] Nistor GI, Totoiu MO, Haque N, Carpenter MK, Keirstead HS. Human embryonic stem cells differentiate into oligodendrocytes in high purity and myelinate after spinal cord transplantation. Glia. 2005 Feb;49(3):385-96. Wolfram Tetzlaff et al

[108] Moviglia GA, Fernandez Viña R, Brizuela JA, Saslavsky J, Vrsalovic F, Varela G, Bastos F, Farina P, Etchegaray G, Barbieri M, Martinez G, Picasso F, Schmidt Y, Brizuela P, Gaeta CA, Costanzo H, Moviglia Brandolino MT, Merino S, Pes ME, Veloso MJ, Rugilo C, Tamer I, Shuster GS. Combined protocol of cell therapy for chronic spinal cord injury. Report on the electrical and functional recovery of two patients. Cytotherapy. 2006; 8(3):202-9.

[109] Kang KS, Kim SW, Oh YH, Yu JW, Kim KY, Park HK, Song CH, Han H. A 37-year-old spinal cord-injured female patient transplanted of multipotent stem cells from human UC blood, with improved sensory perception and mobility, both functionally and morphologically: a case study. Cytotherapy 2005 7(4):368-73.

[110] Deda H, Inci MC, Kureckei A, et al. Treatment of chronic spinal cord injured patients with Autologous bone marrow –derived hematopoietic stemcell transplantation. Cythotherapy:6:551-64,2008.

[111] Jung DI, Ha J, Kang BTm et. A comparison of autologous and allogenic bone marrow-derived mesenchymal stem cell transplantation in canine spinal cord injury. J Neurol Sci ;285:67-77, 2009

[112] Neuhuber B, Brashinger AL, Paul C, et al.Stem cell delivery by lumbar puncture as a therapeutic alternative to direct injection into injured, spinal cord.J Neurosurg Spine: 9:390-9,2008.

[113] Mai Q, Yu Y, Li T, Wang L, Chen MJ, Huang SZ, Zhou C, Zhou Q. Derivation of human embryonic stem cell lines from parthenogenetic blastocysts. Cell Res. 2007 Dec; 17(12):1008-19.

[114] Pal R, Gopinath C, Rao NM, Banerjee P, Krishnamoorthy V, Venkataramana NK, Totey S. Functional recovery after transplantation of bone marrow-derived human mesenchymal stromal cells in a rat model of spinal cord injury.

[115] Harrop JS, Naroji S. Maltenfort MG, Rathiff JK, Tjoumakaris SI, Frank B, etal: Neurologic improvement after thoracic, thoracolumbar and lumbar spinal cord (conus medullaris)injuries. Spine (Phila Pa 1976)36:21-25,2011.

[116] Burns AS, Lee BS, Ditunno JF Jr, Tessler A: Patient selection for clinical trials: the reliability of the early spinal cord injury examination. J Neurotrauma 20:477-482,2013.

[117] Kirshblum S, Millis S, McKinley W, Tulsky D: Late neurologic recovery after traumatic spinal cord injury. Arch Phys Med Rehabil 85:1811-1817,2004.

[118] Marino RJ, Ditunno JF Jr. Donovan WH. Maynard F Jr: Neurologica recovery after traumatic spinal cord injury: data from the Model Spinal Cord Injury:data from the Model Spinal Cord Injury Systems. Arch Phys Med Rehabil 80:1391-1396.1999.

[119] Mehta T, Feroz A, Thakkar U, Vanikar A, Shah V, Trivedi H: Subarachnoid placement of stemcells in neurological disorders. Transplatn Proc 40:1145-1147, 2008

[120] Cristante AF, Barros – Filho TE, Tatsui N. Mendrone A, Caldas JG, Camargo A, et al: Stemcells in the treatment of chronic spinal cord injury: evaluation of somatosensitive evoked potentials in 39 patients. Spinal Cord 47:733-738, 2009.

[121] Saberi H, Firouzi M, Habibi Z, Moshayedi P, Aghayan HR, Arjmand B, et al: Safety of intramedullary Schwann cell transplantation for post rehabilitation spinal cord injuries: 2 year follow up of 33 cases. Clinical article. J Neurosurg Spine 15:515-525,2011.

[122] Yoon SH, Shim YS, Park YH, Chung JK, Nam JH, Kim MO, et al: Complete spinal cord injury treatment using autologous bone marrow cell transplantation and bone marrow stimulation with granulocyte macrophage-colony stimulating factor: Phase I/II clinical trial. Stem Cells 25:2066-2073, 2007.

[123] Kumar AA, Kumar SR,, Narayanan R, Arul K, Baskaran M: Autologous bone marrow derived monomuclear cell therapy for spinal cord injury: a pahse I/II clinical safety and primary efficacy data. Exp. Clin Transplant 7:241-248,2009.

[124] Yoon SH, Shim YS, Park YH, Chung JK, Nam JH, Kim MO, et al: Complete spinal cord injury treatment using autologous bone marrow cell transplantation and bone

marrow stimulation with granulocyte macrophage-colony stimulating factor: Phase I/II clinical trial. Stem Cells 25:2066-2073, 2007.

[125] Tetzlaff W, Okon EB, Karmi-Abdolrezaee S, Hill CE, Sparling JS, Plemel JR, et al; A systemic review of cellular transplantation therapies for spinal cord injury. J Neurotrauma 28:1611-1682,2011.

[126] Park SS, Byeon YE, Ryu HH, Kang BJ, Kim Y, Kim WH, et al: Comparison of canine umbilical cord blood-derived emsenchymal stemcell transplantation times: Involvement of astrogliosis, inflammation, intracellular actin cytoskeleton pathways and neurotrophin. Cell Transplant (epub ahead of print), 2011.

[127] Jung DI, Ha J, Kang BTm et. A comparison of autologous and allogenic bone marrow-derived mesenchymal stem cell transplantation in canine spinal cord injury. J Neurol Sci ;285:67-77, 2009.

[128] Kishk N A, Gabr H, Hamdy S, Afifi L, Abokresha N. mahmoud H, eta l: case control series of intrathecal autologous bone marrow mesenchymal stem cell therapy for chronic spinal cord injury. Neuro rehabil Neural Repair 24:702-708, 2010.

Chapter 12

35 Years in Research on Spinal Cord Lesions and Repair

Giorgio Brunelli

Additional information is available at the end of the chapter

http://dx.doi.org/10.5772/56988

1. Introduction

Paraplegia by spinal cord lesion is a severe condition which cannot be cured.

It is known since the ancient times as figured figured in the Ninive basrelief (fig 1) and described in the Smith papirus (fig 2). Since those times it is known that the spinal cord, after severance does not allow healing.

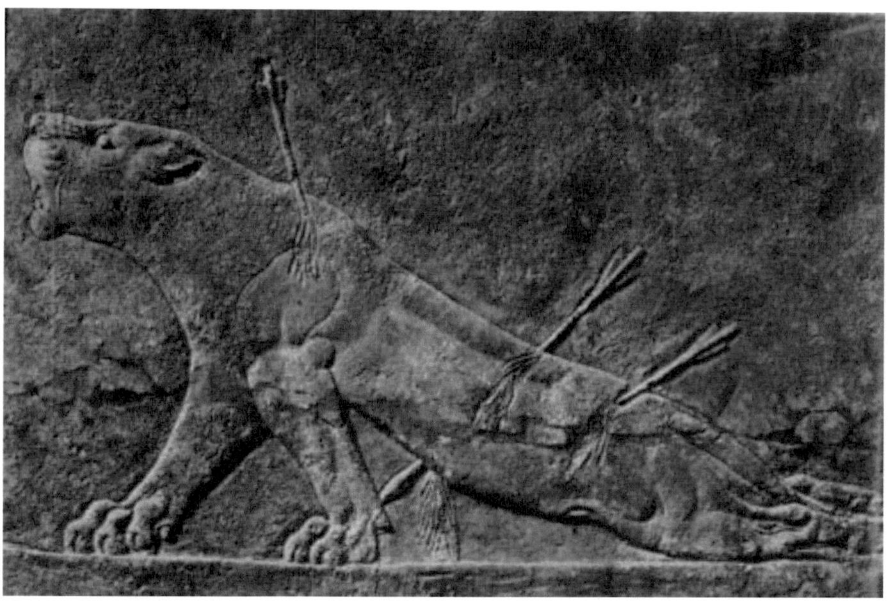

Figure 1. Dying lioness with paraplegia (Ninive bas relief)

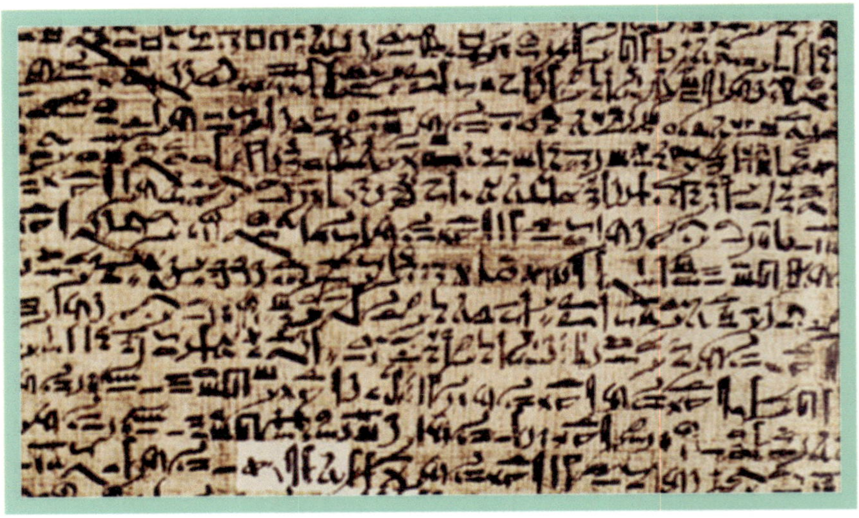

Figure 2. Smith papirus describing the symptoms of cord lesion

It is due to the *nonpermissiveness* of the cord for the advancement of the axons that regrow from the brain neurons.

Not only walking is hindered but there is compromission of all the vegetative function and pression sores (fig 3) not to say the psicological damage of the patient and of his/her relatives and the social heavy burden for assistance and architectural modifications.

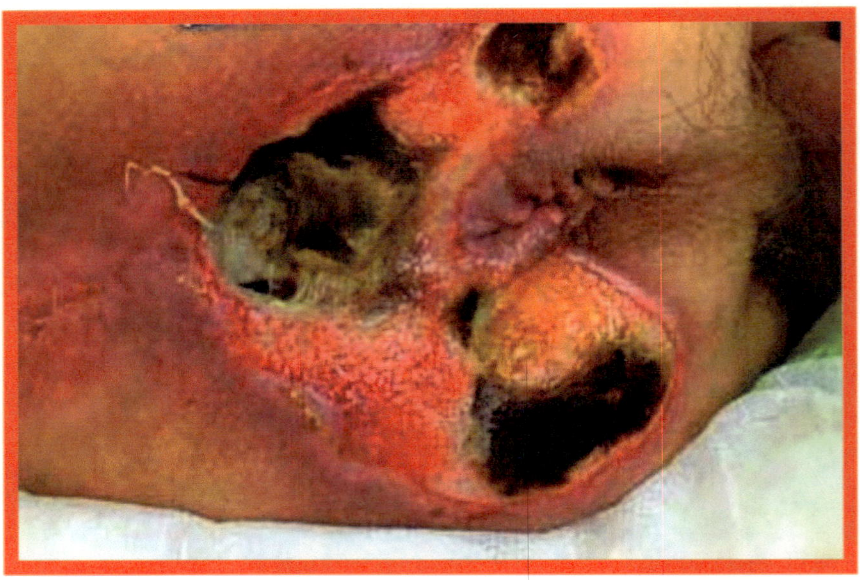

Figure 3. Ptressure sores in a paraplegic

http://dx.doi.org/10.5772/56988

Paraplegia by S.pinal Cord Injury is a very heavy burden:

a. for patients who at the age of their most productive capacity are put in a weelchair for life and undergo severe physical, economical and psycological problems.

(More than 2000 new cases a year occur in Italy and 18/20 cases every milion of inhabitants in the world),

2. for the families which must assist their relative from the economical, physical and psycological point of view and

3. for society and the country which have to supply medical assistance, economical support and architectural facilities.

Non permissiveness and incurability of paraplegia are a DOGMA.

Various explanations of this dogma have been tried without solution.

My research on spinal cord started in 1978 when, thinking that microsurgery had solved almost all the problems related to peripheral nerves lesions, I wondered why no surgical treatment was able to help regeneration of the spinal cord.

One of the hypotetical reason (besides the scar formation) was the lack (in the cord) of Schwann cells which support the regeneration of the nerve fibres in peripheral nerves.

This semplicistic idea pushed me to resect one centimeter of cord in rats and to put in the resulting gap several grafts of peripheral nerves (sciatic n.) which contain Schwann cells. (fig.4)

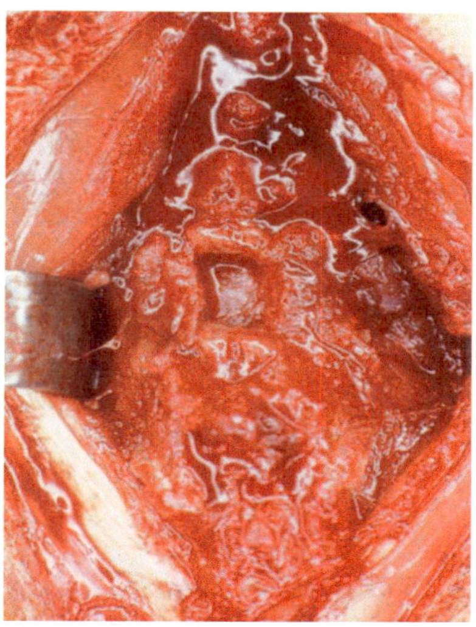

Figure 4. Removal of 1 cm of spinal cord in a rat

As a result I found that the grafts were reinhabited by the axons descending from the brain but that at the very end of the grafts the axons stopped progressing. (fig 5 and 6)

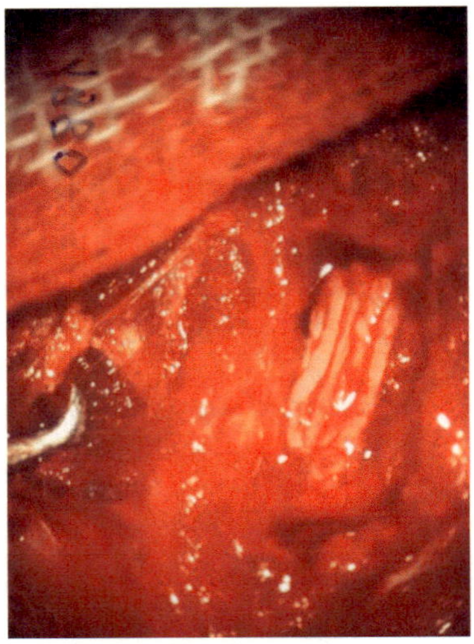

Figure 5. Grafts of sciatic nerve put in the cord of a rat after removal of 1 cm of cord.

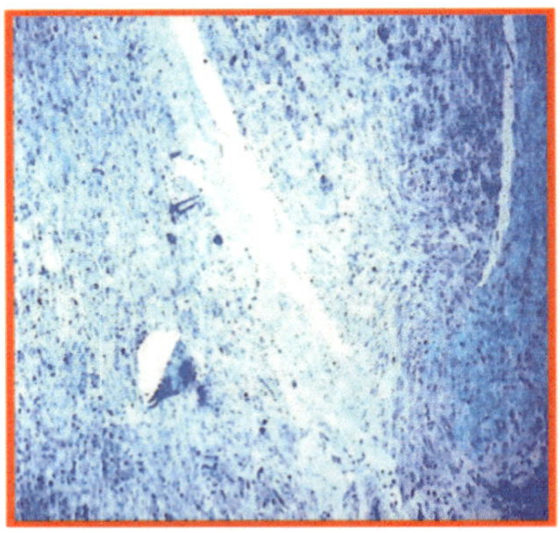

Figure 6. The graft has been reinhabited by the axons regrowing from the upper neurons but axons stopped progressing as soon as in contact again with the C.N.S. (cord). Only a few micron of progession was observed due to the exit of Schwann cells.

This fact confirmed the idea that the central nervous system (C.N.S. of which the cord is part) is "non permissive" for the regrowing axons progression inside it (perhaphs due to specific "no-go" molecules).

Also I took part in the C.A.L.I.E.S. (Computer Assisted Locomotion by means of Implanted Electrical Stimulation) and S.U.A.W (Stand Up And Walk) (European programs intended to obtain walking by means of implanted electrical stimulation of muscles). (fig. 7) The electrical stimulation of the muscles was given by electrodes implanted in 8 muscles of each inferior limb by means of a control-unit implanted under the abdominal skin that received impulses from a computer through a transcutaneous antenna. (fig 8)

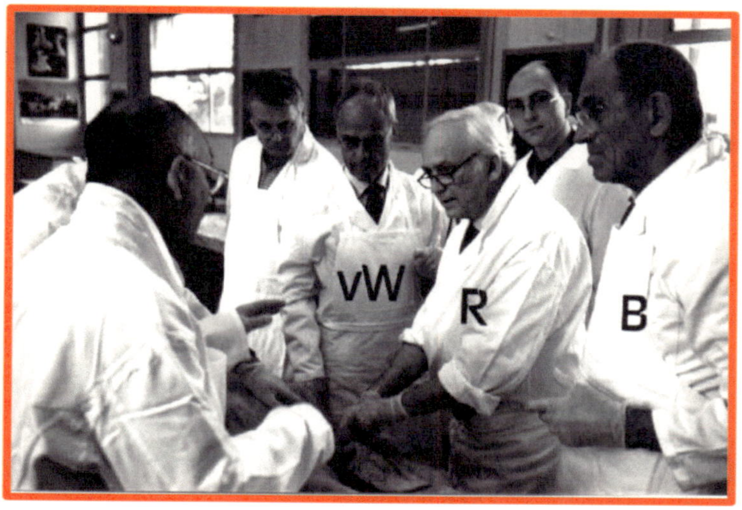

Figure 7. The team of the C.A.L.I.E.S program in Montpellier: VW: Von Wild, R: Rabishong, B:Brunelli

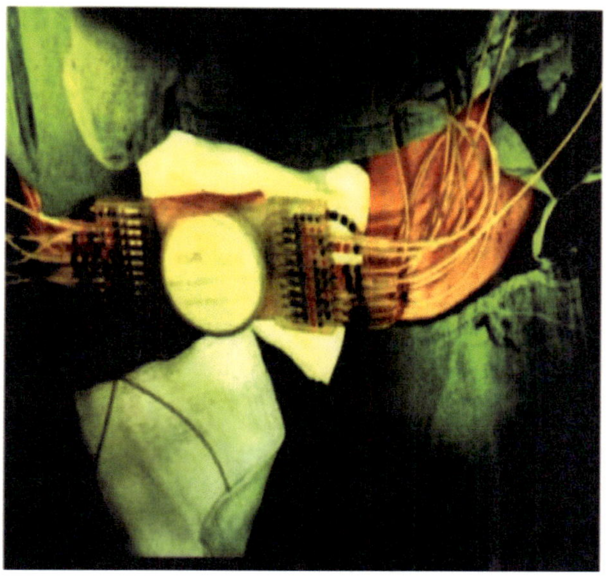

Figure 8. The multichannel control unit of the CALIES, to be implanted under the skin of the abdomen, connected with 8 muscles of the legs and stimulated transcutaneously by an antenna connected with the computer for stimulation of the muscles.

These experimental operations had to be abandoned due to the high cost of the electronic devices (not to say to the necessity for the paraplegics to pull a trolley with batteries and the computerized program that had been studied by means of a meticulous gait analysis that could not anyway change the recorded program of the computer in front of unanticipated obstacles).

My second step (1981) was the connection of the above the lesion cord (by means of a graft of peripheral nerve) to peripheral nerves and muscles. (fig 9 and 10).

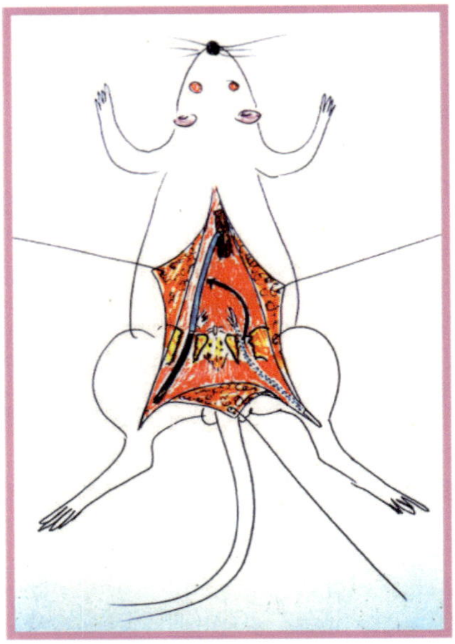

Figure 9. Connection of the C.S,T, to peripheral nerves

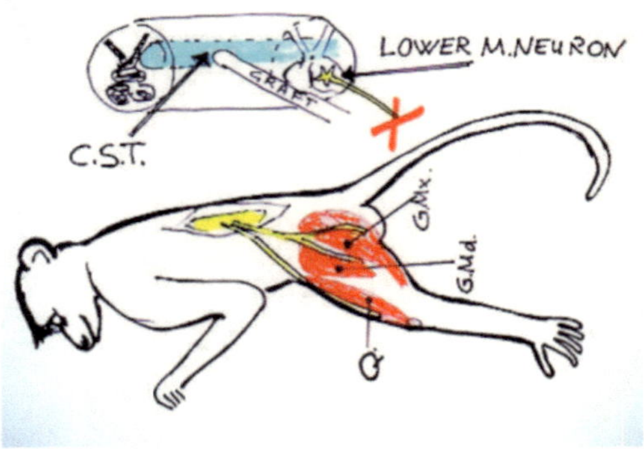

Figure 10. Sketch of the connection.

The regrowing axons elongated up to the muscle forming new motor end-plates and functional connections. (fig 11).

By this connection the result was effective and rats could walk, even if, of course, with some limitation. The presentation of theses results at an international meeting (in San Antonio) stired up a lot of skepticism: *"rats could walk even without any attempt of repairing the cord"* (whic is not true).

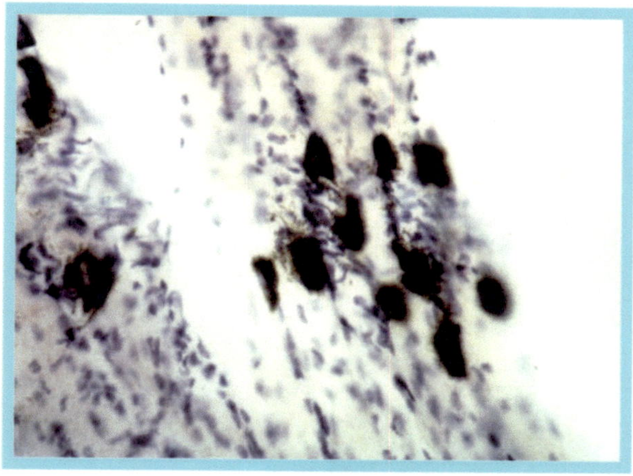

Figure 11. Motor-end plates newly formed at the contact of the graft with the muscle.

The advise was: go to primates. At that time I had not the facilities nor the permission for operating monkeys in Italy. Therefore I was compelled to go abroad and I found the friendy help of dr Carlstedt who hosted me in the primatology institute of the Karolinska Institutet in Solna (Stockolm). I and my staff operated on, over there, 20 "macaca fascicularis" connecting the above the lesion cord with peripheral nerves by means of autologous grafts and checking the results by means of clinical observation, electromyography, magnetic stimulation of both the nerve going to muscles and of the brain (after craniotomy) and histology of the cord and of the graft. (Fig 12,13, 14). Magnetic stimulation of the brain, external and after craniotomy as well as E.M.G. of the grafts and the muscles showed good muscle responses with different latency times according to the distance from the recording electrode (fig 15) The monkeys were able to move the reinnervated muscles.

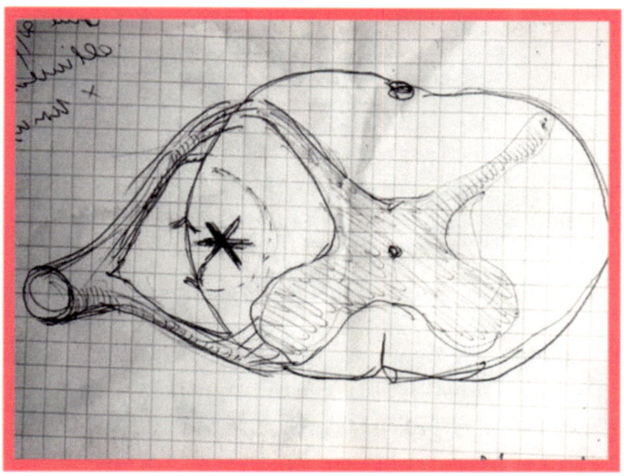

Figure 12. Sketch of the place where the graft is inserted.

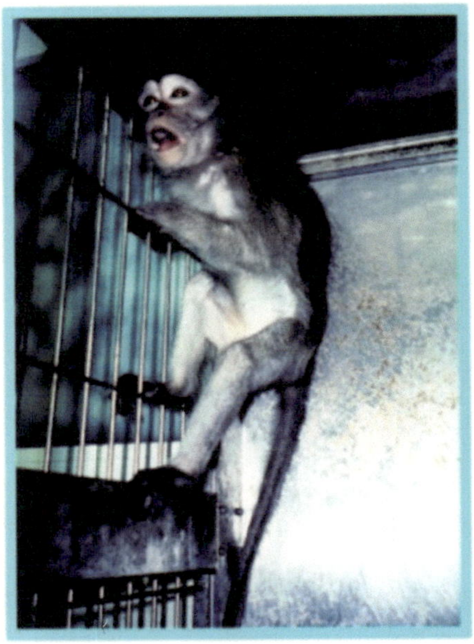

Figure 13. An operated monkey grasping the bars of its cage with its foot

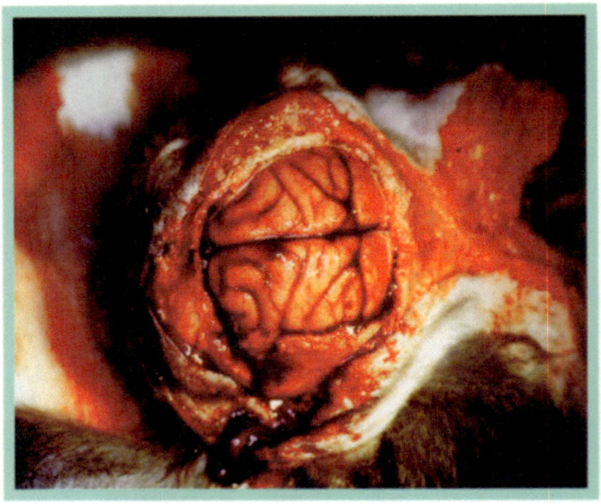

Figure 14. Craniotomy done for magnetography of the graft and muscles.

As at that time we had no effective treatment for spinal cord injury (S.C.I.) I thought, (and the Ethical Committee of the Italian Health Organisation agreed) that it could be ethically justified to operate on *fully informed volunteer patients* by means of surgical procedures already in current use, tried and checked in animals and human beeings as, for instance, the transfer of nerves (ulnar nerves from upper to lower limbs, fig 16 and 16 bis) or the grafting from the corticospinal tract of the cord to peripheral nerves of the lower limbs by means of autologous nerve-grafts.

http://dx.doi.org/10.5772/56988

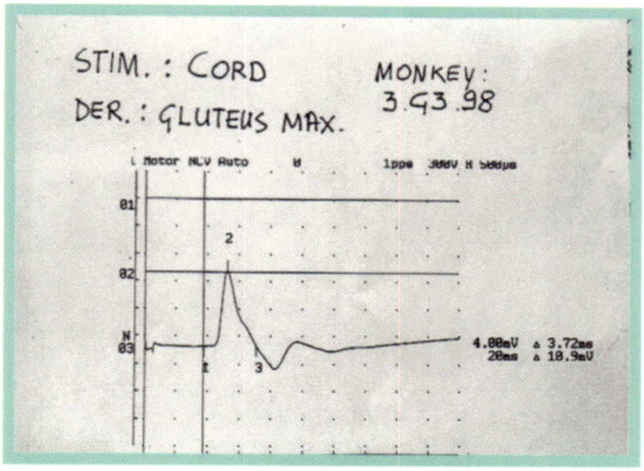

Figure 15. Emg: different latencies according to the distance of the recording electrode.

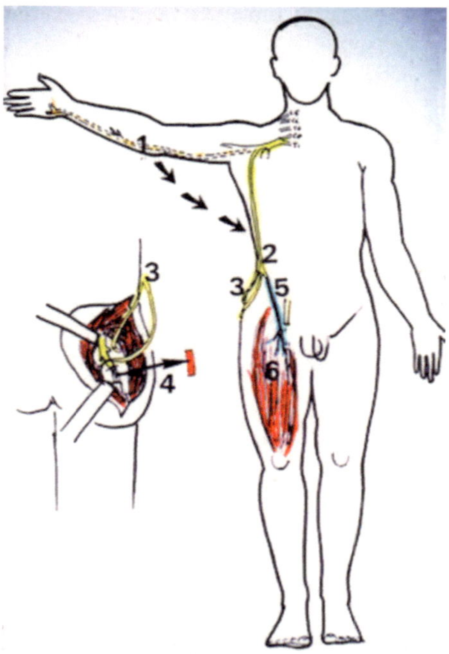

Figure 16. Sketch of the transfer of the ulnar nerve from the upper to the lower limb.

(The damage at the donor hands due to ulnar nerve removal, was repaired by the S.Bunnell and D.Smith procedures. (fig 17) which are well-known procedures of tendon transfers for palsyes of the hand).

Later on in my own laboratories (in the private hospital "saint Rocco of Franciacorta" in Ome), in the following four groups of monkeys operated on with immobilisation in plaster and resuscitation, I got better survival rate and functional results.

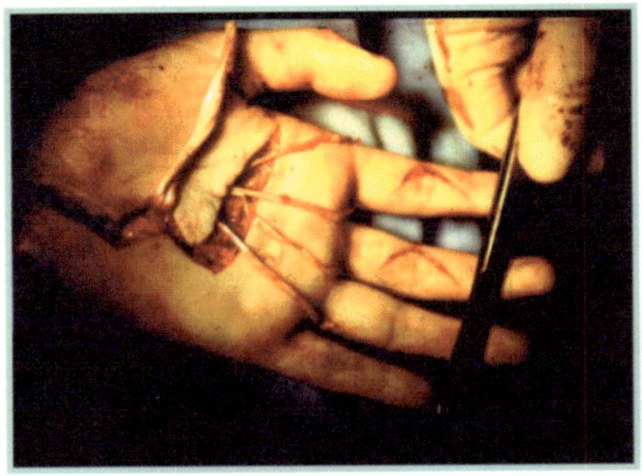

Figure 17. Repair of the damage done at the hands by means of Bunnel and Smith operations

Muscles were first completely disconnected from central nervous system (C.N.S.) and then reconnected to it by means of an autologous nerve graft inserted into the cortico spinal tract (C.S.T.), with exclusion of the lower motoneuron (fig 18).

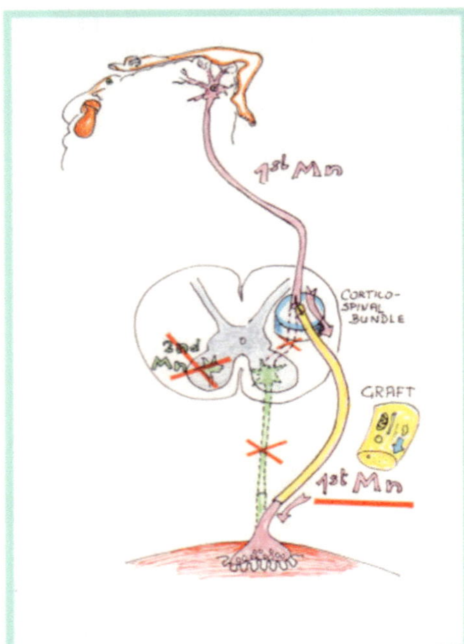

Figure 18. Through this operation the muscle receives innervation by the upper motoneurons and by glutamate instead of acetilcholine

A question arose: how could the muscles (the receptors of which normally respond to acetilcholine) respond to a different neurotransmitter, i.e. glutamate?

http://dx.doi.org/10.5772/56988

In order to understand how this was possible a multidisciplinary research with various institutes of the University of Brescia has been done, in rats, to check which neurotransmitter was really rensponsible for the muscle response:

Vecuronium (nicotinic receptors antagonist) was injected i.v. in the saphen vein (after tracheostomy for artificial ventilation) obtaining the palsy of all the muscles except the reinnervated one. Then GYKY 52466 (antagonist of the glutamate receptors) was injected intraperitoneally obtaining the disappearance of the response of the reinnervated muscle.

Immunoblot analysis of Choline acetyltransferase, Vesicular acetylcholine transporter and vesicular glutamate transporter, demonstrated that the markers for Acetilcholine were present in controls whereas those for Glut were present in the reinnervated muscle. (fig 19).

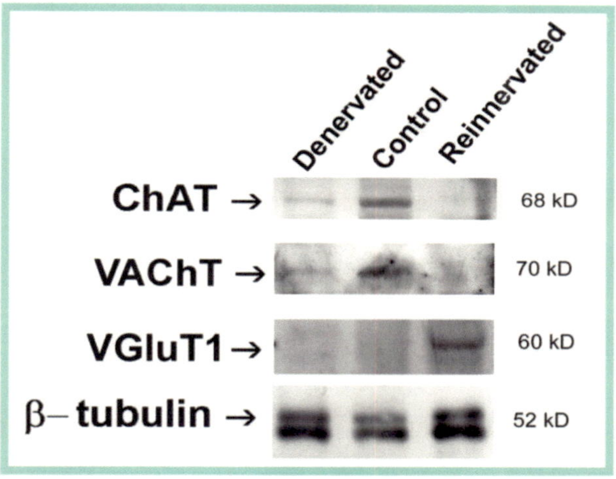

Figure 19. Immunoblot demonstrating that in control muscles are present the markers for ACh whereas in the reinnervated muscles the Glut markers are present.

CTB retrograde tracing of reticular formation and red nucleus neurons was positive.

This research was able to demonstrate that the receptors of the motor end plates, stimulated by the presynaptic nerve fibres (glutamatergic) were able to change one of the molecules of theyr jonic canals so accepting the glutamate transmitter (Proceeding of the National Academy of Science - P.N.S.A).

Going back to the operation of connecting the muscles to the cortico spinal tract by means of autologous nerve grafts, the peroneal component of the sciatic nerve (bilaterally) was used to graft from the C.S.T. of the cord to the muscles (glutei and quadriceps) (fig).

Two teams of microsurgeons, aneasthesiologists and nurses were at work for 12 hours.

The operated patients stayed 4 to 6 days in the intensive care unit and then started a long program of re-education.

After 5 months the first voluntary movements appeared which became functional after one year (fig.20 and 21).

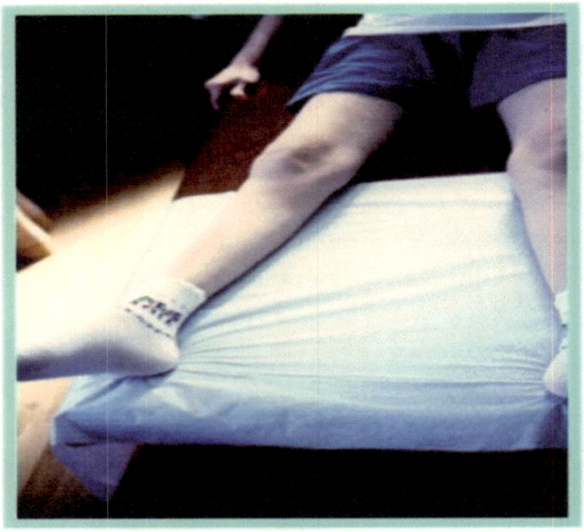

Figure 20. Active abduction

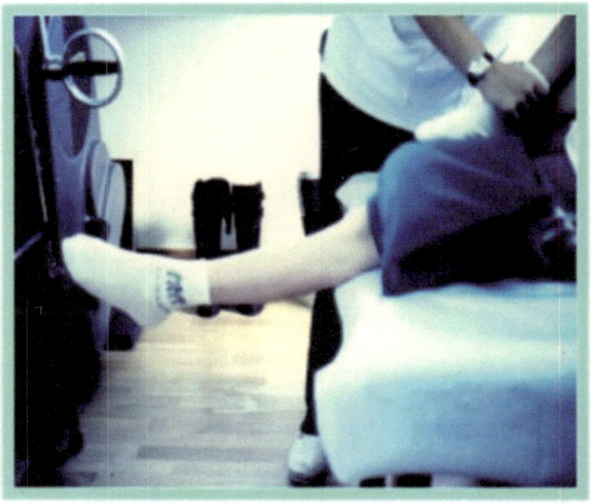

Figure 21. Active extension of the knee without co-contractions

Soon after the patient was able to walk with the help of an ambulator or of quadripode sticks. (fig.22) (cortico spinal tract) by means of nerve grafts, the peroneal nerve (bilaterally) was used to graft from the cortico spinal tract of the cord to the muscles.

Through this operation the muscles receive the innervation by the presynaptic neurons by means of glutamate transmitter (fig 18).

This result has been published in 2006 in the P.N.A.S.

http://dx.doi.org/10.5772/56988

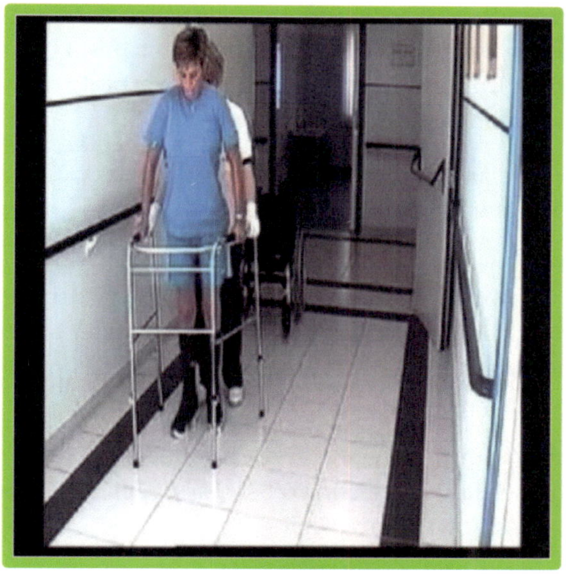

Figure 22. The patient walking with the help of an ambulator. (She had undergone a guillottine severance of the cord at T8 and grafts from the C.S.T. to the glutei and quadriceps).

This occurs probably due to a partial remodelling of the molecules of the trans-membrane channels of the motor end-plates which go back to an embrionic type of channels changing one of their 5 molecular constituents.

Our research demonstrated 5 novelties:

1. the upper motoneuron can build up a cytoskeleton longer than that of the lower motoneuron (up to the muscles)
2. functional connection with muscles occurs,
3. also selective voluntary activation of the muscles occurs,
4. alteration of the motor end-plates from cholinergic to glutamatergic takes place
5. brain plasticity by multiple single neurons, (not only by cortical areas) is demonstrated

But once explained this mistery, one more mistery became evident:

The connection of the graft was inevitably random with the descending axons of the lateral bundle of the cord: the cortico-spinal-tract.

In the C.S.T. thousans and thousands of motor axons run coming from neurons of different areas of the brain cortex having different functions, destined to different muscles having different and even contrasting movements.

The least we could expect should have been co-contractions with severe hindrance of function. All the muscles connected with the C.S.T. should contract contemporarily with no useful function.

On the contrary only the muscles that the patient wanted to move were active. The explanation may be that there must be some until now unknown mechanism of feed back by which the mental command coming from the frontal lobe is able to acticate only those neurons that at the periphery have been connected to the wanted muscles.

This means that the single and selective movements depend on the activation of milion of single motorneurons scattered in various areas of the cortex and not on neurons of a given cortical area.

This means that there is a brain plasticity by multiple (milions) single neurons scattered in different places of the brain cortex that fire simultaneously under the mind command for the desired movement due to theyr peripheral connection even if theyr previous function was different. (fig 22)

Connections of the cord with peripheral nerves have been tried also with other different surgical protocols with the aim of correcting other types of palsies as, for instance, those due to total brachial plexus avulsions in paraplegics.

Total avulsions of the roots of the brachial plexus cannot be repaired by sutures or nerve grafts but can only be treated by extraplexual neurotisations i.e. transfers of extraplexual donor nerves.

In rare cases these lesions occur simultaneously with traumatic paraplegia (or in patients with previous paraplegia) (3 to 5 %).

With the aim of restoring function to the paralized arm in paraplegics I have set up a research in rats by cutting the radial nerve at the armpit and connecting it by means of an autologous graft to the cortico-spinal tract of the spinal cord at level of T3 – T4. (fig 23, 24 and 25)

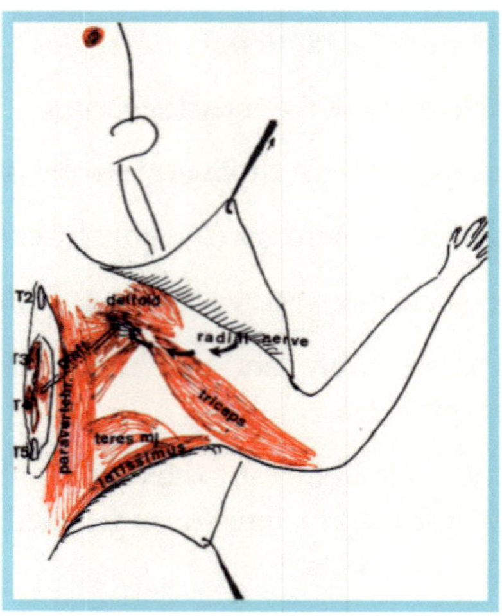

Figure 23. Sketch of the experimental connection of the C.S.T. of the cord below T3 with the radial nerve at the armpit to re innervate the brachial plexus in paraplegics.

http://dx.doi.org/10.5772/56988

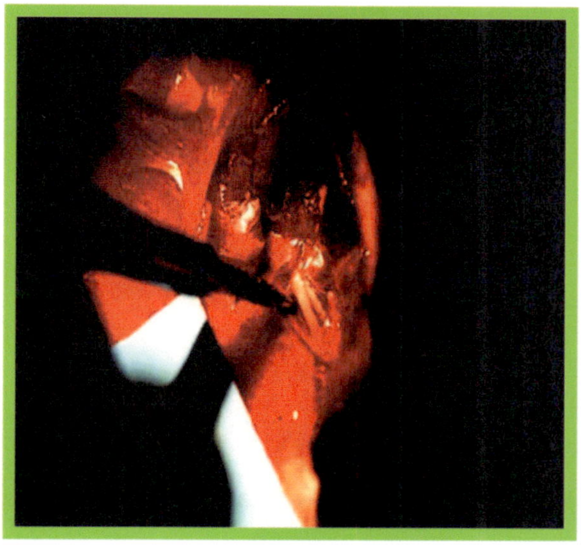

Figure 24. Connection of the brachial plexus of a rat to the c.s.t.

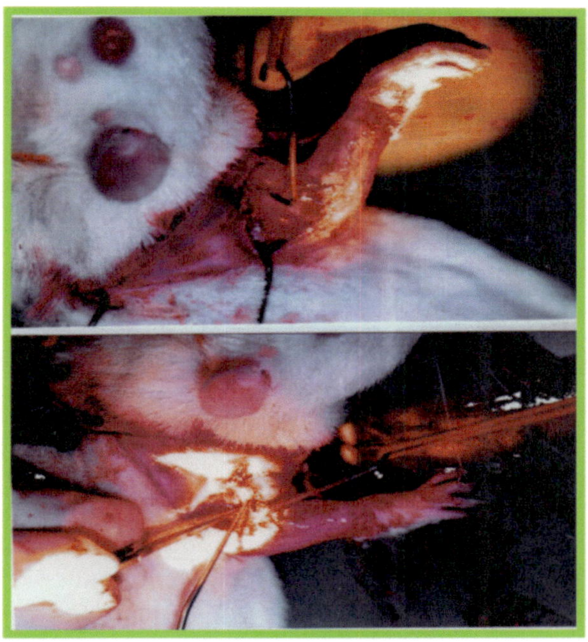

Figure 25. Extension of the elbow,wrist and fingers after connection ocf the radial nerve to the C.S.T.

After 5 months the extension of the wrist and of the digits was recovered.

In human beings with paraplegia no additional damage at the lower limbs can occur.

Author details

Giorgio Brunelli*

Address all correspondence to: giorgio.brunelli@midollospinale.com

Medical School of the University of Brescia, Italy

References

[1] Brunelli: 1983, Innesti sperimentali per lesioni del midollo spinale:G.I.O.T, 9, 53-57.

[2] Aguayo A, 1981.Mc Gill, Montreal. Non permissiveness for regrowing axons in the central nervous sistem.

[3] Brunelli: 1983, Studio sperimentale sulla rigenerazione assonale nel midollo.Policlinico, 90,1334-1336.

[4] Chiasserini: 1944, Compendio di traumatologia del sistema nervoso. Ed Humanitas Nova, Roma.

[5] Brunelli: 1984, Acquisizioni recenti sulle possibilità di riparazione chirurgica delle lesioni midollari.ATTI II° SIMP.intern. pietra Ligure

[6] Brunelli: 1988, Experimental spinal cord repair. In Textbook of microsurgery. Ed Brunelli, Masson ed, 547-554.

[7] Brunelli: 1988, Experimental repair of spinal cord lesions by grafting from C.N.S. to P.N.S. jour, recstr. microsurg.4, 2455-250

[8] Brunelli: 1996 Results in experimental spinal cord repair. Proc 12th Symposium I.S.R.M., Singapore, 3-6.

[9] Brunelli: 1996, Experimental surgery in spinal cord lesions by connecting upper motoneurons directly to peripheral targets. J.periph.nerv.system 1, 111-118.

[10] Brunelli et al: 1996, Sperimentazione sulla possibile riparazione delle lesioni del midollo spinale: gli innesti dal SNC al SNP producono connessioni funzionali. Monograph, Delfo,Brescia 1-56.

[11] Brunelli: 1997: Experimental spinal cord repair.Surgical tecnology 391-395.

[12] Brunelli: 1999: Restoration of walking in paraplegia by transfering the ulnar nerve to the hip. Microsurgery,223-226

[13] Brunelli: 2002: The future: surgery of the spinal cord?. Hand clinic: 18,541-546.

http://dx.doi.org/10.5772/56988

[14] Brunelli et al: 2005: Glutamatergic reinnervation through peripheral nerve grafts dictates assembly of glutamatergic synapses at rat skeletal muscle. P.N.A.S. 102,8752-8757.

[15] Brunelli: 2005: Les reparations chirugicales des lesions de la moelle epiniere. Bull, Acad.Natle med, Paris, 189.n.6.1135-1149.

[16] Pizzi M., Brunelli G.A. et al: 2006: Glutamatergic innervation of rat skeletal muscles by supraspinal neurons. Current Opinion neurobiol 16,323-328

[17] von Wild K.R., Brunelli G.A.: 2003: restoration of locomotion in paraplegics with aid of autologous bypass grafts for direct neurotisation of muscles by upper motoneuron. The future surgery of the spinal cord?. Acta Neurochir suppl. 87, 107-112.

[18] Brunelli G and von Wild K: Unsuspected plasicity of single neurons after connection of the C.S.T.with peripheral nerves in spinal cord lesion. J.Korean neurosurg.society, 46, 1, 1-4.